Medical Education
A Dictionary of Quotations

KIERAN WALSH

MB, BCH, BAO, DCH, FHEA, FRCPI, FAcadMed
Clinical Director, BMJ Learning

Foreword by
DR FIONA GODLEE

Editor, *BMJ*

Radcliffe Publishing
London • New York

Radcliffe Publishing Ltd
33–41 Dallington Street
London
EC1V 0BB
United Kingdom

www.radcliffepublishing.com

British Library Cataloguing in Publication Data

A catalogue record for this book is available from the British Library.

ISBN-13: 978 184619 548 8

The paper used for the text pages of this book
is FSC® certified. FSC (The Forest Stewardship
Council®) is an international network to promote
responsible management of the world's forests.

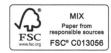

Typeset by Darkriver Design, Auckland, New Zealand
Printed and bound by TJI Digital, Padstow, Cornwall, UK

Contents

Teaching   200

Foreword

Time may be gained by the simple and common-sense process of striking out of the curriculum teaching that oppresses and bewilders the student, that distracts his attention from the real object of his study, that loads his memory without training his intellect.

—Robert Barnes

Robert Barnes' words are likely to ring true with any twenty-first century medical educator. Ideas for creating a leaner curriculum, developing students' intellects, and thinking about the real objectives of a course could all spring from a modern primer on medical education. So it's a surprise that Barnes, Obstetric Physician to St George's Hospital, was writing in 1875, and it's tempting to ask why innovation in medical education can take so long. The quotes in this book give some answers.

One reason for the way medical education has developed over the past 100 years is that heads of traditional medical school departments – anatomy, physiology, biochemistry – clung to their share of the curriculum at all costs. Curriculum reform became a war. But as John Last wrote (p. 9) 'the war for time and students' minds is a sad, futile, self destructive activity in many medical schools.' The pace of reform wasn't helped by the inability of many medical educationalists to manage change and drive forward innovations, especially in the UK. According to George Pickering (p. 101) 'no country has produced so many excellent analyses of the present defects of medical education as has Britain, and no country has done less to implement them.' Another problem may have been that we were working on the wrong raw materials. Selection for medical school has always been a bone of contention (and always will be) but as Nicholas Gold points out (p. 18) selection has tended to lay too much emphasis on pure academic ability. 'By recruiting intelligent strivers with retentive memories medical schools may acquire some lateral thinkers with a capacity for empathy, but they would be there by accident rather than by design.'

Change came eventually and brought with it many of the features we now take for granted. After the 1970s problem-based learning spread quickly throughout medical schools in the Western world and further afield. With it came small group teaching and as Yvonne Steinert says (p. 116) 'the opportunity for students to become actively involved in the process of learning.' Modern technologies have also brought high fidelity simulation and e-learning. And research into medical education has started to build an evidence base so we now know much more about what works and what doesn't. Medical educational research has had to fight its corner against scepticism from those with a background in scientific research. Jill Morrison (p. 106) articulates this particular battleground when she asks: 'why do clear thinking clinicians and researchers sometimes apply illogical thought to education?' The growing number of medical education journals and a burgeoning literature will hopefully see such illogical thinking consigned to history.

This book gives a fascinating insight into medical education – directly from the pens of many leaders who have shaped it. It's heartening that many of the quotes come from late twentieth and twenty-first century educators. As Jennifer Leaning wrote (p. 232) 'Hippocrates and Maimonides still abide, but the vast changes in situation and circumstance since they spoke create the need for other canons.' Let me end with one of them: Peter Richards, Dean of St Mary's Medical School, London from 1979 to 1995 (p. 42):

> *The greatest challenge is to inspire students to curiosity, to fan the flames of their own enthusiasm and the empathy which goes with it. All else will then fall into place.*

Dr Fiona Godlee
Editor, *BMJ*
April 2012

About the author

Dr Kieran Walsh is Clinical Director of BMJ Learning, the education service of the BMJ Group. He is responsible for the editorial direction of the online learning service and for BMJ Masterclasses (face-to-face learning meetings) and onExamination (the assessment division). He has written over 200 articles for publication, mainly in the field of medical education, and he has written the first-ever book on cost and value in medical education. He has worked in the past as a hospital doctor, specialising in neurology and the care of the elderly.

To Sarah Jane, Tommie Jack and Catie Sue, without whom this book would not have been written

Introduction

The wisdom of the wise and the experience of the ages are perpetuated by quotations.

—Benjamin D'Israeli

Medical education is a vitally important discipline. Today's students are tomorrow's doctors and the quality of education that they receive will have a key influence on healthcare of the future. Medical education has developed enormously in the past decade with the emergence of evidence-based teaching techniques, outcomes-based curricula and valid and reliable assessment methods. Yet medical education will never be an exact science – it will always depend on enthusiastic teachers and ambitious learners who are hungry for new knowledge and skills. At a time when doctors and other healthcare professionals bemoan low morale in the profession, the one thing that can still generate enthusiasm among doctors is teaching and learning. This book is intended to encourage and inspire teachers and learners alike. If it makes even just one teacher or learner smile with recognition and return to a burgeoning curriculum or problem-based tutorial with renewed vigour, then it will have succeeded in its aim.

Medical education has had a long history. Teachers have handed down knowledge and learning for millennia and many have captured the essence of medical education in the written and spoken word. The past 30 years have seen a blossoming of medical education research and we may be on the verge of truly evidence-based practice. However, it can be useful to remind ourselves of the timeless nature of many of the problems we continue to struggle with, and we can often do this through reading the words of the old masters. This alone is reason enough to put together a compendium of quotes on medical education.

Quotations from any field of interest can be tricky and medical quotations are no exception. Rick never did say 'play it again, Sam', nor did Marie Antoinette say 'let them eat cake'. People inevitably get misquoted or quoted out of context, and it can sometimes be difficult to tell if someone is being serious or ironic. In this book I have done my best to make the quotes as accurate as possible and to attribute them to the original source. If there are any failures in accuracy, they are my own. If there are successes that make you laugh or raise an eyebrow or have a light-bulb moment, they are down to the many speakers, authors, editors and publishers without whom this book could not have been written. Particular praise must go to the publishing staff of the *BMJ*, *Journal of the American Medical Association*, *Medical Education*, *Medical Teacher* and Radcliffe, all of whom were generous with both quotes and encouragement. Thanks also to Edward Farrow for his help with categorising the quotes.

This book was written in three phases. The first phase involved writing a proposal and making the case for the first book of quotations dedicated to the subject of medical education. My pitch was simple, being that medical education has always been and always will be about one thing: people. The purpose of the book is to celebrate all those involved in medical education, be they teachers, learners or patients. People are defined by their words and it is to be hoped that the quotes in this book show the humanity of all those involved in medical education, as well as showing their wit and insight and occasional frustration and anger.

The second phase involved writing and editing. That started easily enough but then gradually became harder. When I first started writing I was happy to take any quote from any source, but as the work progressed I started to get choosy. Is a quote still a quote when it comes from a committee or a learned council or a college? Is it still a quote when it comes from two authors rather than just one? Midway through writing I decided that I would exclude all examples of writing by committee and any examples suffering from multiple author syndrome. Committees tend to produce worthy but turgid prose, and the more authors involved, the more conservative and guarded statements tend to be. What all the quotes in this book have in common – whether you agree with them or not – is that they are examples of individuals who have raised their head above the parapet, saying something controversial or funny or just plain obvious.

The third and final phase involved adding finishing touches and, as with any labour of love, there is a tinge of sadness at its conclusion. As the project has drawn to a close, people have inevitably started to ask me who is my favourite medical educator and what is my favourite quote. One particular educator whom I have grown fond of is Egerton Yorrick Davis. Davis was a retired US Army surgeon living in Caughnawauga, Quebec, from where he conducted a prolific correspondence with medical societies until his untimely death in a drowning accident at the Lachine Rapids in 1884. He authored a controversial paper on the obstetric habits of Native American tribes (the paper was suppressed and remains unpublished), and he was the first to report a case of penis captivus, indeed only 3 weeks after the first reported case of vaginismus. If all this is starting to sound increasingly bizarre, it is because none of this is true. Egerton Yorrick Davis was the invention of William Osler, who wrote and published several pieces under this pseudonym and further propagated the myth by signing Davis's name to various medical conference attendance lists. Osler is quoted over 30 times throughout this book and it came as a surprise that the father of modern medical education, the man who stares rather po-faced out of sepia-tinged photographs, was in fact an inveterate prankster. Osler would have perhaps approved of Mark Albanese when he said, 'We are all human, and we have been human for much longer than we have been professionals'. Osler is my favourite educator but my favourite quote comes from Francis Peabody. In 1927 Peabody gave his famous lecture on the care of the patient – he was only 47 years old and was dying of metastatic cancer. In a wide-ranging address he spoke of the need to individualise medical care, to make hospitalisation a less dehumanising experience and to care better for patients with symptoms for which an organic cause cannot be found. Here is how Peabody ended this lecture:

One of the essential qualities of the clinician is an interest in humanity, for the secret of the care of the patient is in caring for the patient.

Curriculum

1. CURRICULUM DEVELOPMENT

> In 1987 and again in 1988 the General Medical Council (GMC) education committee reported that British medical schools were having difficulty in achieving their educational objectives. (The claim that medical schools actually had educational objectives came as a considerable surprise to many working within them.)
>
> **Robin Fraser**

For two generations we have been loading and loading this brief curriculum as if we desired to teach many things ill rather than a few things well.

Thomas Clifford Allbutt

Allbutt TC. An address on medical education in London: delivered at King's College Hospital on October 3rd, 1905, at the opening of the medical session. *BMJ.* 1905; 2(2337): 913–18.

Although there is no reason to suppose that learner-centred teaching cannot occur in a curriculum-based teaching programme, there is a tendency for the curriculum to influence how things are taught in that it may structure teaching to 'chosen' areas and so may lead to 'convergent thinking' rather than true exploration and learner centredness.

Tahir Awan

Awan T. Structured, curriculum-based group teaching or unstructured, learner-centred group approaches? *Educ Prim Care.* 2009; 20(6): 462–7.

Any curriculum plan which disregards the nature of learning, and of the learners, is bound to be ineffective.

Raja Bandaranayake

Bandaranayake RC. How to plan a medical curriculum. *Med Teach.* 1985; 7(1): 7–13.

Time may be gained by the simple and common-sense process of striking out of the curriculum teaching that oppresses and bewilders the student, that distracts his attention from the real object of his study, that loads his memory without training his intellect.

Robert Barnes

Barnes R. An address on obstetric medicine and its position in medical education. *BMJ.* 1875; 2(758): 33–5.

What applies to the design of the curriculum as a whole applies to the individual studies.

W Gordon Byers

Byers WG. The place of ophthalmology in the undergraduate medical curriculum. *BMJ.* 1922; 2(3209): 4–6.

I would suggest that, as the majority of us are destined to be general practitioners, general practitioners of good standing should be well represented on our teaching bodies, and the advantage of their experience be applied to the curriculum.

Ernest Carmody

Carmody EP. Education for general practice. *BMJ*. 1932; 2(3734): 224–5.

At present there is no method. The curriculum is the accidental result of multiple collisions between vested interests in a variety of departments, held in check by the inertia of tradition.

Bruce Charlton

Charlton BG. Practical reform of preclinical education: core curriculum and science projects. *Med Teach*. 1991; 13(1): 21–8.

Reforms such as increasing generalist training, increasing ambulatory care exposure, providing social science courses, teaching lifelong and self-learning skills, rewarding teaching, clarifying the school mission, and centralizing curriculum control have appeared almost continuously since 1910.

Nicholas Christakis

Christakis NA. The similarity and frequency of proposals to reform US medical education: constant concerns. *JAMA*. 1995; 274(9): 706–11.

I think that the emphasis laid on the division of the curriculum into pre-clinical and clinical is unfortunate. The division is perhaps convenient in many ways, but it is wholly artificial and educationally unsound.

GA Clark

Clark GA. The medical curriculum. *BMJ*. 1942; 2(4260): 259.

The various subjects of the curriculum have developed as autonomous independent compartments of knowledge; yet for medical education they must be viewed primarily as different facets of the same subject.

Henry Cohen

Cohen H. Medicine, science, and humanism. *BMJ*. 1950; 2(4672): 179–84.

The Malthusian problem for the curriculum is that the length of the curriculum is fixed (or can grow by only slight linear increments) while the subject matter it could cover grows exponentially.

Ken Cox

Cox K. Knowledge which cannot be used is useless. *Med Teach*. 1987; 9(2): 145–54.

To incorporate special study with general medical education is, therefore, to do injustice to both; for general medical education, which already fully occupies the time set apart for it, must be detrimentally curtailed or compressed to make room for the special study; and the special study cannot be advantageously carried on while the foundations on which it ought to rest have not been wholly laid down nor thoroughly consolidated.

James Crichton Browne

Crichton Browne J. The address delivered in the section of psychology. *BMJ*. 1880; 2(1024): 262–7.

If it is this "Jack-of-all-trades" that is wanted, let us by all means go on as we are doing, adding another year to the curriculum every now and again.

Hugh Crichton-Miller

Crichton-Miller H. "The student in irons". *BMJ.* 1932; 1(3718): 680–1.

Now, the average student is a gentleman admitted to society; drinking, card-playing, and midnight rioting, are no longer essentials in his curriculum; frequently he has secured for himself the status of graduate or undergraduate of a university; more often he has been reared in a public school, and entering upon his technical education with all the rawness and inexperience of a schoolboy, has nevertheless an intellect prepared for theoretical instruction.

Edward Crossman

Crossman E. An address on the maintenance of the honour and respectability of the medical profession. *BMJ.* 1883; 2(1176): 61–7.

Will the [Edinburgh] declaration change medical education? Anyone familiar with the kind of wranglings that precede the transfer of even a week of curricular time in an established medical school will not be optimistic.

Colin Currie

Currie C. Global village fête. *BMJ.* 1988; 297(6648): 630.

There is abundant justification, however, for the plea that the real object of the medical curriculum, perhaps more than of any other educational discipline, should be to train the student to observe, to think, and to form a reasoned judgement, and not to make confused and evanescent records on his memory.

Henry Dale

Dale H. An address on the relation of physiology to medicine, in research and education. *BMJ.* 1932; 2(3753): 1043–6.

The expansion of knowledge is also not a new problem. Medical curricula of 100 years ago also lamented that five years was not long enough to learn all that is needed.

Matt Doogue

Doogue M. Debunking one myth and perpetuating another. *BMJ.* 2002 January 20. Available at: www.bmj.com/content/324/7330/173.1/reply#bmj_el_18941?sid=d5e693ea-0765-423d-ac1d-1c98624d8fdf (accessed 10 July 2011).

In my beginning is my end.

TS Eliot

East Coker, from *Four Quartets.* 1940.

Educational experiences designed to develop the intellect are not commonly offered except in an additional year of study – though some schools make time for them by a horizontally integrated curriculum which enables a core of basic knowledge to be acquired quickly.

John Ellis

Ellis J. Editorial: 2. The present state of medical education in Britain. *Med Teach.* 1987; 9(3): 243–6.

The great worry is that premed requirements and much of what is taught in medical school has simply persisted without good justification by inertia and the potential energy barrier that discourages curricular changes, no matter how meritorious.

Ezekiel Emanuel

Emanuel EJ. Changing premedical requirements: reply. *JAMA.* 2007; 297(1): 38–9.

Objectives are no more than a means to an end, but they are essential for an analytical, logical and systematic approach to the education of future doctors.

Charles Engel

Engel CA. Controversy: for the use of objectives. *Med Teach.* 1980; 2(5): 232.

In the school curriculum of the medical student more emphasis should be given to the prevailing dangers arising from the too-ready acceptance of the action and clinical value of medicines conveyed through the pressing salesmanship by representatives of drug houses, or convened in colourful advertisements which arrive by mail at unwarranted prodigious cost.

William Evans

Evans W. Addiction to medicines. *BMJ.* 1962; 2(5306): 722–5.

In curricular innovation, as in the rest of life, I would contend that the way something is done is often even more important that the act itself.

David Findlay

Findlay DJ. How to do it: strategy and tactics in curricular innovation. *Med Teach.* 1988; 10(2): 147–8.

One of the most difficult problems in revising course content in any discipline is the establishment and maintenance of some systematic approach.

Lawrence Fisher

Fisher LA. What can be done about curriculum. *Arch Dermatol.* 1966; 93(5): 536–8.

What sound reason can be given for requiring the able and the less able, the industrious and the less industrious, to complete practically the same course of instruction in the same period of time?

Abraham Flexner

Flexner A. Medical education, 1909–1924. *JAMA.* 1924; 82(11): 833–8.

In 1987 and again in 1988 the General Medical Council (GMC) education committee reported that British medical schools were having difficulty in achieving their educational objectives. (The claim that medical schools actually had educational objectives came as a considerable surprise to many working within them.)

Robin Fraser

Fraser RC. Undergraduate medical education: present state and future needs. *BMJ.* 1991; 303(6793): 41–3.

Progress in medical education occurs slowly because it is generally envisaged in a fixed framework; the effort to find more room for more subjects is frustrated by the difficulties of omitting or contracting others.

Hugh Gainsborough

Gainsborough H. Medical education. *BMJ.* 1958; 2(5099): 795.

The teaching of professionalism in undergraduate medical education has traditionally been entrusted to the hidden curriculum through transmission via respected role models.

John Goldie

Goldie J. Integrating professionalism teaching into undergraduate medical education in the UK setting. *Med Teach.* 2008; 30(5): 513–27.

The strength of medical education is its integration of service and training.
Janet Grant

Grant J. The Calman report and specialist training: Calman report builds on the status quo. *BMJ.* 1993; 306(6894): 1756.

Then, in the latter part of the curriculum, it is nothing less than a scandal that a man may be fully qualified and yet be absurdly ignorant of the most elementary principles of hygiene, medical jurisprudence, and psychology.
Alfred Gubb

Gubb AS. The colleges and the M.D. degree. *BMJ.* 1885; 2(1299): 996.

At the present time, therefore, when the medical curriculum is being overhauled and improvements made, not only as to the means of acquiring knowledge, but also as to the tests of acquirement, it would be well to have the claims of public health attended to.
John Haddon

Haddon J. The teaching of public medicine. *BMJ.* 1890; 2(1542): 178–9.

To date much of the attention in OBE [outcome-based education] has focussed on the specification of learning outcomes and less on the implementation of an OBE approach in practice.
Ronald Harden

Harden RM. Learning outcomes as a tool to assess progression. *Med Teach.* 2007; 29(7): 678–82.

All training programmes should have some form of documented curriculum, ideally developed with the assistance of a range of stakeholders and interest groups, and therefore reflecting reasonable consensus on what the graduate of the training programme should know and do.
Richard Hays

Hays R. An overview of clinical teaching issues. In: Hays R. *Teaching and Learning in Clinical Settings.* Oxford: Radcliffe Publishing; 2006. pp15–28.

Another advantage gained from the study of medical history is the additional incitement and encouragement it gives us in the scientific pursuit of our profession.
Alexander Henry

Henry A. Lectures on the history of medicine. *BMJ.* 1860; 1(169): 219–23.

Yet, strange though it may seem, the teaching of the history of medicine is a novelty in England.
Alexander Henry

Henry A. Lectures on the history of medicine. *BMJ.* 1860; 1(169): 219–23.

Social networks often underpin educational activities, especially those which are peer led, but these may be disrupted by competition, and differences across the UK may lead to divisions on curricula and training models.
Amanda Howe

Howe A. Thinking ahead: GP educators in England need to be planning for the NHS reforms. *Educ Prim Care.* 2010; 21(6): 352–3.

Undergraduate medical education is supposed to prepare the future doctor for their role and its responsibilities, but the curriculum neglects teaching the doctors of tomorrow how to teach.

Judith Jade

Jade J. Shouldn't we all be medical educators? *BMJ.* 2010 May 26. Available at: www.bmj.com/content/340/bmj. c2351/reply#bmj_el_236070?sid=31b7420e-2cd9-4337-8329-2f40df508216 (accessed 21 September 2011).

The relentless march of quality controllers into the earliest stages of the undergraduate curriculum promises to rob what's left of UK medical education of its transformative value, and should be resisted at all costs.

William James

James WS. Education fit for professional and public life. *BMJ.* 2005 October 9. Available at: www.bmj.com/content/331/7520/791/reply#bmj_el_118642?sid=cb764c2a-ad1a-4f84-a8c4-88b3568c267c (accessed 10 July 2011).

In most innovative schools there is an inherent mechanism to check 'curricular ossification', but the risk of 'iatrogenic curriculitis' is on the increase.

PT Jayawickramarajah

Jayawickramarajah PT. The analysis of medical curriculum. *Med Teach.* 1987; 9(2): 167–78.

The first step in integration is coordination.

Reg Jordan

Lowry S. Strategies for implementing curriculum change. *BMJ.* 1992; 305(6867): 1482–5.

Role models and the hidden curriculum are a much more powerful learning force than is the formal curriculum.

Max Kamien

Kamien M. Radical versus traditional schools: are the graduates different? *Med Teach.* 1983; 5(3): 104–6.

Changes in curricular models in medical education have historically been introduced without documentation of value.

Hans Karle

Karle H. International trends in medical education: diversification contra convergence. *Med Teach.* 2004; 26(3): 205–6.

Undergraduate curriculum bashing has been a diverting pastime for diverse doctors for at least the past half century (my father used to say that they were hard at it well before the health service came in), and it is all too easy for those of us involved in "core teaching" to allow such criticisms to pass by default.

MJ Kelly

Kelly MJ. Undergraduate medical education. *BMJ.* 1991; 303(6796): 245–6.

There is no justification in blaming modern curricula as being responsible for the difficulty in recruiting to certain disciplines – the present day shortage of pathologists reflects a lack of interest from graduates taught along traditional and didactic lines that so often divorced pathology from the clinical setting.

Peter Kopelman

Kopelman PG. Undergraduate medical teaching: evangelism, puritanism or clinical common sense? *BMJ.* 2004 July 26. Available at: www.bmj.com/content/329/7457/92/reply#bmj_el_68675?sid=3f545f3a-8b62-4679-979a-2c0b244a4cd7 (accessed 11 August 2011).

The war for time and students' minds is a sad, futile, self destructive activity in many medical schools.

John Last

Last JM. Personal view. *BMJ (Clin Res Ed)*. 1985; 290(6485): 1900.

Although formally the functions of medical education are to convey medical knowledge, skills and attitudes, in addition the covert processes of professional socialisation are equally important, and it is in this domain that the hidden curriculum particularly appears to operate.

Heidi Lempp

Lempp H. Qualitative research in understanding the transformation from medical student to doctor. *Educ Prim Care*. 2005; 16(6): 648–54.

In considering the usual medical curriculum of to-day, and asking where in it clinical science is to play its part, I would start from the statement that this curriculum is already overloaded.

Thomas Lewis

Lewis T. The Huxley lecture on clinical science within the university. *BMJ*. 1935; 1(3873): 631–6.

No one can assume that the effects of a teaching programme run parallel with the thoughts and efforts put into it.

Tsung-Yi Lin

Lin TY. Teaching of psychiatry at National Taiwan University. *BMJ*. 1960; 2(5195): 345–8.

I would beg the student to proceed with order and regularity in his studies, and not to be led off from one subject to another, made more inviting by its novelty, for this has caused many to regret the dissipation of great abilities in a boundless multiplicity of pursuits, and to lament the inaccuracies and deficiencies of their acquirements, by aiming at too much.

James Long

Long J. Introductory lecture delivered at the Liverpool Royal Institution: October 1, 1841. *Prov Med Surg J.* 1841; s1–3(54): 23–9.

The uncertainty of our duration ought at once to set bounds to our designs, and add incitements to our industry; and when we find ourselves inclined either to immensity in our designs, or to sluggishness in our endeavours, we may either check or animate ourselves by recollecting, with the Father of Physic, "that art is long, and life short."

James Long

Long J. Introductory lecture delivered at the Liverpool Royal Institution: October 1, 1841. *Prov Med Surg J.* 1841; s1–3(54): 23–9.

Most people accept that the way in which a subject is taught can have as much impact on what students learn as the content of the course.

Stella Lowry

Lowry S. Strategies for implementing curriculum change. *BMJ*. 1992; 305(6867): 1482–5.

The low status of teachers in medical education, the departmental organisation of many courses, and the traditional divide between the basic sciences and the clinical course were identified as major barriers to change.

Stella Lowry

Lowry S. Curriculum design. *BMJ.* 1992; 305(6866): 1409–11.

The General Medical Council first expressed concern about curriculum overload at the end of the nineteenth century.

Stella Lowry

Carnall D. Sweeping reforms recommended for medical education. *BMJ.* 1995; 311(7001): 345.

In the length of the course and the variety of its elements is its strength, for the curriculum is constructed so as to afford a base wide enough to be an adequate foundation for your life-work, and neglect of any part is sure to prove a source of weakness; for if the foundation be not well and truly laid in each particular, it will inevitably lead to subsequent settlements and dislocations in the superstructure.

Alexander Macalister

Macalister A. An address on fifty years of medical education: delivered at the opening of the winter session at King's College, London. *BMJ.* 1908; 2(2492): 957–60.

There is nothing novel about the deceptive allure of a core curriculum, but those tempted by it should be aware of generic arguments against this particular solution or of voices that counsel moderation in the definition of foundation medical knowledge.

Stuart MacLeod

MacLeod SM. Undergraduate medical education: too many facts not enough innovation. *BMJ.* 1993; 307(6918): 1565.

As the failure of medical witnesses is most frequently manifested in trials concerning mental sanity, the study of mental disease should be inculcated and insisted upon by the several Colleges of Physicians and Surgeons, and form a part of the curriculum of medical education.

Stephen Macswiney

Macswiney SM. Medico-legal evidence. *BMJ.* 1867; 2(361): 492–4.

It is not new curriculae that reform medical education, but new teachers.

Marshall Marinker

Marinker M. The way we teach . . . general practice. *Med Teach.* 1980; 2(2): 63–70.

The main criticisms levelled against the use of objectives are that they are restrictive and inflexible, incompatible with opportunistic teaching and prone to trivialisation (the more trivial the objective, the easier it is to express).

Brian McAvoy

McAvoy BR. How to choose and use educational objectives. *Med Teach.* 1985; 7(1): 27–35.

Protagonists of the use of objectives claim that they encourage clear and original thinking, enhance communication and make values and assumptions explicit.

Brian McAvoy

McAvoy BR. How to choose and use educational objectives. *Med Teach.* 1985; 7(1): 27–35.

The function of the curriculum is to provide logic, a rationale for what students learn, how they learn it and how that learning is assessed.

Anne McKee

McKee A. The exercise of professional judgement in the context of the curriculum: the role of general practice trainers; a new challenge for GP specialised training. *Educ Prim Care.* 2007; 18(5): 558–63.

With more integrated and student-centred curricula, where students are exposed to the medical profession early in their studies, perhaps even in the first year, clinical role models, on whom the profession has relied for generations, now assume a more important role than in a traditional programme.

Michelle McLean

McLean M. Clinical role models are important in the early years of a problem-based learning curriculum. *Med Teach.* 2006; 28(1): 64–9.

Medical knowledge has accumulated very rapidly in recent years, and as each major advance has come to be accepted we have included it in the medical curriculum. But I fear that we have not always discarded much, and certainly not a corresponding amount, of the old material.

Arthur Morgan Jones

Morgan Jones A. Medical progress and medical education. *BMJ.* 1952; 2(4782): 466–9.

A medical curriculum should constantly develop in response to the needs of students, institutions, and society.

Jill Morrison

Morrison J. ABC of learning and teaching in medicine: evaluation. *BMJ.* 2003; 326(7385): 385–7.

Whenever there is a change in the examination pattern, or change in curriculum, students complain that it happened only with them and they are the experimental batch.

Satheesha Nayak

Nayak S. What is the reason for yawning in the class? *BMJ.* 2005 July 10. Available at: www.bmj.com/content/331/7508/105.2/reply#bmj_el_111907?sid=cb764c2a-ad1a-4f84-a8c4-88b3568c267c (accessed 10 July 2011).

Assess the products of differing medical schools as you wish but do not assume a 'one size fits all' curriculum will improve standards.

Roderick Neilson

Neilson R. Undergraduate medical teaching. *BMJ.* 2005 October 11. Available at: www.bmj.com/content/331/7520/791/reply#bmj_el_118842?sid=cb764c2a-ad1a-4f84-a8c4-88b3568c267c (accessed 20 June 2011).

It is clear that the Commonwealth does not require two standards of medical men, one having received an inferior form of training and the other a superior form. All medical education should be fundamentally one and the same in regard to basis, technique, and spirit. All practitioners require a minimum of comprehensive training, the same elements of scientific method, a similar scientific inspiration.

George Newman

Starling EH. Medical education in England: the overloaded curriculum and the incubus of the examination system. *BMJ.* 1918; 2(3010): 258–9.

The purpose of the medical curriculum is the training not of specialists, but of general practitioners.
George Newman
Gregory A. The G.P. and the curriculum. *BMJ*. 1932; 2(3753): 1078–9.

This strange medley of a curriculum is worth retaining if it can give in our own time a Lister, a Hughlings Jackson, a Michael Foster, and a James Mackenzie.
John Nixon
Nixon JA. The art and science of medicine in relation to professional training. *BMJ*. 1928; 2(3530): 363–4.

Any effort to "revitalise" medical education ought to begin at the beginning, i.e., with the question, why do we educate people to function as physicians?
Lawrence O'Brien
O'Brien LJ. A task from hell. *BMJ*. 2004 March 14. Available at: www.bmj.com/content/328/7440/597/reply#bmj_el_53179?sid=3f545f3a-8b62-4679-979a-2c0b244a4cd7 (accessed 10 July 2011).

Curriculum pressures and a decline in hospital autopsy rates have reduced the opportunity for medical students to learn from autopsy findings.
Gregory O'Grady
O'Grady G. Death of the teaching autopsy. *BMJ*. 2003; 327(7418): 802–3.

Conferences should be about learning and change (never mind job seeking, flirtation, tax breaks, drinking, and the rest of the conference's hidden curriculum).
Jules Older
Older J. Personal view. *BMJ (Clin Res Ed)*. 1985; 290(6472): 930.

Luck usually plays a larger part in what students learn than does curricular planning.
Nigel Oswald
Oswald N. Where should we train doctors in the future? *BMJ*. 1991; 303(6794): 71.

Do not have any illusions about being able to organize and run joint and integrated teaching in the same way as you would with students from a single department.
Neville Owen
Owen N. How to: organize and conduct joint and integrated teaching. *Med Teach*. 1982; 4(2): 47–55.

As a medical student, it is generally accepted that you will sometimes (or often, depending on your consultant) be made to look stupid in front of friends, doctors and patients, and the 'hidden curriculum' teaches you to accept this early on.
Philip Peacock
Peacock P. Culture change is needed. *BMJ*. 2004 October 10. Available at: www.bmj.com/content/329/7469/770/reply#bmj_el_77707?sid=3f545f3a-8b62-4679-979a-2c0b244a4cd7 (accessed 11 September 2011).

Once the learning aim is defined, then the most appropriate teaching method can be employed.
Philip Pemberton
Pemberton P. Joint consultations revisited: getting to the point. *Educ Prim Care*. 2008; 19(4): 408–15.

A philosophical framework and a set of defined outcomes are essential if a medical educa-tion system is to meet social or institutional goals and serve the needs of a community.

Susan Phillips

Phillips SP. Models of medical education in Australia, Europe and North America. *Med Teach.* 2008; 30(7): 705–9.

While we know through strong supportive evidence about aspects of teaching and learning that work 'best' in particular circumstances and intentions, this also cannot be dogmatised without taking into account that individual learners can be shown to vary in their approaches to learning, motivation and reasoning; there can be managerial and political pressures over curriculum topics, and the issue of resources is very real, due to funding and pressures of the high service commitment.

John Pitts

Pitts J. 'Judging educational research' and the selection of papers for publication. *Educ Prim Care.* 2004; 15: 143–9.

The curriculum must be in a form that can be communicated to those associated with the learning institution, should be open to critique, and should be able to be readily transformed into practice.

David Prideaux

Prideaux D. ABC of learning and teaching in medicine: curriculum design. *BMJ.* 2003; 326(7383): 268–70.

Rather than work harder; trainees, and those responsible for their training, need to find ways to work smarter. There needs to be a more efficient and effective training pathway.

Lucy Radmore

Radmore L. Surgical trainees need to work smarter not harder. *BMJ.* 2009 November 23. Available at: www.bmj.com/content/339/bmj.b4260/reply#bmj_el_224782?sid=c01598e6-7fa7-4552-bbff-d3bc10847fd9 (accessed 10 August 2011).

Teachers should be informed of and have easy access to written learning outcomes for their courses so that they can plan their teaching strategies and methods.

Subha Ramani

Ramani S. Twelve tips to promote excellence in medical teaching. *Med Teach.* 2006; 28(1): 19–23.

The ideals of the physician's role and the doctor-patient relationship must be afforded as much emphasis in the medical school curriculum as is anatomy, pathology, and internal medicine.

Stephen Reingold

Reingold S. How important is role model education in making good doctors? *BMJ.* 2002 September 28. Available at: www.bmj.com/content/325/7366/707/reply#bmj_el_25851?sid=d5e693ea-0765-423d-ac1d-1c98624d8fdf (accessed 16 August 2011).

Designing and planning a medical curriculum – or, in most cases, redesigning and replan-ning – is a chess game.

Peter Richards

Richards P. Book review: medicine and books. *BMJ.* 1990; 300: 1146.

The hapless student finds himself compelled to be learning in one and the same period the most incongruous subjects, to be listening to harangues on natural science which have little or no bearing on the great object of his studies at a hospital and medical school, to be attending courses of instruction on diseases and injuries affecting parts of the body of which he scarcely knows the names, much less the composition and structure; and to prove practically the error of one of Euclid's cardinal axioms by being in several places at the same time.

Walter Rivington

Rivington W. Medical education. *BMJ.* 1879; 2(970): 168–70.

Planning for the elective attachment should be an integral part of any medical school curriculum. Despatching medical schools have a responsibility to ensure that students are as well prepared as possible prior to their elective attachments.

Andrew Rowland

Rowland AG. Education concerning HIV & elective attachments is the responsibility of medical schools. *BMJ.* 2003 February 10. Available at: www.bmj.com/content/326/7384/338.2/reply#bmj_el_29544?sid=7f27ee1c-bc1e-486c-bc82-03a5164885cc (accessed 14 July 2011).

Performance review can form the basis of a curriculum for continued education but will be useful only if all the important aspects of practice are included and not just those that are easily measured – for instance, record keeping.

TPC Schofield

Schofield TPC. Continued medical education must not be an optional extra. *BMJ (Clin Res Ed).* 1987; 294(6571): 526–7.

Constant changes have been one of the most striking features of the curriculum in the last twenty years, but the men responsible for these changes have been drawn too much from one class, and that a small class of the profession; so that it is not surprising that complaints are made that the curriculum becomes less and less suitable for the education of the profession generally.

Lauriston Shaw

Shaw LE. Presidential addresses to the branches of the British Medical Association: Metropolitan countries branch: the true aim of a united medical profession and the handicap of the trade union bogey. *BMJ.* 1910; 2(2585): 121–4.

If one school needs only two hours to teach omphalology and produces average and adequate doctors, isn't St Brides-in-the-Bath grossly overdoing it with 117 hours? Sadly, such data never seem to be used to support the wholesome activity of reducing curriculum content.

Michael Simpson

Simpson MA. Educational inflation. *Med Teach.* 1981; 3(1): 5–8.

Students learn surgery which they will never practise, and will practise midwifery which they have never learned.

Japp Sinclair

Routley TC. Lest we forget. *BMJ.* 1955; 1(4929): 1489–93.

Although the undergraduate medical curriculum is a good time to introduce medical ethics, students may learn best when faced with ethical dilemmas in clinical practice.

Peter Singer

Singer PA. Recent advances: medical ethics. *BMJ.* 2000; 321(7256): 282–5.

The medical curriculum has reached the limit of human endurance, and it is only the genius of the medical student for clearing his brain completely after every examination that enables him to preserve his sanity.

Henry Souttar

Langdon-Brown W. The medical curriculum and present-day needs. *BMJ*. 1938; 2(4052): 481–4.

"Integration" (pax to the Old Guard!) in the curriculum, about which there has been much hue and cry in the 'fifties, is a topic which still arouses both cynicism and fanaticism.

John Spillane

Spillane JD. New American medical schools. *BMJ*. 1960; 2(5201): 778–85.

Medical schools often neglect the teaching of public health and population-based approaches as part of the medical curriculum, and medical schools that boast public health departments rarely undertake research and teaching in global health.

Alfred Spira

Spira AV. Global public health. *BMJ*. 2002 February 21. Available at: www.bmj.com/content/324/7333/309/reply#bmj_el_19866?sid=d5e693ea-0765-423d-ac1d-1c98624d8fdf (accessed 17 August 2011).

And those of us who admit that examinations are a valuable and, in fact, the only way of testing our young men may also without inconsistency deplore the present tendency of the medical curriculum, the strictly student's curriculum, which leans towards over-examination.

Samuel Squire Sprigge

Squire Sprigge S. An address on prizes and performances: delivered at the opening of the medical session at St. George's Hospital, on October 1st. *BMJ*. 1910; 2(2597): 1024–7.

Perhaps the most recent change in undergraduate medical education relates to the realization of the power of the informal curriculum.

Alex Stagnaro-Green

Stagnaro-Green A. Personal view: applying adult learning principles to medical education in the United States. *Med Teach*. 2004; 26(1): 79–85.

The primary objective in any scheme for the improvement of medical education should be to get away from the idea that it is necessary to train a doctor to do everything.

GA Stanton

Stanton GA. Medical education. *BMJ*. 1962; 2(5306): 737.

The arguments for and against changes in medical curricula are similar to arguments for and against change in medical practice itself. Change must occur in response to changes in society, medical knowledge, and of course even consumerism.

Jill Thistlethwaite

Thistlethwaite JE. Evidence based medical education. *BMJ*. 2004 July 10. Available at: www.bmj.com/content/329/7457/92/reply (accessed 14 July 2011).

Deans and professors organise curricula, deans and professors sit on the committee, the committee makes recommendations, it seeks the views of other deans and professors and approves curricula, and so it goes round and round with little intervention from the outside world.

Richard Wakeford

Smith R. Profile of the GMC: medical education and the GMC; controlled or stifled? *BMJ*. 1989; 298(6684): 1372–5.

For among the many anomalies of the existing system of medical education the absence of proper instruction in psychological medicine is perhaps the most glaring and chronic.

George Walker

Walker GF. The springs of neurosis. *BMJ.* 1935; 1(3867): 296–9.

Curriculum, teaching and learning and assessment should all match, and all 'blueprint' onto each other.

David Wall

Wall D. The official curriculum teacher. In: Mohanna K, Chambers R, Wall D. *Your Teaching Style: a practical guide to understanding, developing and improving.* Oxford: Radcliffe Publishing; 2008. pp41–51.

By excluding unnecessary factual detail and by concentrating on principle rather than comprehensiveness, overcrowding in the curriculum can be reduced and has indeed been reduced by many medical schools with advantage to the learning process.

John Walton

Walton J. Educating the doctor: basic medical education. *BMJ.* 1985; 290(6483): 1719–22.

We need open debate on the feasibility of setting a national competency based curriculum for medical schools to achieve a correct balance between scientific knowledge and patient centred care.

Val Wass

Wass V. Ensuring medical students are "fit for purpose". *BMJ.* 2005; 331(7520): 791–2.

A major fault in our present medical education is the lack of cohesion between those responsible for welding the individual parts of the finished machine.

Beckwith Whitehouse

Whitehouse B. The British tradition and the new outlook. *BMJ.* 1942; 2(4264): 357–9.

The traditional method of apprenticeship teaching by clinical experience requires a continual expansion of the curriculum as ad hoc knowledge in a wide variety of subjects increases. The inevitable result, now seen in many teaching hospitals, is an overburdened curriculum and an unseemly wrangle among a variety of specialties for their piece of the cake.

CWM Whitty

Whitty CWM. Medical education. *BMJ.* 1962; 2(5311): 1058.

It is nowhere denied that we ask impossible tasks of students, who are bewildered by hours of listening, and that we stamp out the habit of reflection by a ceaseless drill.

Charles Wilson

Wilson CM. "The student in irons": the curriculum. *BMJ.* 1932; 1(3714): 485–7.

2. SELECTION

I wondered for some time afterwards how he had been able to discover from these questions that I had the attributes of a successful doctor, but I later found out that even this brief interview was superfluous, as the Dean always took the advice of his old secretary and told applicants this man disliked the look of that there were no vacancies.

Richard Gordon

Why is the cry of medical school expansion so shrill in a time of actual and impending medical unemployment?

Michael Allen

Allen M. An act of madness? *BMJ (Clin Res Ed)*. 1981; 282(6275): 1551.

It is no wonder the selection and training of medical students has a long way to go. I believe the desired end product should be a compassionate, vocationally dedicated, culturally literate individual who has a healthy cynicism for scientific dogma and who recognises that medicine will always be more an art than a science.

Roger Allen

Allen RKA. Selection of medical students. *BMJ*. 2002 May 18. Available at: www.bmj.com/content/324/7347/1170/reply#bmj_el_22616?sid=d5e693ea-0765-423d-ac1d-1c98624d8fdf (accessed 14 September 2011).

In the training of medical personnel there is a considerable time-lag before the products reach the market in any substantial numbers.

Gunnar Biörck

Biörck G. The next ten years in medicine: attempt at an analysis of factors determining medical and social development. *BMJ*. 1965; 2(5452): 7–11.

In trying to predict the likely manpower requirements of the health services in the next century it is necessary to make an assumption about the role which they will be required to fulfil.

Stephen Brearley

Brearley S. Manpower. *BMJ*. 1992; 304(6830): 832–4.

It is inevitable that training standards in Europe will converge, but they start from a point of great diversity and progress is likely to be slow.

Stephen Brearley

Brearley S. Medicine in Europe: medical education. *BMJ*. 1992; 304(6818): 41–4.

I advocate the rights of women, both with respect to academic degrees and the practice of the learned professions.

Frederick Brown

Brown FJ. Female medical education. *BMJ*. 1873; 1(650): 690–1.

Our profession continues to have as many means of entry as a cup-tie final.

Hugh Crichton-Miller

Crichton-Miller H. "The student in irons". *BMJ*. 1932; 1(3718): 680–1.

The old system of apprenticeship, with all its drawbacks, had this benefit – that it was an obstacle to the indiscriminate admission of youths, for every candidate was bound to find a master willing to stand sponsor for him.

Edward Crossman

Crossman E. An address on the maintenance of the honour and respectability of the medical profession. *BMJ*. 1883; 2(1176): 61–7.

What is a doctor, anyway? What does a general practitioner have in common with a forensic pathologist, or a neurosurgeon with a clinical biochemist? Increasingly little in these days of specialisation, yet their basic medical training and qualifications are likely to be similar.

John Dickinson

Dickinson J. Twelve new doctors for Nepal. *BMJ (Clin Res Ed)*. 1984; 289(6460): 1715–7.

Must it always be only in rueful valedictory repentance that the gatekeepers of medical education come to see what they have been doing?

Henry Dicks

Dicks HV. Medical education and medical practice. *BMJ*. 1965; 2(5465): 818–19.

The medical education for women is now so far organised in England that there is very little to say about it. It is almost as easy at this moment for a woman to get a complete medical education in England, Scotland, or Ireland, as it is for a man.

Elizabeth Garrett Anderson

Garrett Anderson E. Medical education of women: the qualification of female practitioners. *BMJ*. 1895; 2(1810): 608–9.

My main argument is that it would be discriminatory to school leavers and to mature non-graduates to limit medical training to people who already have a degree in the absence of any convincing evidence of benefit.

Charles George

George C. Should all medical students be graduates first? NO. *BMJ*. 2007; 335(7629): 1073.

By recruiting intelligent strivers with retentive memories medical schools may acquire some lateral thinkers with a capacity for empathy, but they would be there by accident rather than by design.

Nicholas Gold

Gold N. Medical education. *BMJ (Clin Res Ed)*. 1984; 288(6431): 1690.

I wondered for some time afterwards how he had been able to discover from these questions that I had the attributes of a successful doctor, but I later found out that even this brief interview was superfluous, as the Dean always took the advice of his old secretary and told applicants this man disliked the look of that there were no vacancies.

Richard Gordon

Doctor in the House.

Aptitude testing for medical school is certainly not the panacea it was once hoped to be, and in fact even as an aid in the evaluation of applicants it must be used judiciously and with due regard for its limitations.

Harrison Gough

Gough HG. Select medical students. *Med Teach*. 1979; 1(1): 17–20.

Judging by the number of students who fail to complete their education, together with those whose after career is a failure, it is manifest that many serious mistakes are made; and that it would have been better for such men had they attempted some other calling in life, more suitable to their capacities, and more congenial to their tastes.

CS Hall

Hall CS. Abstract of an address on the aspects of medicine as a profession, and on the training and work of medical men. *BMJ*. 1885; 2(1281): 94–100.

Is it good for the profession to demand that pupils should decide on medicine at the age of 13? Is it really a requirement of medical education that pupils should be so engaged in theoretical science from such a tender age?

MC Hime

Hime MC. The national curriculum and medical education. *BMJ*. 1989; 298(6673): 601–2.

There are amongst us, I believe, a few who really regard it as a thing to be desired, for the good of society, that women should be admitted to our medical schools, and become qualified to practise; but I suspect that the number of these is exceedingly small, and that it includes scarcely any who are actually engaged in practice.

Jonathan Hutchinson

Hutchinson J. A review of current topics of medical and social interest. *BMJ*. 1876; 2(816): 231–5.

Lowering entrance requirements for medical school is not the answer – medical school (and subsequent medical practice) requires intellect and application. An under-qualified profession will soon be devalued and will not serve its patients well.

Robin Ireland

Ireland R. Don't despise excellence. *BMJ*. 2006 August 29. Available at: www.bmj.com/content/333/7565/453.2/ reply#bmj_el_140577?sid=20523c27-2e0d-443d-a7db-86e43c2767d3 (accessed 14 July 2011).

Trying to get into medical school is like playing bridge with a silent partner: you're never sure what to bid because your partner refuses to declare his interests. And so prospective candidates continue to mutter nervously about their "strong motivation" or their "love of people" or "Daddy who's a professor of medicine" while wondering what their interviewers are really looking for.

Bobbie Jacobson

Jacobson B. Personal view. *BMJ*. 1978; 2(6152): 1638.

The Edinburgh School of Medicine for Women has now twenty-three students.

Sophia Jex-Blake

Jex-Blake S. Medical education of women. *BMJ*. 1888; 2(1453): 1023.

It is a mistake to restrict education to professional subjects so early in life as 16.

Walter Langdon-Brown

Langdon-Brown W. The medical curriculum and present-day needs. *BMJ*. 1938; 2(4052): 481–4.

To ensure that examinations are fair, most examination boards have a rigorous selection process for examiners which includes essential examiner specifications.

Anthea Lints

Lints A. Legal perspectives of assessment. In: Jackson N, Jamieson A, Khan A, editors. *Assessment in Medical Education and Training: a practical guide*. Oxford: Radcliffe Publishing; 2007. pp159–62.

I feel that medical students choose to do medicine for a great variety of reasons; and it cannot be seen as any reflection on those students, or the persons who select them, that all of those students do not follow a medical career for the whole of their working lives.

Ian Logan

Logan IS. Out in the cold. *BMJ (Clin Res Ed)*. 1983; 286(6372): 1216.

Despite the time, effort, and money that many schools invest in their selection processes, few have staff who are properly trained in selection theory and techniques, and in many cases the processes are amateurish and depend more on luck than design for their success.

Stella Lowry

Lowry S. What's wrong with medical education in Britain? *BMJ*. 1992; 305(6864): 1277–80.

If we could clearly identify the aims of undergraduate medical education we could begin to decide how best to select medical students.

Stella Lowry

Lowry S. Student selection. *BMJ*. 1992; 305(6865): 1352–4.

Students at US medical schools in the early decades of the 20th century had attrition rates of 5% to 50%, which represented a huge waste of human capital, individual and family aspirations, faculty time and energy, and misspent tuition money.

William McGaghie

McGaghie WC. Assessing readiness for medical education: evolution of the medical college admission test. *JAMA*. 2002; 288(9): 1085–90.

It is easier to criticise the present selection procedure than to design a better one.

Thomas McKeown

McKeown T. Personal view. *BMJ (Clin Res Ed)*. 1986; 293(6540): 200.

Yet few medical schools would now consider seriously an applicant who had an A in biology, C in chemistry, D in physics and an intense interest in natural history and foreign travel, the credentials that Darwin, a slow starter, might have offered.

Thomas McKeown

McKeown T. Personal view. *BMJ (Clin Res Ed)*. 1986; 293(6540): 200.

Students admitted to medicine in the United Kingdom do not match the national profile of social and ethnic diversity.

John McLachlan

McLachlan JC. Outreach is better than selection for increasing diversity. *Med Educ*. 2005; 39(9): 872–5.

Ideally we should be selecting medical students who have the attitudes and learning styles that will help them to continue lifelong education.

Chris McManus

Lowry S. Student selection. *BMJ*. 1992; 305(6865): 1352–4.

Despite occasional casual claims that A levels do not predict performance at medical school, evidence shows the opposite.

Chris McManus

McManus IC. Medical school applications: a critical situation; the supply of medical students may not meet the demands of medical school expansion in the United Kingdom. *BMJ*. 2002; 325(7368): 786–7.

A levels should not be the sole basis for the selection of students.

Chris McManus

McManus IC. Do school exams predict doctors' success? Author's reply. *BMJ.* 2003; 327: 810.

We should certainly broaden selection criteria if we wish to include students from poorly represented groups such as indigenous, financially disadvantaged and rural students, but we should be extremely cautious about screening applicants on the basis of personality factors or specific skills, other than previously demonstrated aptitude in knowledge, skills and reasoning.

Malcolm Parker

Parker M. Assessing professionalism: theory and practice. *Med Teach.* 2006; 28(5): 399–403.

Precise knowledge about production of doctors is important for planning, but existing data make satisfactory analysis difficult.

James Parkhouse

Parkhouse J. Intake, output, and drop out in United Kingdom medical schools. *BMJ.* 1996; 312(7035): 885.

Although commonality exists across all specialties and levels, selection criteria for each are distinct, with evidence supporting different priorities between specialties.

Fiona Patterson

Patterson F. Response: Fiona Patterson replies to Parashkev Nachev. *BMJ.* 2007; 335(7624): 802.

Selection is a different matter when students have had a chance to prove themselves independently, meeting the challenges of a university setting, and perhaps those of the workplace.

Ed Peile

Peile E. Head to head: should all medical students be graduates first? Yes. *BMJ.* 2007; 335(7629): 1072.

We must stop the headlong rush of pupils going straight from school into five year long medical courses.

Ed Peile

Peile E. Head to head: should all medical students be graduates first? Yes. *BMJ.* 2007; 335(7629): 1072.

Those who would improve the profession by narrowing its portal of entrance by adding strictures to the preliminary examination would bend to fashion's mood, and, like the "emancipated" woman wither the body to fatten the mind – an over-wise and ridiculous taxation.

Dobson Poole

Poole D. Medical education. *BMJ.* 1902; 2(2171): 426.

It is a topic that has been debated for years: Is it useful to include assessment of personal qualities in the selection procedure for future health professionals?

David Powis

Powis D. Personality testing in the context of selecting health professionals. *Med Teach.* 2009; 31(12): 1045–6.

Selection criteria for medical schools should not be solely based on grades but personality and aptitude.

Umesh Prabhu

Prabhu U. Modernisation must be for better! *BMJ.* 2004 May 15. Available at: www.bmj.com/content/328/7449/1158.7/reply#bmj_el_59513?sid=3f545f3a-8b62-4679-979a-2c0b244a4cd7 (accessed 14 July 2011).

The most compelling justification for race-based medical school admissions programs is the need for culturally competent physicians.

James Ryan

Ryan J. Affirmative action in medical school admissions. *JAMA.* 2003; 289(23): 3085.

Equal opportunity policies fail to deliver equity in access to medicine.

Judy Searle

Searle J. Equal opportunity does not produce equity: (not) getting into medical school. *Med Educ.* 2003; 37(4): 290–1.

Frustration, even despair, cannot be far from the minds of those who, over the years, have tried to formulate a reasonable basis for the staffing structure of hospitals.

Thomas Holmes Sellors

Sellors TH. Hospital career structure. *BMJ.* 1968; 3(5616): 496.

Of all the professions into which women might seek to be admitted, that of medicine is, in my opinion, the least suitable.

Septimus Sibley

Sibley SW. Remarks on some current medical topics. *BMJ.* 1877; 2(870): 283–6.

Every doctor will know somebody who would have given his right arm to become a doctor and yet was never accepted for medical school.

Richard Smith

Smith R. St George's University School of Medicine, Grenada: benefit or liability? *BMJ (Clin Res Ed).* 1982; 285(6337): 276–7.

Provided, of course, the grounds are sound, early exclusion not only benefits the school but may benefit the unsuccessful student also, in that he may be given an early opportunity to change to some other, less demanding course of study in which he may have a much better chance of success.

William Trethowan

Trethowan WH. Assessment of Birmingham medical students. *BMJ.* 1970; 4(5727): 109–11.

The selection criteria for medical education should be based on a rigorous analysis of what makes for the best possible doctors of the future.

Nigel Turner

Turner N. Medical schools and racial discrimination: recruiting ethnic minority medical students. *BMJ.* 1995; 310(6993): 1532.

If I were to draw up a code of laws for the regulation of medical education, I would make every student undergo a preliminary examination before he entered the profession, to test his scholastic and general attainments; this he should go through before a competent board of examiners; and if found eligible, he should be admitted as a medical student.

Thomas Turner

Turner T. Mr. Turner's introductory lecture: to the students at the Royal School of Medicine and Surgery, Pine-Street, Manchester, for the winter session of 1840–41. *Prov Med Surg J.* 1840; 1(3): 33–8.

The phenomenon of reversal of the gender ratio in medical schools, and eventually in the practice of medicine, is just about universal.

Leo van der Reis

van der Reis L. Causes and effects of a changed gender ratio in medicine. *Med Teach.* 2004; 26(6): 506–9.

Scientific reports are uncommonly conclusive on the use of interviews in selection. In finding candidates who are going to make better doctors or medical students they are, as typically used, useless.

Richard Wakeford

Medicine and the media. *BMJ.* 1986; 293: 127.

Give the places to the brightest students who have professed a desire to enter the most noble of professions.

William Watson

Watson W. Re: Evidence-based admissions procedures for medical students. *BMJ.* 2006 March 23. Available at: www.bmj.com/content/332/7548/1005/reply#bmj_el_130320?sid=20523c27-2e0d-443d-a7db-86e43c2767d3 (accessed 14 July 2011).

Why, only last term we sent a man who had never been in a laboratory in his life as a senior Science Master to one of our leading public schools. He came wanting to do private coaching in music. He's doing very well, I believe.

Evelyn Waugh

Decline and Fall. 1928.

I would appoint trainees only if there were a prospect of offering them a career post at the end of their training.

PW Wenham

Wenham PW. Personal view. *BMJ (Clin Res Ed).* 1981; 282(6277): 1701.

Looking at the overcrowded state of the profession, one cannot wish to see the entrance made easier; on the contrary, one would rather see it made more difficult, and should consider it an omen of better days for the science of medicine, and the status of its practitioners, if there were a more general falling off in the numbers of new entries, except where the standard of literary, scientific, and professional knowledge is pitched the highest, and the means for its acquisition are most complete.

Edward Willoughby

Willoughby EF. The London University and the medical schools. *BMJ.* 1885; 1(1263): 566–7.

3. BASIC SCIENCES

> There is no such thing as chemistry for medical students! Chemistry is chemistry!
>
> **Alfred Werner**

Medicine needs to be scientifically based, but physicians need to be engaged through their passions and emotions.

Robert Brook

Brook RH. A physician = emotion + passion + science. *JAMA*. 2010; 304(22): 2528–9.

Bee never without some institution or the like of physick whereof you may daylie or often read, and so continue in mind the method and doctrine of physick, which intention upon varietie or objects of other subjects may make you forget.

Thomas Browne

Shaw AB. Sir Thomas Browne: the man and the physician. *BMJ*. 1982; 285(6334): 40–2.

In medical and paramedical education, the Biological Sciences (anatomy and physiology particularly) are problematical areas because they are taught not just for the acquisition of facts, but rather in order that the student may acquire medical knowledge, understand disease processes and treatment rationale, and attain competent clinical skills.

Jennifer Butler

Butler JA. Use of teaching methods within the lecture format. *Med Teach*. 1992; 14(1): 11–25.

That skeleton is the skeleton of one of the prettiest girls I ever saw.

Joseph Constantine Carpue

D'Arcy Power. British Medical Association: Sixty-Third Annual Meeting of the British Medical Association in London, 1895; the medical institutions of London; the rise and fall of the private medical schools in London. *BMJ*. 1895; 1(1799): 1388–91.

The curriculum, teaching, and assessment must encourage the learning of clinically meaningful anatomy.

John Collins

Collins JP. Modern approaches to teaching and learning anatomy. *BMJ*. 2008; 337: a1310.

A parcel of lazy, idle fellars, that are always smoking and drinking and lounging . . . a parcel of young cutters and carvers of live people's bodies, that disgraces the lodgings.

Charles Dickens

The Pickwick Papers

At the early part of the century, with some few exceptions, very few surgeons, even of large hospitals, had personally dissected the human body; and the demand then for subjects became so great that a disreputable association had to be entered into between the teachers of anatomy and a class of men who were termed "Resurrectionists," to supply them with subjects.

William Alfred Elliston

Elliston WA. President's address: delivered at the Sixty-Eighth Annual Meeting of the British Medical Association. *BMJ*. 1900; 2(2066): 273–80.

Believing, as I do, that physiology is the one great basis of rational medicine, I argue that a very accurate study of it should be considered essential on the part of all those who desire to enter the profession of medicine – a far more accurate study, I mean, than has yet been deemed possible.

Arthur Gamgee

Gamgee A. An address delivered at the opening of the section of physiology. *BMJ*. 1877; 2(869): 239–43.

There is ample evidence that medical schools can and should do a better job in leveraging basic science training to facilitate the development of clinical decision-making skills.

Joseph Grande

Grande JP. Training of physicians for the twenty-first century: role of the basic sciences. *Med Teach*. 2009; 31(9): 802–6.

Medicine is what you are to profess. Medical practitioners you are intended to become. Most of you are not to be pure physicists, chemists, physiologists, or pathologists, but all these subjects have to be correlated with the great aim of your life.

David Hamilton

Hamilton DJ. An address on the study of pathology. *BMJ*. 1882; 2(1142): 977–80.

Ideally it would clearly be better for all medical research workers to have the background of a medical education. In practice this object cannot be achieved so long as it remains unusual for medically qualified men and women to devote sufficient time to the study of a scientific subject such as chemistry or physics to be able to carry out serious research work in it.

Charles Harington

Harington C. Medical research in the laboratory. *BMJ*. 1948; 2(4574): 459–62.

Animal dissection and/or "study" has no place in modern medical education. We treat people, not animals.

Kent Hoffman

Hoffman K. Use of animals in medical education. *JAMA*. 1991; 266(24): 3422.

Doubtless, the careful study of anatomy, regarded merely as entailing the acquisition of a certain number of facts, as acquiring a cognisance of the structure and relations of the several parts of the body, is a good mental exercise, inasmuch as it cultivates, among other qualities, those of attention, accuracy, and painstaking, which are the very foundation stones of the educational building.

George Humphry

Humphry GM. The address delivered in the section of anatomy and physiology. *BMJ*. 1882; 2(1128): 269–70.

There must always be a conflict in university medical education between the ideal of a broad education in science and the technical demands of a medical career.

Alastair Hunter

Hunter A. Medical education and medical practice. *BMJ*. 1965; 2(5461): 552–7.

Were I to place a man of proper talents, in the most direct road for becoming truly great in his profession, I would chuse a good practical anatomist, and put him into a large hospital to attend the sick, and dissect the dead.

William Hunter

Lecture 2, from *Last Course of Anatomical Lectures*.

Gentlemen may have an opportunity of learning the art of dissecting during the whole winter season, in the same manner as at Paris.

William Hunter

Tweedy J. The Hunterian oration: delivered before the Royal College of Surgeons of England, February 14th, 1905. *BMJ*. 1905; 1(2303): 341–5.

Dissection is the only perfect way of learning anatomy, which has been even defined as a "doctrine learned by dissections".

Henry Morris

Morris H. A lecture introductory to the course on anatomy. *BMJ*. 1876; 2(825): 515–17.

If the physician be ignorant of anatomy, how is he to diagnose disease?

Henry Morris

Morris H. A lecture introductory to the course on anatomy. *BMJ*. 1876; 2(825): 515–17.

No one can emerge from a medical degree having achieved a comprehensive knowledge of the basic sciences: biochemical and genetic knowledge is expanding faster than anyone can retain it.

Joshua Payne

Payne JDR. Reform of undergraduate medical teaching in the United Kingdom: "problem based learning" v "traditional" is a false debate. *BMJ*. 2004; 329(7469): 799.

In view of the extensive demands on the medical student it has been suggested that the time spent on anatomy and physiology should be curtailed by altering the teaching so as to insist on those details only which are of obvious practical use in medicine and surgery.

Humphry Rolleston

Rolleston HD. Introductory address on universities and medical education: delivered at the opening of the medical session of the Victoria University of Manchester on October 1st, 1912. *BMJ*. 1912; 2(2701): 886–7.

Many teachers of anatomy, physiology, and pathology (and perhaps this obtains more particularly at the universities devoid of clinical schools) instruct their students as though they, too, were destined to become anatomists, physiologists, and pathologists, whereas nine out of ten of them are destined to be doctors.

John Ryle

Ryle JA. "The student in irons". *BMJ*. 1932; 1(3716): 587.

I strive that in public dissection the students do as much as possible so that if even the least trained of them must dissect a cadaver before a group of spectators, he will be able to perform it accurately with his own hands; and by comparing their studies one with another they will properly understand this part of medicine.

Andreas Vesalius

De Humani Corporis Fabrica Libri Septem. 1543.

Widespread experience in the field of pathological anatomy must be the foundation, unless the whole procedure is to eventuate in deception.

Karl von Rokitansky

Handbuch der Pathologischen Anatomie. 1842.

Few people would disagree that two years spent in the company of a corpse is not the most imaginative introduction to a profession that, more than any other, needs to develop the skills of talking to distressed people.

David Weatherall

Weatherall DJ. The inhumanity of medicine. *BMJ.* 1994; 309(6970): 1671–2.

There is no such thing as chemistry for medical students! Chemistry is chemistry!

Alfred Werner

Kauffman GB. *Alfred Werner: founder of coordination chemistry.* 1966. p60.

Although medicine requires a thorough knowledge of biology, chemistry, physics, mathematics, pharmacology, physiology, histology, anatomy, biochemistry, pathophysiology and microbiology and then experience in surgery, medicine, obstetrics and pediatrics, it is a field of endeavor which must somehow be accessed through the heart as much as through the mind. For if a physician does not love to care, to empathize, to treat and assuage suffering then all of his or her knowledge will have been for naught. Caring in its broadest sense is what medicine is about.

Paul Winchester

Personal correspondence, 30 June 2011.

4. UNDERGRADUATE MEDICAL EDUCATION

> A first year medical student recently commented to me that in every lecture he attended he fell asleep after 45 minutes or so. Of course, with my years of experience of medical education I reassured him that with time and some effort he would be able to achieve this in as little as ten minutes or less.
>
> **Eugene Milne**

Hear instruction, and be wise, and refuse it not.

Prov. 8.33.

God help you all. What will become of you?

John Abernethy

Havard JD. One hundred and fifty years of service. *BMJ (Clin Res Ed).* 1982; 285(6334): 5–6.

But it is of the utmost importance, before this contraction of field comes about, that the youth should be trained in his imagination, a faculty which at school lies almost dormant.

Thomas Clifford Allbutt

Allbutt TC. The training of the medical student. *BMJ.* 1922; 2(3218): 407–9.

We need reprobates, beer swillers, card sharps, bong puffers, the irreverent and the like in medical students. It is their job.

Roger Allen

Allen RKA. Bring me your reprobates. *BMJ.* 2010 May 12. Available at: www.bmj.com/content/340/bmj.c1677/reply#bmj_el_235971?sid=31b7420e-2cd9-4337-8329-2f40df508216 (accessed 14 July 2011).

Natural abilities are like natural plants, that need pruning by study.

Francis Bacon

Of Studies, from *Essays*. 1625.

Medical schools will produce more doctors who will survive to practise medicine till retirement age if their graduates do not smoke cigarettes.

Keith Ball

Ball K. Medical students and smoking. *BMJ*. 1970; 4(5731): 367.

It is well to remember that a degree, apart from certain academical privileges – such as talking in convocation and voting for a member of Parliament – is simply a start in a career, and that real distinction is only acquired by subsequent honourable work.

Robert Barnes

Barnes R. The relations of the graduates and convocation of the University of London to the proposed reform of the university. *BMJ*. 1890; 1(1518): 267–8.

Medical schools are confronted by problems which increase in number, dimension, and complexity. There is no unanimity about what a good doctor is. Therefore, the objectives of medical education are oriented toward an insecurely visualized, if not uncertain, target.

William Bean

Bean WB. A study of twenty medical schools. *AMA Arch Intern Med*. 1960; 105(6): 979–80.

Medical undergraduate education traditionally has been a process bound by pedagogy, lacking in support structures and fuelled by a sense of achievement rather than understanding.

Ajay Bedi

Bedi A. An andragogical approach to teaching styles. *Educ Prim Care*. 2004; 15(1): 93–108.

When I was at medical school, I dreaded the ward round as I knew that I would be made to appear a fool, but maybe it was my desire to avoid that fate that ultimately made me a better doctor.

Jonathan Belsey

Belsey JD. Belittlement and harassment of medical students. *BMJ*. 2006 October 14. Available at: www.bmj.com/content/333/7572/809.2/reply#bmj_el_143938?sid=20523c27-2e0d-443d-a7db-86e43c2767d (accessed 14 July 2011).

Abiding by the dictates of best practice recommendations when obtaining consent for teaching will protect patients and students and promote good practice for students to emulate.

Susan Bewley

Bewley S. The law, medical students, and assault. *BMJ*. 1992; 304(6841): 1551–3.

When combining treatment with teaching doctors have dual roles and must guard against conflict between them.

Susan Bewley

Bewley S. The law, medical students, and assault. *BMJ*. 1992; 304(6841): 1551–3.

GRAVE, n. A place in which the dead are laid to await the coming of the medical student.

Ambrose Bierce
The Devil's Dictionary

HYENA, n. A beast held in reverence by some oriental nations from its habit of frequenting at night the burial-places of the dead. But the medical student does that.

Ambrose Bierce
The Devil's Dictionary

As medical students, when we finished the basic sciences and started clinics, there was a pleasurable difference noted immediately, as we no longer had to cram dull theory like in the basic sciences. The patient was our greatest teacher of medicine as much as the dead body had been in anatomy.

Rakesh Biswas
Biswas R. On being a medical student. *BMJ*. 2001 August 7. Available at: www.bmj.com/content/322/7288/709/reply#bmj_el_13530?sid=bfae656f-d7d3-4ae5-abb6-1b0e432b89b5 (accessed 14 July 2011).

The primary responsibility of medical schools is to prepare their students for their careers. In the interests of their students, therefore, medical schools must take note of employers' views.

Nick Black
Black N. Research, audit, and education. *BMJ*. 1992; 304(6828): 698–700.

How wonderful it would be if from the beginning of their clinical course medical students were expected to concern themselves with people, their home background, family worries, and anxieties about hospital treatment.

Isabel Boag
Boag I. Medical education. *BMJ*. 1958; 2(5103): 1042.

As the numbers of medical students increase and the numbers of staff to educate and train them decrease, one of the casualties of this phenomenon is a reduction in the provision of opportunities for medical students to learn about research methods.

Christine Bundy
Bundy C. Research training should be viewed as core business to medical education. *BMJ*. 2006 April 19. Available at: www.bmj.com/content/332/7546/863/reply#bmj_el_132065?sid=20523c27-2e0d-443d-a7db-86e43c2767d3 (accessed 14 July 2011).

Many students seem to believe that purchasing texts in addition to the required/recommended texts will somehow translate into learning the content.

Robert Burns
Burns R. Learning syndromes afflicting beginning medical students: identification and treatment: reflections after forty years of teaching. *Med Teach*. 2006; 28(3): 230–3.

Half of what you are taught as medical students in 10 years has been shown to be wrong. And the trouble is, none of your teachers knows which half.

Sydney Burwell
Pickering GW. The purpose of medical education. *BMJ*. 1956; 2(4985): 113–16.

To be an effective practitioner at endoscopic manipulations in the knee joint is there any justification for the traditional training of six years plus an additional preregistration year covering subjects which will have not the remotest practical relevance to the OK surgical techniques?

Roy Calne

Calne R. OK surgical technology. *BMJ.* 1990; 301(6766): 1479–80.

By the age of 17, a youth would have had time to procure a good preliminary education, and the subsequent six years would admit of a good medical education, including a period – not of five years, but of some months – occupied in something analogous to the apprenticeship of the present day.

Charles Carter

Carter CT. Observations on the clauses and provisions of Sir James Graham's Medical Bill. *Prov Med Surg J.* 1844; s1–8(38): 593–5.

It seems of late years to have been settled that four years are enough wherein to prepare a student for the duties of medical practice – aye, and for the degree of M.D. Surely this is too short a term of study. Six years at least should be exacted.

Charles Carter

Carter CT. Observations on the clauses and provisions of Sir James Graham's Medical Bill. *Prov Med Surg J.* 1844; s1–8(38): 593–5.

Research interests of medical schools and their parent university may take precedence over teaching commitments and clinical duties.

Graeme Catto

Catto G. Interface between university and medical school: the way ahead? *BMJ.* 2000; 320(7235): 633–6.

The beds are filled, indeed, but necessarily with obscure, chronic, and convalescent cases, who doubtless are proper objects for charity, but not useful for illustration. Advanced pupils may often with advantage puzzle out these enigmas, but to juniors they are insoluble.

Thomas Chambers

Chambers TK. Shall Oxford teach medicine? *BMJ.* 1878; 1(891): 140.

Above all else, caring for the dying requires good communications skills and these must be instilled at the time of entering medical school.

Rodger Charlton

Charlton RC. Using role-plays to teach palliative medicine. *Med Teach.* 1993; 15(2–3): 187–93.

The profession which you have chosen is one of the noblest, the most important, and the most interesting of all those occupations to which the highest human endeavours are turned. But it is also the most self-denying and the most arduous.

Andrew Clark

Clark A. Introductory address delivered at the Medical School of the London Hospital. *BMJ.* 1876; 2(823): 453–8.

If something is to be done about doctors' widespread ignorance of the special needs of disabled people then medical school is the logical place to start.

Alleyna Claxton

Claxton A. Teaching medical students about disability. *BMJ.* 1994; 308(6932): 805.

Addressing the reasons for the somewhat higher risk of attrition among minority medical students is yet another critical element in the effort to close the racial and ethnic diversity gap in our profession.

Jordan Cohen

Cohen JJ. Increasing medical school matriculation for minority students: reply. *JAMA*. 2007; 297(3): 265.

Medical schools must reduce significantly their dependence on high tech hospitals and find ways to educate their students in community settings, where patients receive the vast majority of their health care.

Jordan Cohen

Roehr B. More medical students should be educated in the community, US report says. *BMJ*. 2009; 338: b431.

The medical student should be clinically trained from the very outset, and the scientific training poured in by degrees as explanatory.

Thomas Corker

Corker TM. The student-apprentice. *BMJ*. 1932; 2(3741): 573.

However prolonged the training, the first year in practice will always be a salutary shock to the system.

EHJ Cotter

Cotter EHJ. Undergraduate medical education. *BMJ*. 1970; 2(5710): 666, 667.

What is wanted in medical education? Is it not a training as complete and thorough as possible in general medicine and surgery for every student?

Arthur Neville Cox

Cox AN. A diploma in tuberculosis. *BMJ*. 1922; 1(3193): 414–15.

The recent tendency has been to blame undergraduate education for inadequacies such as alleged deficiencies in clinical skills when it may be that the preregistration and early specialist training phases are more culpable.

Arthur Crisp

Crisp AH. Initiatives in the preregistration year (general clinical training). *BMJ (Clin Res Ed)*. 1985; 290(6484): 1764–5.

We must not fail to recognise that the medical student of the present day is a very different character from his predecessor. No further back than the days of Mr. Pickwick he was sui generis; the materials out of which the profession was then formed were rude and unhewn in the extreme.

Edward Crossman

Crossman E. An address on the maintenance of the honour and respectability of the medical profession. *BMJ*. 1883; 2(1176): 61–7.

Physicians-in-training always have learned at the bedside of the poor, and today's physicians must be brought there again.

Bob Cutillo

Cutillo B. Teaching professionalism to medical students. *JAMA*. 2000; 283(2): 197–8.

I am reminded of my medical student days, when my colleagues who could rattle off 50 causes of hepatomegaly, including many exotic ones which most would never see in their lifetimes, were considered academic stars as compared with those who were more interested in the "mundane" issues related to applying simple approaches successfully to improve health systems and population health.

Lalit Dandona

Dandona L. Public health sciences need strengthening in developing countries. *BMJ.* 2003 November 4. Available at: www.bmj.com/content/327/7422/1000/reply#bmj_el_39559?sid=7f27ee1c-bc1e-486c-bc82-03a5164885cc (accessed 14 July 2011).

The discipline of the University has appeared to me to offer not only the best, but the only safe, ground, on which to raise the school of our art.

Henry Dayman

Dayman H. Medical education. *Prov Med Surg J.* 1845; s1–9(11): 166–7.

The medical student pipeline is fundamental to keeping the complex adaptive system that is health services on track.

Ken Donald

Donald K. Medical schools: do they add value? *Med Teach.* 2007; 29(1): 1.

If a newly qualified doctor cannot resuscitate a patient, it does not say very much for Western medicine and, in particular, those who organise and run undergraduate courses.

AB Drake-Lee

Drake-Lee AB. Resuscitation needed for the curriculum? *BMJ.* 1985; 290(6486): 1986.

An energetic teaching program in the clinic can contribute materially to the learning experience of medical students, interns, and residents, and can be highly rewarding to the teacher.

Hugo Dunlap Smith

Dunlap Smith H. Essays in medical education II: the pediatric outpatient department as a pedagogical challenge. *Am J Dis Child.* 1965; 110(2): 185–8.

The most obvious advantage of a large school is the capacity to carry the teaching team required, but perhaps equally valuable is the ability to mount a variety of courses.

John Ellis

Ellis J. The Flowers report: three views. *Med Teach.* 1980; 2(3): 111–15.

Academic freedom has many aspects but one of the most important is freedom for the student to develop his full potential at university without being moulded into a particular kind of practitioner.

John Ellis

Ellis J. Editorial: 2. The aim of the undergraduate medical course. *Med Teach.* 1986; 8(2): 99–102.

It's surprising how patients tend to accept medical student's [*sic*] presence in a consultation if they are addressed as 'student doctor' or 'trainee doctor' – as opposed to 'the medical student'.

Hany El-Sayeh

El-Sayeh HG. 'Student Doctor', if you please. *BMJ.* 2003 August 12. Available at: www.bmj.com/content/327/7410/326/reply#bmj_el_35607?sid=7f27ee1c-bc1e-486c-bc82-03a5164885cc (accessed 14 July 2011).

Successful innovation in undergraduate education will presuppose sympathetic collaboration by the profession at large, first as role models and teachers and subsequently as supportive senior colleagues.

Charles Engel

Engel CA. Editorial: 2. Curricula for change. *Med Teach.* 1989; 11(1): 5–7.

Medical students in a traditional programme fill folders with lecture notes giving the currently accepted "facts," but this method of learning is unavailable after graduation.

Richard Farrow

Farrow R. Problem based learning at medical school: some people think it's thrilling . . . *BMJ.* 1995; 311(7020): 1642–3.

The effect of giving workers control over certain aspects of their jobs has been reported as mediating the effects of high demands, and in medical education this has been partly achieved by the introduction of staff student committees that can examine for change the rules governing difficult aspects of jobs.

Jenny Firth

Firth J. Levels and sources of stress in medical students. *BMJ (Clin Res Ed).* 1986; 292(6529): 1177–80.

The undergraduate and house officer learn more from the example of the general physicians and surgeons whom they serve and respect than from any instruction.

Francis Fraser

Fraser FR. The challenge to the medical profession. *BMJ.* 1960; 2(5216): 1821–6.

The main problem is that British medical schools are attracting some of the most able young people in the country and simply boring them to death.

Robin Fraser

Fraser RC. Undergraduate medical education: present state and future needs. *BMJ.* 1991; 303(6793): 41–3.

Unfortunately, some medical schools are less than fully committed to teaching.

Robin Fraser

Fraser RC. Undergraduate medical education: present state and future needs. *BMJ.* 1991; 303(6793): 41–3.

The present thrust of medical education and activity is away from "specialism" and "medical science" toward bringing good medical care to those who do not have it.

Daniel Funkenstein

Funkenstein DH. Medical students and surgery 1970. *AMA Arch Surg.* 1971; 102(1): 81–6.

There is a difference between an examination that a medical student would carry out and that by a qualified doctor. We therefore specifically advise medical students to explain to patients if they would like permission to examine them as part of their medical education, rather than for the patients' benefit.

John Gilberthorpe

Gilberthorpe J. Student doctors and consent. *BMJ.* 2005 September 7. Available at: www.bmj.com/content/331/7515/522.2/reply#bmj_el_116003?sid=cb764c2a-ad1a-4f84-a8c4-88b3568c267c (accessed 14 July 2011).

The medical student is likely to be one son of the family too weak to labour on the farm, too indolent to do any exercise, too stupid for the bar and too immoral for the pulpit.
Daniel Coit Gilman
Attributed.

Unfortunately there are troubling, if inconclusive, data that suggest that during medical school the ethical behaviour of medical students does not necessarily improve; indeed, moral development may actually stop or even regress.
Shimon Glick
Glick SM. Cheating at medical school: schools need a culture that simply makes dishonest behaviour unacceptable. *BMJ*. 2001; 322(7281): 250–1.

The ultimate aim of medical education is to transform students from members of the lay public to members of the profession.
John Goldie
Goldie J. Integrating professionalism teaching into undergraduate medical education in the UK setting. *Med Teach*. 2008; 30(5): 513–27.

Physicians demonstrate their concern for the future of the medical profession in their commitment to the education of medical students, residents, fellows, peers, and themselves.
Robert Golub
Golub RM. Medical education 2006: beyond mental mediocrity. *JAMA*. 2006; 296(9): 1139–40.

It is true that undergraduate medical training instructs rather than educates and both creates and rewards tunnel vision.
Trisha Greenhalgh
Greenhalgh T. Medical education. *BMJ (Clin Res Ed)*. 1984; 288(6431): 1689–90.

Due to the rapidly increasing amount of knowledge, within the constraints of a university degree or diploma, the relative time allocated to the teaching of university courses is decreasing remarkably.
Clayton Grieve
Grieve C. Knowledge increment assessed for three methodologies of teaching physiology. *Med Teach*. 1992; 14(1): 27–32.

How will it benefit these services and society if the recent increase in numbers of medical student is maintained but they are trained to a lower standard?
Anne Grüneberg
Grüneberg A. University budgets and medical education. *BMJ*. 1981; 282(6280): 1987–8.

Concept learning is the process in which subjects learn to categorize objects, processes or events.
Jan Gulmans
Gulmans J. The effect of prototype-based versus attribute-based presentation forms on the acquisition of a medical concept. *Med Teach*. 1990; 12(3–4): 329–37.

Medical students must come to understand that much of medical knowledge is a function of time and place, that medicine is a profoundly social enterprise and that the practice of medicine is a value-laden undertaking.

Edward Halperin

Halperin EC. Preserving the humanities in medical education. *Med Teach.* 2010; 32(1): 76–9.

Undergraduate teaching hospitals should be staffed mainly by junior consultants, providing the students with young enthusiastic teachers who have no conflict of interest with private practice.

DF Hawkins

Hawkins DF. System of postgraduate training. *BMJ.* 1970; 2(5703): 240.

Teaching is a peculiar activity; if the student fails to learn, teaching, existentially speaking, does not exist.

Harley Haynes

Haynes HA. What do medical students need and what do they want? *Arch Dermatol.* 1998; 134: 731–2.

One response to the global shortage of medical work-forces has been a rapid expansion of undergraduate medical education into new secondary and primary care facilities, where service loads are high and educational resources are stretched.

Richard Hays

Hays R. Foundation programme for newly qualified doctors. *BMJ.* 2005; 331(7515): 465–6.

Medical students, it has been said, are partially committed iatroblasts. Medical schools have the responsibility of providing them with the ethical receptors and expressors which prepare them to enter the medical body with due knowledge of the ethical self of the profession.

Gonzalo Herranz

Herranz G. An meaningful omission. *BMJ.* 1998 June 15. Available at: www.bmj.com/content/316/7145/1623/reply#bmj_el_210?sid=6a4ef178-62d7-4865-ac37-192d0fd43924 (accessed 14 July 2011).

Medical students require the individual attention and personal influence of their teachers, as exerted in small classes, and the esprit de corps of a hospital; they would not benefit by being herded into vast central lecture halls.

Leonard Hill

Hill L. London university and medical education. *BMJ.* 1905; 1(2305): 510–11.

Rather than simply acquiring factual knowledge, medical students need to acquire the following professional skills of a physician: problem solving and critical thinking, independent self-directed learning, and communication skills.

Robert Hilliard

Hilliard RI. The good and effective teacher as perceived by pediatric residents and by faculty. *Am J Dis Child.* 1990; 144(10): 1106–10.

I have no doubt that teaching ethics to medical students, if done well, will hasten the process of effective self-regulation amongst doctors.

Jeremy Hobson

Hobson J. Medical students and self-regulation. *BMJ.* 1998 September 21. Available at: www.bmj.com/content/317/7161/811/reply#bmj_el_817?sid=6a4ef178-62d7-4865-ac37-192d0fd43924 (accessed 16 July 2011).

It is impossible not to suspect that the assault on the round is a vicarious exercise: the real target is the academic centre itself, which must be exposed as an overprivileged, overspecialized ivory tower, lacking relevance to the community at large and diverting the medical student from the problems of primary health care.

HJK Hodgson

Hodgson HJK. Controversy: the case for the medical grand round. *Med Teach.* 1980; 2(2): 98–9.

Medical students learn much by apprenticeship and one of the things they learn from their seniors is a generalised (in the broadest sense) approach to patients.

Graham Howarth

Howarth GR. Informal curriculum. *BMJ.* 2003 January 31. Available at: www.bmj.com/content/326/7383/268/reply#bmj_el_30287?sid=7f27ee1c-bc1e-486c-bc82-03a5164885cc (accessed 16 July 2011).

[A]nd I am quite sure a very considerable number of young men spend a large portion of their first session simply learning how to learn in a fashion that is entirely new to them.

Thomas Huxley

Huxley T. Introductory address on the intervention of the state in the affairs of the medical profession. *BMJ.* 1883; 2(1189): 709–11.

Some of the medical schools enumerated, while giving equal opportunities to men and women as far as graduation, do not realize their further responsibilities, and have made no effort to throw open to their women graduates the resident posts in their own hospitals.

Frances Ivens

Ivens F. Women doctors. *BMJ.* 1925; 1(3343): 192.

It is generally conceded that the ideal in teaching is to have the student see personally as many clinical problems as possible, with an opportunity to take a history and examine and closely follow the patient with the aid and counsel of the teaching staff.

Hilger Perry Jenkins

Jenkins HP. Motion pictures in medical education, with particular reference to the undergraduate phase. *AMA Arch Surg.* 1958; 77(3): 303–12.

My thesis is essentially that every medical student should have an opportunity to see in good color motion picture photography every disease or condition about which he should be expected to know something, accompanied by discussion from his teacher appropriate to the importance of the subject.

Hilger Perry Jenkins

Jenkins HP. Motion pictures in medical education, with particular reference to the undergraduate phase. *AMA Arch Surg.* 1958; 77(3): 303–12.

The thesis that international social forces are affecting undergraduate medical education hardly needs defending. When one considers the liberalization of curricular structure in many medical schools, the freeing-up of greater and greater amounts of truly elective time, the lowering of costs of international travel, the affluence of our society which makes grants and fellowships available so that international travel is more readily possible as well as the great number of medical schools which have formal or informal ties with medical centers in other parts of the world, it is easy to understand why there has been such a marked increase in international travel by undergraduate medical students and by faculties since the Second World War.

C Henry Kempe

Kempe CH. International social forces affecting undergraduate medical education. *Am J Dis Child.* 1967; 114(5): 538–44.

After 35 years of dealing with medical students and residents as programme director, the greatest recent deficiency in applying educational theory in practice seems to be personal entitlement and the lack of autodidacticism.

Robert Knuppel

Knuppel RA. Perhaps medicine should now be considered a trade. *BMJ.* 2003; 326(7396): 986.

Concept maps that integrate and relate concepts in a nonlinear fashion are widely accepted as an educational tool that can underpin meaningful learning in medical education.

David Laight

Laight DW. Attitudes to concept maps as a teaching/learning activity in undergraduate health professional education: influence of preferred learning style. *Med Teach.* 2004; 26(3): 229–33.

Medical students are continually being asked to do things they think of as wrong. Under the guise of teaching them how to be physicians, they are asked to forget that they are human beings.

Stephen Lammers

Lammers SE. Are these dilemmas or something more? *BMJ.* 2001 March 26. Available at: www.bmj.com/content/322/7288/709/reply#bmj_el_13530?sid=bfae656f-d7d3-4ae5-abb6-1b0e432b89b5 (accessed 16 July 2011).

So unlike all other things in the world are medicine and the practice of it, that indications of treatment (simple things, but great mysteries) need to be pointed out to the most intelligent student with the care and patience that you would teach his letters to a child.

Peter Mere Latham

Latham PM. A word or two on medical education: and a hint or two for those who think it needs reforming. *BMJ.* 1864; 1(162): 141–3.

Till now, just when the medical student was throwing off the school-boy, and putting on the young man, with a young man's ardent aspirations – a young man's peculiar sensitiveness – a young man's quick perceptions, he has been bound down by the apprentice system, with its degrading offices and menial employments.

James Thomas Law

Law JT. Address, delivered at the opening of the present session of Queen's College, Birmingham. *Prov Med Surg J.* 1846; s1–10(41): 485–8.

No matter how many degrees or diplomas you obtain, you can never cease being medical students.

Alexander Macalister

Macalister A. An address on fifty years of medical education: delivered at the opening of the winter session at King's College, London. *BMJ.* 1908; 2(2492): 957–60.

The London student has the benefit of the fact of 25,000 beds being in the hospitals of the English metropolis, and the hungry man consumes the whole roast.

Angus Macdonald

Macdonald AD. A teaching university for London. *BMJ.* 1885; 1(1264): 622.

Implicit in the core and options approach is the acceptance of an illusory degree of homogeneity in medical education and practice.

Stuart MacLeod

MacLeod SM. Undergraduate medical education: too many facts not enough innovation. *BMJ.* 1993; 307(6918): 1565–6.

Medical students are the enemy of larger lists.

Geoffrey Marsh

Handysides S. Enriching careers in general practice: building morale through personal development. *BMJ.* 1994; 308(6921): 114–16.

I can conceive no other remedy than that the student should have a responsible master or masters; for instance, should be absolutely required to become dresser (for surgery), and clinical clerk (for medicine).

Samuel Martyn

Martyn S. Medical education. *BMJ.* 1864; 1(165): 247.

While no one would deny that severe bullying and harassment can have a negative effect on medical students, I cannot help but wonder where one draws the line between abrasive, if effective, teaching methods and outright bullying and whether the behaviour of my own consultants would constitute such objectionable behaviour?

David McKean

McKean D. Beware censoring our best teachers. *BMJ.* 2006 October 2. Available at: www.bmj.com/content/333/7570/682?tab=responses (accessed 19 November 2011).

It took me 10 years of medical practice to realise that the skills in history taking that I had been taught at medical school were severely limited in terms of the information that they uncovered.

Janet Menage

Menage J. Undergraduate medical education. *BMJ.* 1991; 303(6796): 245.

All physicians have unique experiences as medical students and residents, but some memories of medical education are universal: camaraderie, miraculous cures, unexpected deaths, inspiring attendings, and on-call terrors.

Tony Miksanek

Miksanek T. Becoming a doctor: from student to specialist, doctor-writers share their experiences. *JAMA.* 2010; 304(11): 1245.

A first year medical student recently commented to me that in every lecture he attended he fell asleep after 45 minutes or so. Of course, with my years of experience of medical education I reassured him that with time and some effort he would be able to achieve this in as little as ten minutes or less.

Eugene Milne

Milne E. Papers and reports: miscellanea; from Mindy's Institute, Broadway. *BMJ (Clin Res Ed)*. 1985; 291(6511): 1822.

I am not one of those who wish to place a strict limit upon the enjoyment of all rational recreations and amusements – far from it – but I do say that a medical student who is to be seen in Covent Garden Theatre when he ought to be found in the theatre of his own medical school, is making a very great fool of himself, to say the least of it.

John Morgan

Morgan J. Clinical lectures in course of delivery during the present session, at Guy's Hospital. *Prov Med Surg J*. 1841; s1–2(28): 21–5.

What dissection is to the anatomical student, hospital practice is to the medical student.

John Morgan

Morgan J. Clinical lectures in course of delivery during the present session, at Guy's Hospital. *Prov Med Surg J*. 1841; s1–2(28): 21–5.

Master conscientiously the precepts of medicine, and labour to carry those precepts with you into action, then, indeed, the allotted days of each one of you will be usefully spent.

John Edward Morgan

Morgan JE. Medicine in 1876: being an inquiry into the effects of experimental researches on the principles and practice of medicine. *BMJ*. 1876; 2(823): 458–63.

The trainer should be regarded as an educational facilitator rather than as a teacher. This is in recognition that medical students and junior doctors are adults and that educational experiences should be learner centred.

Martyn Neil

Neil MW. Doctors need to be taught how to teach. *BMJ*. 2005 September 6. Available at: www.bmj.com/content/331/7515/465/reply#bmj_el_115867?sid=cb764c2a-ad1a-4f84-a8c4-88b3568c267c (accessed 16 July 2011).

It will be a sorry day if the education of the medical student divides too soon, so that the training for general practice becomes divorced from the training for research work.

John Nixon

Nixon JA. The art and science of medicine in relation to professional training. *BMJ*. 1928; 2(3530): 363–4.

When a medical student is first qualified he has to recall what he has learnt of the experience of others, but presently he must rely on his own, and he soon finds that experience must be actively earned; it does not fall into the lap unsought.

John Nixon

Nixon JA. The art and science of medicine in relation to professional training. *BMJ*. 1928; 2(3530): 363–4.

It used to be said that you could tell the difference between medical and science students very simply. You walked into a room and said "Good morning": the science students said "Good morning" and the medical students wrote it down. Nowadays, the medical students look down to see if you put it in the handout.

R Alan North

North RA. Personal view. *BMJ*. 1975; 2(5970): 555.

Fear of litigation from unsuccessful students, explosive growth of evidence based medicine, risk management and protocol driven medicine have attempted to and to a considerable extent have succeeded in reducing medicine to binary notation.

Makarnd Oak

Oak MK. A well argued case. *BMJ.* 2008 June 3. Available at: www.bmj.com/content/336/7655/1250/reply#bmj_ el_196557?sid=b74f0c68-fddb-4ccf-81b2-5e2a3899315c (accessed 16 July 2011).

Medical education has been described as a process of socialization in which students are taught to acquire the beliefs and behaviors that will identify them as physicians.

Michael O'Connor

O'Connor MM. The role of the television drama ER in medical student life: entertainment or socialization? *JAMA.* 1998; 280(9): 854–5.

Would undergraduate medical students benefit from a non-clinical as well as a clinical elective? This non-clinical elective could be a compulsory period as a restaurant waiter or similar position where students would be exposed to customers, some of whom will be anxious and may seem rude and unreasonable. This would form the basis for further education on effective interaction with patients and colleagues.

William O'Neill

O'Neill WM. Patients' complaints: students must learn communication skills. *BMJ.* 1993; 307(6916): 1427.

We are in a transition stage in our methods of teaching, and have not everywhere got away from the idea of the examination as the "be-all and end-all" so that the student has constantly before his eyes the magical letters of the degree he seeks.

William Osler

Osler W. An address on the master-word in medicine: delivered to medical students on the occasion of the opening of the new laboratories of the Medical Faculty of the University of Toronto, October 1st, 1903. *BMJ.* 1903; 2(2236): 1196–200.

He who studies medicine without books sails an uncharted sea, but he who studies medicine without patients does not go to sea at all.

William Osler

Osler W. *Aequanimitas, With Other Addresses to Medical students, Nurses and Practitioners of Medicine.* New York: McGraw Hill; 1906. p211.

I desire no epitaph . . . than the statement that I taught medical students in the wards, as I regard this as by far the most useful and important work I have been called upon to do.

William Osler

Osler W. *Aequanimitas, With Other Addresses to Medical students, Nurses and Practitioners of Medicine.* 4th ed. London: Keynes Press; 1984.

A candidate was asked by an examiner in physiology a simple question, the answer to which involved an elementary knowledge of the brain. Thereon the candidate politely informed the examiner that he did not know anything about the anatomy of the brain, that he was "only up for physiology" on that occasion.

Edmund Owen

Owen E. Abstract of an address on the medical student and his environment. *BMJ.* 1888; 1(1413): 175–6.

The medical student of today is crammed with a store of teaching which would do credit to a nineteenth century Solomon.

Edmund Owen

Owen E. Abstract of an address on the medical student and his environment. *BMJ.* 1888; 1(1413): 175–6.

Medicine at its best translates to physicians with patient-oriented minds of the finest caliber finding answers to disease, training students in the practice of medicine derived from that research, and ensuring that the product of that effort results in better, more responsive patient care.

Herbert Pardes

Pardes H. The perilous state of academic medicine. *JAMA.* 2000; 283(18): 2427–9.

Age and ageing are medical challenges which demand a response not only in the planning of the undergraduate course but at all stages of medical education, and above all from those who aspire to teach.

Kenneth Parry

Parry KM. Editorials. *Med Teach.* 1983; 5(4): 124–6.

Education demands the active participation of the student's mind.

George Pickering

Pickering G. Postgraduate medical education: the present opportunity and the immediate need. *BMJ.* 1962; 1(5276): 421–5.

The students have one great ground for complaint – namely, that the educational system to which they are subjected is out of date.

George Pickering

Pickering G. Postgraduate education and society: the lesson from medicine. *BMJ.* 1969; 3(5667): 375–8.

Undergraduate medical education is always victim to the syndrome that the teachers are often from a system that taught differently.

Sebastien Pillon

Pillon SL. Desirability & practicality. *BMJ.* 2006 December 21. Available at: www.bmj.com/content/333/7580/1226/reply#bmj_el_151876?sid=20523c27-2e0d-443d-a7db-86e43c2767d3 (accessed 21 September 2011).

It seems incredible that what we have accepted for a few hundred years as the basic training for medicine should exclude almost any reference to the unconscious mind and human behaviour; for, although most universities give some lectures in psychology to their medical students, academic departments of psychology are all too often concerned with precise methods of measuring the irrelevant rather than with exploring the origins of human emotion.

Robert Platt

Platt R. Thoughts on teaching medicine. *BMJ.* 1965; 2(5461): 551–2.

The task of an undergraduate medical school is to train generalists, not specialists.

Adrian Pointer

Pointer AE. The nature of academic medicine. *BMJ.* 2001 June 18. Available at: www.bmj.com/content/322/7300/1442.1/reply#bmj_el_15143?sid=bfae656f-d7d3-4ae5-abb6-1b0e432b89b5 (accessed 21 August 2011).

Students with disabilities account for 0.2% of medical school graduates.
Michael Reichgott

Reichgott MJ. The disabled student as undifferentiated graduate: a medical school challenge. *JAMA*. 1998; 279(1): 79.

The farewell thank you by the medical students at the end of the day is sufficient.
Adel Resouly

Resouly A. St George's University School of Medicine, Grenada: benefit or liability? *BMJ (Clin Res Ed)*. 1982; 285(6341): 574.

Undergraduate, general professional, and specialist education are run as virtually separate entities.
Philip Rhodes

Rhodes P. Profile of the GMC. *BMJ*. 1989; 298(6688): 1641.

With regard to the Medical Council, it appears to me an anomaly that, while nine-tenths of the medical men in this country are general practitioners, they are not represented on the Council, and have no voice in the management of the education of the medical students.
John Richards

Richards J. Remarks on current medical topics. *BMJ*. 1876; 2(821): 394–5.

The greatest challenge is to inspire students to curiosity, to fan the flames of their own enthusiasm and the empathy which goes with it. All else will then fall into place.
Peter Richards

Richards P. Clinical competence and curiosity. *BMJ (Clin Res Ed)*. 1986; 292(6534): 1481–2.

Programming students for today's medicine is important but insufficient; students must also emerge able to adapt to a succession of revolutions in medicine within their working lifetime.
Peter Richards

Richards P. Departmental divisions and the crisis in undergraduate medical education. *BMJ (Clin Res Ed)*. 1988; 296(6632): 1278–9.

University medicine in Britain had a difficult birth, a retarded wartime childhood, and an adolescence full of promise and expectation. Is it to die on the threshold of its maturity, at a time when a traditional craft education was never less fitted to prepare for the future?
Peter Richards

Richards P. Departmental divisions and the crisis in undergraduate medical education. *BMJ (Clin Res Ed)*. 1988; 296(6632): 1278–9.

Yes, of course, there are a few, sometimes likable, scallywags who behave like prodigal sons; despite repeated offers of advice and help they squander their intellects, fail degree exams, and are discontinued as medical students.
Ian Richardson

Richardson IM. Personal view. *BMJ (Clin Res Ed)*. 1982; 284(6321): 1039.

The image created years ago of the well heeled, yellow checked waistcoated, MG Midget owning, beer swilling medical student, with more interest in rugby and nurses than in clinical studies, was and still is utterly false.

Ian Richardson

Richardson IM. Personal view. *BMJ (Clin Res Ed).* 1983; 287(6400): 1215.

The modern student never learns anything about a thorough and full physical examination, but relies entirely on reports from special departments.

Henry Robinson

Robinson H. Limitations of current medical training. *BMJ.* 1944; 2(4367): 382–3.

It is more satisfactory to combine research and the teaching and training of university students by whole-time professors and their skilled assistants than to make special arrangements for original work alone, because the scientific spirit is thus more widely diffused.

Humphry Rolleston

Rolleston HD. Introductory address on universities and medical education: delivered at the opening of the medical session of the Victoria University of Manchester on October 1st, 1912. *BMJ.* 1912; 2(2701): 886–7.

It is widely accepted that communication skills can be taught but practical experience of teaching undergraduates indicates that students' abilities to understand and communicate with their patients varies enormously.

Virginia Royston

Royston V. How do medical students learn to communicate with patients? A study of fourth-year medical students' attitudes to doctor-patient communication. *Med Teach.* 1997; 19(4): 257–62.

I have recently seen medical students play their part as naturally and effectively and with as good a humour when their hospital was bombed and patients had to be moved by difficult routes to safety as if that were the occasion for which they had been particularly trained. For the moment, however, you must accept that your first line of national service is to learn as much as you can of the sciences essential to the equipment of a good doctor.

John Ryle

Ryle JA. To-day and to-morrow. *BMJ.* 1940; 2(4167): 657–9.

The whole future of medical education depends on the foundations being properly laid, but if the general practitioner is to fulfil his functions properly it will be necessary to curtail his later undergraduate studies in certain directions while extending them in others.

Harold Sanguinetti

Sanguinetti HH. "The student in irons". *BMJ.* 1932; 1(3725): 1011.

You may not learn here how to diagnose measles or to treat whooping-cough, but you ought to acquire what is of far more importance, those habits of scientific thought which will make you accurate diagnosticians and rational practitioners.

Robert Saundby

Saundby R. An address on modern universities: delivered at the opening of the medical school of University College, Cardiff. *BMJ.* 1898; 2(1971): 1034–8.

Students mistrust and misunderstand the purpose of pastoral care and avoid seeking help for fear of jeopardising their careers.

Melissa Sayer

Sayer M. Stopping medical students going off the rails. *BMJ.* 2002 September 15. Available at: www.bmj.com/content/325/7364/556?tab=responses (accessed 19 November 2011).

Momentum for fundamental change in the education of American medical students is mounting. Alterations of training are suggested as a logical solution for uneven quality of care, lack of primary physicians, and even widespread disability from long-term disease.

Irwin Schatz

Schatz IJ. Changes in undergraduate medical education: a critique. *Arch Intern Med.* 1993; 153(9): 1045–52.

Medical schools need to climb down from their lofty perches and recognise that they are training doctors for the community – not for their own ranks.

James Sherifi

Sherifi J. Medical students are overqualified to be GPs. *BMJ.* 2002 October 18. Available at: www.bmj.com/content/325/7368/786/reply#bmj_el_28867?sid=7f27ee1c-bc1e-486c-bc82-03a5164885cc (accessed 16 July 2011).

Regarding the essential clinical and operative training, apparently of less importance than the university training, the regional hospitals are being utilized for this work. Surely this is a far better place for training the students than sitting in classrooms or watching animal experiments in university hospitals specializing in rare research subjects, most of which are unfortunately time-wasting and unproductive.

John Shipman

Shipman J. Medical education for the future. *BMJ.* 1968; 4(5627): 392.

Most medical students start by wanting to take care of patients but end more interested in the mechanisms and diagnosis of disease.

Andrew Smith

Smith A. Learning the practical art. *BMJ.* 1975; 1(5951): 219.

A main problem with undergraduate medical education is that it is too full.

Richard Smith

Smith R. Profile of the GMC: medical education and the GMC; controlled or stifled? *BMJ.* 1989; 298(6684): 1372–75.

Medical education was learning by humiliation, with naming, shaming, and blaming. Now, students are encouraged to question received wisdom.

Richard Smith

Smith R. Thoughts for new medical students at a new medical school. *BMJ.* 2003; 327(7429): 1430–3.

A child begins with the alphabet and some years later may appreciate Shakespeare. Similarly, medical students need to be given the facts first so that they may develop to confidently tackle challenging medical problems.

Thomas Smith

Smith TE. Learning problems. *BMJ.* 2006 February 15. Available at: www.bmj.com/content/332/7537/365.1/reply#bmj_el_128164?sid=20523c27-2e0d-443d-a7db-86e43c2767d3 (accessed 16 July 2011).

It is my firm conviction, however – and I speak from some considerable experience – that the teaching of medicine cannot be too severely practical, and that the most successful teacher is the one who shows his students how to observe the obvious.

Henry Souttar

Souttar HS. Educational number, session 1932–3: the education of the medical student. *BMJ.* 1932; 2(3739): 427–9.

Nobody who has not examined in surgery can conceive that a medical student can in a few short months forget so completely every shred of anatomy he has ever learned.

Henry Souttar

Souttar HS. Educational number, session 1932–3: the education of the medical student. *BMJ.* 1932; 2(3739): 427–9.

The student logically proceeds through his different blocks of preliminary science, he advances to anatomy and physiology, and then he proceeds to the wards, and so far as I can judge from a fairly extensive examination experience, it takes him about six weeks to forget everything he has learned in the preceding block.

Henry Souttar

Souttar HS. Educational number, session 1932–3: the education of the medical student. *BMJ.* 1932; 2(3739): 427–9.

Learning in the community benefits all, not least future hospital specialists.

John Spencer

Spencer J. What can undergraduate education offer general practice? In: Harrison J, van Zwanenberg T, editors. *GP Tomorrow.* 2nd ed. Oxford: Radcliffe Medical Press; 2002. pp49–66.

The matron, on the subject of married medical students (70% of the final year), says, "Why, there are a dozen here who would marry me to-morrow – if I'd put them through college!"

John Spillane

Spillane JD. New American medical schools. *BMJ.* 1960; 2(5201): 778–85.

The teachers of medical students are at present confronted by a dilemma, which they are attempting to solve by the use of worn-out machinery invented at a time when medicine was little more than a craft entrusted to a guild jealous of its privileges and its perquisites.

Ernest Starling

Starling EH. Medical education in England: the overloaded curriculum and the incubus of the examination system. *BMJ.* 1918; 2(3010): 258–9.

A pupil who is pure, obedient to his preceptor, applies himself steadily to his work, and abandons laziness and excessive sleep, will arrive at the end of the science he has been studying.

Susruta

Sutrasthanam (ch. 3), from *Sushruta-Samhita*

While it is true that most if not all students who enter on a medical course are impelled to do so by a desire to alleviate human suffering, they differ widely in the ways in which they picture themselves doing it – through scientific or clinical research, specialist or general practice, and so on.

Alexander Todd

Todd A. The doctor in a changing world. *BMJ.* 1968; 4(5625): 207–9.

Only a few days since, a fully fledged M.B. and M.R.C.S., who had taken the highest honours at an especially medical university, and whose clinical notes on cases were deserving of the highest praise, assured me, that during the four years spent in medical study, he had not seen a case of measles.

Thomas Underhill

Underhill T. Medical education, past and present. *BMJ*. 1868; 2(410): 509–10.

We accept racehorses and turn out asses.

Unknown

As a researcher in basic medicine after graduation, I felt bitter, and still do, about those classes which had so little pertinence to medicine.

Daizo Ushiba

Ushiba D. My medical education: its relevance to my career. *Med Teach*. 1980; 2(5): 238–40.

A stimulating hypothesis is that bright, undiagnosed learning-disabled medical students are unable to compensate for their learning disability on standardized examinations.

Jane Uva

Uva JL. Performance on the NBME Part I Examination. *JAMA*. 1995; 273(8): 617.

One of the most frustrating things for medical students is knowing what is wrong with their medical education but not being able to do much about it.

Tiago Villanueva

Villanueva T. The future for medical education. *BMJ*. 2005; 331(7508): 105–6.

Medical instruction does not exist to provide individuals with an opportunity of learning how to make a living, but in order to make possible the protection of the health of the public.

Rudolf Virchow

Address to medical students in Berlin.

Can the mind of a medical student be made as supple, effective, strong, and available an instrument for his purposes – so far as Nature has endowed him with faculties – by no education unless it includes Latin?

Willoughby Francis Wade

Wade WF. President's address, delivered at the Fifty-Eighth Annual Meeting of the British Medical Association. *BMJ*. 1890; 2(1544): 259–62.

It is impossible as an undergraduate to predict your future career course. The end of your medical training is a time when you have acquired your metaphorical set of basic tools for the rest of your career.

David Walker

Walker DA. Reform of undergraduate medical teaching in the United Kingdom: a triumph of evangelism over common sense. *BMJ*. 2004 September 16. Available at: www.bmj.com/content/329/7457/92/reply#bmj_el_74479?sid=3f545f3a-8b62-4679-979a-2c0b244a4cd7 (accessed 16 July 2011).

Any demoralisation that we may feel as professionals must not be apparent to those we are teaching.

James Walker

Walker JD. Medical students demoralised by teachers. *BMJ*. 2002 January 23. Available at: www.bmj.com/content/324/7330/173.1/reply#bmj_el_18941?sid=d5e693ea-0765-423d-ac1d-1c98624d8fdf (accessed 16 July 2011).

Medicine, the law, and theology have traditionally been called the learned professions.

Richard Wilbur

Wilbur RS. Continuing medical education: past, present, and future. *JAMA*. 1987; 258(24): 3555–6.

Facts the student must have – they are the food on which he must live; but a system which has become concerned too narrowly, too exclusively, with their mechanical acquisition is surely a misconception.

Charles Wilson

Wilson CM. "The student in irons": the curriculum. *BMJ*. 1932; 1(3714): 485–7.

Despite a renewed emphasis on defining and developing professionalism, recent studies indicate that attributes typically associated with professional virtue often decline during undergraduate medical education, a most worrisome reality.

Alexander Wong

Wong A. Relationships and respect: keys to addressing the "hidden curriculum". *BMJ*. 2004 October 12. Available at: www.bmj.com/content/329/7469/770/reply (accessed 16 July 2011).

Surely it is time to stop arguing about the process and ensure that diversity in undergraduate educational provision is related to declared graduate outcomes and delivers doctors who have the required competencies for good medical practice.

Diana Wood

Wood DF. Problem based learning. *BMJ*. 2008; 336(7651): 971.

It might be argued that the purpose of undergraduate education is to produce a healthy stem cell which can differentiate later.

Verna Wright

Wright V. The consultant rheumatologist and postgraduate education. *BMJ (Clin Res Ed)*. 1983; 287(6400): 1158–9.

Furthermore, with the media and the public regarding medical students as a group with significant earning potential, medical students have little say in influencing government budgets. Instead, medical graduates are voicing their dissent through migrating to other countries.

Catherine Yang

Yang CJ. Migration of health professionals: not just a problem for developing countries. *BMJ*. 2005 February 2. Available at: www.bmj.com/content/330/7485/210/reply#bmj_el_95146?sid=1e069fc1-8837-4789-925c-3c1714669644 (accessed 1 August 2011).

5. POSTGRADUATE MEDICAL EDUCATION

BODY-SNATCHER, n. A robber of grave-worms. One who supplies the young physicians with that which the old physicians have supplied the undertaker.

Ambrose Bierce

Why does a caring profession cast its babies out into the cold when it's spent years of time, patience, patients, and money on them?

Joe Andrews

Medicopolitical digest. *BMJ.* 1992; 304(6831): 920–2.

[A]ll training programmes (and other conditions of service, including the provision of hospital creches) should consider the needs of women, who are likely to marry and have children.

Tom Arie

Arie T. Married women doctors as part-time trainees. *BMJ.* 1975; 3(5984): 641–3.

Reading maketh a full man; conference a ready man; and writing an exact man.

Francis Bacon

Of Studies, from *Essays.* 1625.

We do not need to further document that scheduled sleep deprivation and chronic fatigue is deleterious to the physical and mental health of residents rather we need to study the current system of graduate medical education.

Bertrand Bell

Bell B. Assess graduate medical education not resident hours of work. *BMJ.* 2002 November 27. Available at: www. bmj.com/content/325/7374/1184/reply#bmj_el_27393?sid=d5e693ea-0765-423d-ac1d-1c98624d8fdf (accessed 1 August 2011).

BODY-SNATCHER, n. A robber of grave-worms. One who supplies the young physicians with that which the old physicians have supplied the undertaker.

Ambrose Bierce

The Devil's Dictionary

If we have learnt anything from the past decade of reform it is that the postgraduate training of doctors can't simply be fitted in round service: it takes planning and hard work.

Graeme Catto

Catto G. Specialist registrar training: some good news at last. *BMJ.* 2000; 320(7238): 817–18.

Academic medicine must continue its fight for a broad-based, all-payer system that explicitly supports graduate medical education, teaching hospitals, medical schools, biomedical and behavioral research, and advanced nursing education.

Jordan Cohen

Cohen JJ. Academic medicine: facing change. *JAMA.* 1995; 273(3): 245–6.

Every surgeon has to do his first appendix.

Lawrence Cohn

Cohn L. Closing the gap between professional teaching and practice. *BMJ.* 2001 April 27. Available at: www.bmj. com/content/322/7288/685/reply#bmj_el_13965?sid=bfae656f-d7d3-4ae5-abb6-1b0e432b89b5 (accessed 1 August 2011).

Designing programs for IMGs [international medical graduates] is a complex task, and programs must be tailored to individuals and local conditions.

Geoff Couser

Couser G. Twelve tips for developing training programs for international medical graduates. *Med Teach.* 2007; 29(5): 427–30.

In a more rational world some of the central processes of medical education and career development would be less mysterious – or at least more subject to rational scrutiny.
Colin Currie
Currie C. Role models and patronage. *BMJ.* 1993; 306(6880): 735–6.

Medical education is in bad shape. That it is nasty, brutish, and long is but the least of its problems.
Carl Elliott
Elliott C. The making of a doctor: medical education in theory and practice. *JAMA.* 1993; 270(11): 1374.

It is unacceptable that ethnicity should be a factor determining the progress of students who enter medical school or qualified doctors who sit professional examinations.
Aneez Esmail
Esmail A. Ethnicity and academic performance in the UK. *BMJ.* 2011; 342: d709.

Over half of all postgraduate medical education in the UK, and much education of nurses, is funded by the pharmaceutical industry from its annual marketing budget of £1.65bn.
Robin Ferner
Ferner RE. The influence of big pharma. *BMJ.* 2005; 330(7496): 855–6.

I learn many things from the residents . . . especially on how to get out of their mess.
Allan Fisher
Personal correspondence, 1 July 2011.

It is a depressing thought that, since 1953, medical graduates in the UK have been undergoing a period of training which is badly organized, has negligible educational content and to which adjectives such as appalling, deplorable and soul destroying have been applied. In such terms has the preregistration year been described.
Peter Fleming
Fleming PR. The preregistration year: need for a national survey. *Med Teach.* 1981; 3(2): 45–6.

During clinical training, emphasis is still centred on disease per se.
Harold Fox
Fox H. Medical education. *BMJ.* 1958; 2(5099): 795–6.

Many more medically qualified persons enter general practice than any other branch of medicine, so that training for general practice is numerically the most important task of postgraduate education.
Francis Fraser
Fraser F. Postgraduate education. *BMJ.* 1952; 2(4782): 455–8.

The remarkable development of postgraduate medical education in regional hospitals in the last 10 years is perhaps the most encouraging advance since the National Health Service was introduced.
George Godber
Godber GE. Future of postgraduate medical centres. *BMJ.* 1972; 2(5814): 654.

The process of maturation from student to resident to skilled physician is gradual and prolonged, sometimes painful, and always accompanied by times of self-examination.
Robert Golub
Golub RM. Are you sure this is right? Insights into the ways trainees act, feel, and reason. *JAMA*. 2010; 304(11): 1236–8.

Globalization requires that the fortunate medical schools in the first world must partner with their colleagues in the less developed parts of the globe to assure that educational standards and basic health care delivery are assured for all.
Jean Gray
Gray JD. Creating a roadmap for academic medicine. *BMJ*. 2004 April 1. Available at: www.bmj.com/content/328/7440/597/reply#bmj_el_55225?sid=3f545f3a-8b62-4679-979a-2c0b244a4cd7 (accessed 1 August 2011).

Doctors who organise postgraduate activities may use them, like their professional journals, as a subtle form of advertising. They may even acquire merit from them (not in the religious but in the highly specific medical sense of the term).
JC Griffiths
Griffiths JC. Personal view. *BMJ (Clin Res Ed)*. 1983; 286(6383): 2058.

If we are able to accept international medical graduates as suitably qualified despite their country of training, it would be a shot in arm for medical training across the world. Medical Schools would compete across the world and not merely nationally.
Maneesh Gupta
Gupta M. International medical curriculum. *BMJ*. 2005 September 11. Available at: www.bmj.com/content/331/7516/561/reply#bmj_el_116308?sid=cb764c2a-ad1a-4f84-a8c4-88b3568c267c (accessed 1 August 2011).

How can satisfactory training be provided in limited time when there are competing demands from clinical workload?
Richard Harling
Harling R. Multimedia: on-the-job training for physicians. *BMJ*. 1999; 318(7180): 405.

There seems to be a reluctance, even among medical administrators, to accept that it is actually in the interests of patients for those who look after them to pursue postgraduate education by research, attending courses or conferences.
David Hide
Hide DW. Christ Church conference on postgraduate education: 25 years on. *BMJ (Clin Res Ed)*. 1987; 294(6572): 643–4.

Medical know-how has attained such a state of specialization that it is impossible to train a doctor in depth for any one of the branches of medicine until the postgraduate stage.
Kenneth Hill
Hill KR. Some reflections on medical education and teaching in the developing countries. *BMJ*. 1962; 2(5304): 585–7.

Life is short,
the art long.
Hippocrates
Aphorisms. I, 1.

It is time to understand and accept that health professionals will succumb to all the factors which affect all other professionals; and that human mobility is part of life in the 21st century. It is time to bury the archaic concept of brain drain, and turn to assessing performance of health professionals and systems, wherever they are in the world.

Adnan Hyder

Hyder AA. Health professionals' mobility in the 21st century. *BMJ.* 2003 July 31. Available at: www.bmj.com/content/327/7407/170.1/reply#bmj_el_34676?sid=7f27ee1c-bc1e-486c-bc82-03a5164885cc (accessed 1 August 2011).

Our overarching conclusion is that the science clearly shows that fatigue increases the chances of errors, and residents often work long hours without rest and regular time off.

Michael Johns

Kuehn BM. IOM: shorten residents' work shifts to reduce fatigue, improve patient safety. *JAMA.* 2009; 301(3): 259–61.

Graduates engaged in post-graduate work are reminded that their Supervisor is a University Officer and when visiting him officially in that capacity they should dress as they would in visiting any other officers of the University or of their own College (e.g. a tutor).

John Edward Lennard-Jones

Note from Lennard-Jones to his PhD student Charles Coulson, 14 July 1933.

Postgraduate medical education is essential, and there should be some measure of compulsion or reward to secure its full benefits, which are considerable in developing a satisfactory Service.

George MacFeat

MacFeat G. The family doctor in the N.H.S. *BMJ.* 1950; 1(4654): 663–4.

We must be very careful, in our insistence on the need for a continuing surveillance of professional standards over an extended period of postgraduate development, that the Government officials who control our destinies do not seize upon the opportunity to relegate the doctor to the social and economic status of a perpetual probationer.

D McClure

McClure D. Doctors of the future. *BMJ.* 1968; 2(5601): 368.

Fundamental questions of equity and justice suggest that if higher medical degrees are important to people in their careers then the degrees should be administered in equivalent fashion in different universities.

Chris McManus

McManus IC. The MD and MS degrees in Britain. *BMJ.* 1988; 297(6641): 115–16.

As an educational experience, a good system of medical audit is worth any number of postgraduate courses.

Ian McWhinney

McWhinney IR. Medical audit in North America. *BMJ.* 1972; 2(5808): 277–9.

Our continuing education is controlled by postgraduate deans and clinical tutors, none of whom are general practitioners, many of whom take no advice from general practitioners, and few of whom seem to have any understanding of the principles and practice of adult education.

David Metcalfe

Metcalfe D. General practice revisited. *BMJ.* 1981; 283(6285): 233–4.

For centuries advances in medicine and surgery had been so slow that a good medical education then sufficed for a lifetime.

Rutherford Morison

Morison R. Post-graduate teaching of surgery: the inaugural address for 1914–15 delivered before the Midland Medical Society. *BMJ.* 1915; 1(2835): 749–56.

Healthcare professionals are trained very well to care for individuals but receive very little, if any, training in how to care for the system of healthcare delivery.

Fiona Moss

Moss F. The clinician, the patient and the organisation: a crucial three sided relationship. *Qual Saf Health Care.* 2004; 13: 406–7.

No training of the surgeon can be too arduous, no discipline too stern, and none of us may measure our devotion to our cause.

Berkeley Moynihan

The approach to surgery, from *Addresses on Surgical Subjects.*

It now remains for me to direct your attention to the present state of obstetric education, which, I regret to be obliged to confess, is deficient in the extreme; so imperfect, so inadequate, that if some expansive and efficient means be not taken to improve it, the accidents will become so frequent; the public so indignant; the coroner so often called upon; the doctor, who parades a diploma, so often exposed, that I fear our whole profession may be dragged down from the honourable pedestal on which it ought to rest, into the deepest abyss of degradation – public contempt.

Edward William Murphy

Murphy EW. Lettsomian lectures for 1853. *Assoc Med J.* 1853; s3–1(15): 323–9.

My colleagues and I deal with the immediate postgraduate training of juniors and know that, regardless of where the doctors have qualified, their practical education starts when they start working with patients for real.

Roderick Neilson

Neilson R. National qualifying exams: authors have missed gap between theory and reality. *BMJ.* 2008; 337: a1783.

But postgraduate medical education should not be restricted to one or two hospitals or institutions; it should be the direct responsibility of every teaching hospital to look after regional peripheral hospital junior staff interests.

Richard Neville

Neville R. Training of specialists. *BMJ.* 1962; 1(5276): 474–5.

That the man who brings to the study of the healing art the greatest store of theoretical knowledge, and skilful practical application, gathered from varied sources, will, ceteris paribus, be the most successful practitioner is self-evident. There is only one other point to which I will direct your attention, and to this I beg your earnest and careful heed. It is to strive to become careful observers and correct reasoners.

Thomas Nunneley

Nunneley T. Introductory lecture: delivered at the Leeds School of Medicine, October 4th, 1852. *Prov Med Surg J.* 1852; s1–16(21): 525–9.

The orientation of medical education in this country has been almost entirely towards the search for a physical pathology to "explain" the occurrence of disease.

Desmond O'Neill

O'Neill D. Stress and disease: a review of principles. *BMJ.* 1958; 2(5091): 285–7.

A chapter of accidents would be unfortunate; a compendium of deliberate mistakes seems like a truer but less excusable epitome of our efforts to deal with the problems of postgraduate training and medical staffing.

James Parkhouse

Parkhouse J. Manpower: compendium of deliberate mistakes. *BMJ.* 1986; 292(6530): 1286–7.

How does the National Health Service reconcile a good service for patients with effective postgraduate training for doctors and a healthy research programme? Until recently a combination of tradition, haphazard evolution, and serendipity has enabled the service to muddle through.

James Parkhouse

Parkhouse J. Hospital medical staffing: our hope for years to come. *BMJ (Clin Res Ed).* 1987; 295(6607): 1157–8.

It has never been true to say – and how much less is it true today – that once a doctor has passed his final examinations and is entering practice his education has been completed.

Kenneth Parry

Parry KM. Educational organizations: the Scottish Council for Postgraduate Medical Education. *Med Teach.* 1979; 1(3): 157–9.

The link between the assessment of medical education and the evaluation of medical care lies at the root of many of the current issues for postgraduate education.

Kenneth Parry

Parry KM. Postgraduate education in Australia and the United Kingdom compared. *BMJ.* 1981; 282(6257): 52–5.

After some years in general practice I found that what I had been taught in the past and what I learnt from attending postgraduate courses could only be applied to about half of the patients seeking my advice.

H Stephen Pasmore

Pasmore HS. Medical education and medical practice. *BMJ.* 1965; 2(5467): 940.

It took British medicine 40 years to do for preregistrands what the Council on Medical Education of the A.M.A. and the Association of the American Colleges did together in 1914 on accreditation of internships. We then failed miserably to ensure preregistration standards were maintained by adequate review procedure.

JW Paulley

Paulley JW. Postgraduate education and training. *BMJ.* 1970; 1(5688): 115.

Postgraduate medical education has been undergoing constant changes over the last decade and so far it is hard to see the end of this process. This instability makes career planning impossible.

Mikolaj Pawlak

Pawlak MA. Money is not the major factor. *BMJ.* 2004 June 2. Available at: www.bmj.com/content/328/7451/1280.2/reply#bmj_el_61295?sid=3f545f3a-8b62-4679-979a-2c0b244a4cd7 (accessed 1 August 2011).

We know that learning takes place in the zone of complexity, yet I know of little evidence about optimal complexity of case material in postgraduate medical education.

Ed Peile

Peile E. Commentary: the value of complexity. *BMJ.* 2009; 338: b796.

Just as the units in undergraduate education are the undergraduate teaching hospitals, and their associated medical schools of the university, so the units for postgraduate education should be the larger hospitals of the regional board.

George Pickering

Pickering G. Postgraduate medical education: the present opportunity and the immediate need. *BMJ.* 1962; 1(5276): 421–5.

Unless the service reaches a certain standard a hospital should not have training-posts at all.

George Pickering

Pickering G. Postgraduate medical education: the present opportunity and the immediate need. *BMJ.* 1962; 1(5276): 421–5.

Reconciling the needs of the service with educating doctors is not always easy. Often the same people are concerned with service and education, but it is valuable and helpful to give formal recognition to education.

Philip Rhodes

Rhodes P. Postgraduate education. *BMJ.* 1983; 286(6378): 1635–6.

The growth of the large institutions, such as universities and medical faculties and schools, the royal colleges and faculties, the General Medical Council, and the councils for postgraduate medical education, may have seemed to put the responsibility for education on more or less defined teachers, allowing others to think that they have been edged out of their traditional roles as masters in charge of apprentices.

Philip Rhodes

Rhodes P. Educating the doctor: postgraduate, vocational, and continuing education. *BMJ.* 1985; 290(6484): 1808–10.

We can all benefit from medical migration, so long as it goes round and back with enhanced skills and opportunities and is not one-way to the detriment of the populations of the less well developed countries of the world.

Jane Richards

Richards J. Suction rather than drainage. *BMJ.* 2002 March 4. Available at: www.bmj.com/content/324/7336/499/reply#bmj_el_20334?sid=d5e693ea-0765-423d-ac1d-1c98624d8fdf (accessed 1 August 2011).

With so many doctors to choose from they prefer to go next door, to the doctor with an MS or MD or maybe an FRCS or MRCP and, no doubt, a good number of other initials after his name. Well it proves he's the better doctor doesn't it?

Tessa Richards

Richards T. Impressions of medicine in India: the push for postgraduate degrees. *BMJ (Clin Res Ed).* 1985; 290(6476): 1196–9.

The deliberate division into "teaching" and "nonteaching" hospitals is artificial and misleading. Many "non-teaching" hospitals, both voluntary and municipal, have a tradition for providing postgraduate training which is widely recognized.

GO Richardson

Richardson GO. Postgraduate medical education. *BMJ.* 1962; 1(5279): 712.

The advantage of using a non-teaching hospital is that, the number of students being relatively small, it is possible to develop a good teacher-student relationship and every form of instruction becomes, in effect, a tutorial.

Edward Rigby

Rigby EP. Postgraduate medical education. *BMJ.* 1962; 1(5292): 1623.

My advice to medical students and residents who wish to work in the third world would be FINISH YOUR TRAINING FIRST, get all experience you can working within your educational system then consider volunteering abroad under the tutelage of more experienced practitioners.

Robert Ripley

Ripley RG. Required reading. *BMJ.* 2000 April 25. Available at: www.bmj.com/content/320/7240/1017.1/reply#bmj_el_7405?sid=7f1b5b2e-7b0c-43f6-8a46-f45951808b4f (accessed 1 August 2011).

Anyone who knows anything about being a medical student and a preregistration house officer recognises that you learn more in a fortnight as a house officer when the chips are down than in six months as a student.

NRC Roberton

Roberton NRC. LMSSA: a back door entry into medicine? *BMJ (Clin Res Ed).* 1987; 294(6579): 1096.

The hospitals without medical schools are responsible through their resident appointments for the practical postgraduate training of the majority of the general practitioners of this country.

Thomas Robson

Robson T. The non-teaching hospital. *BMJ.* 1945; 1(4386): 131.

Before qualification few men realize that there will be much more to learn when once the portal is safely passed; when, however, this has been negotiated, they soon begin to see that, like the preliminary subjects of the so-called ancillary sciences, the hospital knowledge of their professional subjects is only a further though more complete preliminary to the efficient practice of the healing art.

Henry Rolleston

Rolleston H. The aims and methods of graduate study. *BMJ.* 1920; 1(3081): 77–9.

Women doctors in training and postgraduate education need opportunities for part-time training in order to get the experience they require.

William Russell

Russell W. Letter from Westminster. *BMJ (Clin Res Ed).* 1981; 282(6282): 2147.

Continuity in care during training schemes should provide follow-up mechanisms, allowing expansion of knowledge of the natural history of illness, recovery time, resolution of clinical signs, assessment of accuracy of diagnostic reasoning, in addition to the valuable insight learned from mistakes, including awareness of heuristics and bias inherent in the development of metacognition.

Wesley Scott-Smith

Scott-Smith W. The development of reasoning skills and expertise in primary care. *Educ Prim Care.* 2006; 17: 117–29.

If clinical work has somehow become dissociated from teaching . . . the primary aims of the institution have become confused.

JD Swales

Swales JD. The Tomlinson report and postgraduate medical education. *BMJ.* 1993; 306(6869): 42–4.

Unlike the other departments of medical education, clinical surgery has not an end as well as a beginning, since its subject is inexhaustible, and limited only by the time allotted for its study.

James Syme

Syme J. Concluding lecture of a winter course on clinical surgery. *BMJ.* 1868; 1(381): 371.

I, for one, desire to raise my voice in protest against the absurd attention to detail and the enormous waste of time involved in the present biological training of the surgeon student.

Lawson Tait

Tait L. Address in surgery. *BMJ.* 1890; 2(1544): 267–73.

Quality of training should be reflected in performance rather than in competence of graduates.

Olle ten Cate

ten Cate O. Medical education: trust, competence, and the supervisor's role in postgraduate training. *BMJ.* 2006; 333(7571): 748–51.

Constructive use of time spent in quality training is important in answering the question of what is effective postgraduate medical education.

Hemal Thakore

Thakore H. Cost effective postgraduate medical education. In: Walsh K, editor. *Cost Effectiveness in Medical Education.* Oxford: Radcliffe Publishing; 2010. pp14–21.

Effective postgraduate medical education produces a competent specialist by the correct utilisation of training time, training experience, trainee assessment, teaching curriculum, learning environment and teachers.
Hemal Thakore

Thakore H. Cost effective postgraduate medical education. In: Walsh K, editor. *Cost Effectiveness in Medical Education*. Oxford: Radcliffe Publishing; 2010. pp14–21.

Exposure to the correct case-mix is vital in providing an effective, quality education programme for trainees.
Hemal Thakore

Thakore H. Cost effective postgraduate medical education. In: Walsh K, editor. *Cost Effectiveness in Medical Education*. Oxford: Radcliffe Publishing; 2010. pp14–21.

Should doctors in general, and specialists in particular, decide for themselves what their needs for postgraduate education are or should politicians, medical associations or the public have a right to demand proof that they keep up to date?
Anvik Tor

Tor A. Around the world: education for primary care in Norway. *Educ Prim Care*. 2003; 14: 277–87.

Cooperation between surgeons and educationalists is essential to improve the quality and the delivery of postgraduate surgical education.
Zaher Toumi

Toumi Z. Gap between educationalists and surgeons. *BMJ*. 2006 September 19. Available at: www.bmj.com/content/333/7567/544/reply#bmj_el_142089?sid=20523c27-2e0d-443d-a7db-86e43c2767d3 (accessed 1 August 2011).

Training based on competency outcomes has flourished in both undergraduate and post-graduate education, in a climate of increasing accountability to the NHS [National Health Service]. But there is scant evidence to support this arguably minimalist and behaviourist approach to clinical learning.
Val Wass

Wass V. What the educators are saying. *BMJ*. 2004; 329(7461): 335.

Because young doctors are constantly rotating through different training programmes, and as a consequence of the new regulations to limit their working hours, there is lack of day to day continuity of care at all junior grades.
David Weatherall

Weatherall DJ. The inhumanity of medicine. *BMJ*. 1994; 309(6970): 1671–2.

Surgical training programs are in the doldrums. Like it or not, "see one, do one, teach one" is no longer acceptable as a tenet of medical learning.
John Weigelt

Weigelt JA. Medical education crisis: not just an issue of work hours. *Arch Surg*. 2003; 138(9): 1027–8.

The unremitting growth in the aggregate number of resident physicians enrolled in GME [graduate medical education] programs, in association with what is viewed as an imbalance in the specialty mix of those programs, has led policymakers once again to express concerns about the adverse impact the GME system has on the size and specialty composition of the physician workforce.

Michael Whitcomb

Whitcomb ME. The role of medical schools in graduate medical education. *JAMA.* 1994; 272(9): 702–4.

Surely the secret of a good apprenticeship is to have a good master, and the basic requirement for being a good master is to work alongside one's apprentices.

David Wilson

Wilson DH. Teaching in casualty. *BMJ (Clin Res Ed).* 1982; 285(6351): 1355–6.

The patient with a serious illness has much to gain from being treated in a teaching hospital, for in addition to the special skills and facilities available to him the presence of undergraduate and postgraduate students in my experience helps to maintain a high standard of patient care. Against this, however, is the fact that in some hospitals there are too many students in relation to the number of patients.

Michael Woodruff

Woodruff MFA. Personal view. *BMJ.* 1968; 3(5613): 311.

The universities are so diverse in their requirements for the degree of M.D. that this now, despite its rank, no longer carries the status it should, and the diploma of M.R.C.P. has become the temperamental prima donna (or ballerina, for what a dance it is!) of the trainee physician stage, and no advances can be tolerated from him until he has gained favour and given satisfaction in it.

H Wykeham Balme

Wykeham Balme. M.R.C.P. (London). *BMJ.* 1962; 1(5279): 710.

Case by case analysis of medical schools in sub-Saharan Africa would show an excellent first 10 years followed by a general downward spiral.

Joseph Yikona

Yikona J. Sustaining medical education is difficult in poor countries. *BMJ.* 2003; 326(7379): 51.

6. CONTINUING PROFESSIONAL DEVELOPMENT

> The kind of doctor that I want is one who, when he's not examining me, is home studying medicine.
>
> **George Kaufman**

If the family physician is to do more than mark time, he must have opportunities of entering, for not inconsiderable vacations, on instruction in new methods and introduction to new principles; also for conversance in his daily work with the scientific methods and equipment of district laboratories.

Thomas Clifford Allbutt

Allbutt TC. Medical education in England: a note on Sir George Newman's memorandum to the president of the Board of Education. *BMJ.* 1918; 2(3005): 113–15.

Continuing medical education is a vital part of good practice by any self respecting professional.

Joseph Ana

Ana J. Caring for older people: launching the Nigerian edition of the *BMJ*: implications for Nigeria's health care. *BMJ*. 1996; 313(7049): 105.

He that will not apply new remedies must expect new evils: for time is the greatest innovator.

Francis Bacon

Of Innovations, from *Essays*. 1625.

Although the number of CME [continuing medical education] offerings has increased enormously since many states have made it mandatory for relicensure, most physicians do not view such licensure regulation as the most important motivation of their pursuit of medical knowledge.

William Barclay

Barclay WR. CME: more than just keeping up-to-date. *Arch Intern Med*. 1981; 141(7): 839.

The education of the doctor which goes on after he has his degree is, after all, the most important part of his education.

John Shaw Billings

Billings JS. Address to the Harvard Medical Alumni Association. *Boston Med Surg J*. 1894; 131; 140–2.

Medical education is, or should be, a lifelong process, and local medical societies play an indispensable part in this, and combine with it the cultivation of friendship between doctors.

Russell Brain

Brain R. Dickensian diagnoses. *BMJ*. 1955; 2(4955): 1553–6.

Patients expect their physicians to have the right answer every time. Does the testing process in medical school or the continuing medical education (CME) process increase the likelihood that patient expectations will be met?

Robert Brook

Brook RH. Continuing medical education: let the guessing begin. *JAMA*. 2010; 303(4): 359–60.

I keepe the sheets of the transactions [of the Royal Society] as they come out monethly.

Thomas Browne

Shaw AB. Sir Thomas Browne: the man and the physician. *BMJ*. 1982; 285(6334): 40–2.

The new CPD [continuing professional development] is based on sound educational principles, such as being relevant to problems encountered at work, based on identified learning need, directed by the learner, shared with peers, using reflection, recording and evaluating outcomes.

Peter Burrows

Burrows P. Continuing professional development: filling the gap between learning needs and learning experience. *Educ Prim Care*. 2003; 14: 411–13.

We need to address the question of helping people to sustain their capacity to learn for, from and at work, and this means helping people to maintain and celebrate their own personal commitment to learning, their creativity and their curiosity.

Jonathan Burton

Burton J. Work based learning in health and social care: innovations and applications, Middlesex University, 25 February 2004. *Work Based Learn Prim Care.* 2004; 2(2): 193–5(3).

The term 'learning trajectory' is used to define the pattern of involvement (or non-involvement) in learning. Learning trajectories are plotted by the retrospective study of the learning experience of individuals or groups of individuals.

Jonathan Burton

Burton J. Self-assessment, peer assessment and third party assessment: significance for work based learning. *Work Based Learn Prim Care.* 2005; 3(1): 1–3(3).

Those truly interested in improving physician performance need to dump CME [continuing medical education] as it presently exists and develop a new model to improve practice quality, once we have decided what quality is.

Christopher Buttery

Buttery CM. Does continuing medical education work? *BMJ.* 2006; 333(7558): 99.

We must see medical education as a continuum, including continuing medical education, and recognise that doctors have an ethical obligation to keep up to date.

Kenneth Calman

Calman K. The profession of medicine. *BMJ.* 1994; 309(6962): 1140–3.

You cannot fail to organise a successful meeting or conference if you choose a subject that addresses people's needs, at a price they can afford, at a convenient time in an accessible location.

Ruth Chambers

Chambers R. Practical tips for organising educational activities efficiently. In: Chambers R, Wall D, editors. *Teaching Made Easy: a manual for health professionals.* Oxford: Radcliffe Medical Press; 2000. pp59–76.

Continuing medical education (CME) is a time-honored but questionable strategy by which physicians update their knowledge of recent scientific developments and in turn apply this knowledge to patient care.

Carolyn Clancy

Clancy C. Commentary: reinventing continuing medical education. *BMJ.* 2004; 328(7445): E291.

Multiple studies have shown that CME does indeed advance physicians' knowledge, but that passive acquisition of information results in only modest – if any – measurable improvements in care.

Carolyn Clancy

Clancy C. Commentary: reinventing continuing medical education. *BMJ.* 2004; 328(7445): E291.

A central tenet of contemporary educational theory is that adult learning is most effective when it is self-directed and based on real problems experienced in the workplace.

Robert Clarke

Clarke R. Foundation programme assessments in general practice. *Educ Prim Care.* 2006; 17: 291–300.

Healthcare practitioners need to be able to demonstrate their ability to capitalise on both formal learning activities and the informal opportunities for development that present themselves in the course of practice.

Mark Cole

Cole M. Capture and measurement of work based and informal learning: a discussion of the issues in relation to contemporary healthcare practice. *Work Based Learn Prim Care.* 2004; 2(2): 118–25(8).

At its heart audit should be concerned with taking note of what we do, learning from it, and changing if necessary. Fundamentally, it is educational.

Colin Coles

Coles C. Self assessment and medical audit: an educational approach. *BMJ.* 1989; 299(6703): 807–8.

Continuation of media-comparative research will only consume resources that would be better spent investigating elements of online CME [continuing medical education] that could make it more effective and efficient, such as specific instructional methods, presentation formats, and approaches to implementation.

David Cook

Cook DA. Internet-based continuing medical education. *JAMA.* 2006; 295(7): 758.

International CME is more than conferences and courses – it includes projects in needs assessment, a wide variety of formats and strategies, and evaluation of doctors' performance and health care outcomes.

Dave Davis

Davis D. Continuing medical education: global health, global learning. *BMJ.* 1998; 316(7128): 385–9.

Rapid changes in today's medicine, both in knowledge and technology, make it difficult and impractical for practicing physicians to rely on more traditional "passive" learning (eg, didactic continuing medical education lectures) to keep current.

Thomas DeWitt

DeWitt T. Can we train a lifelong learner? *Arch Pediatr Adolesc Med.* 2001; 155(6): 637–8.

The vast majority of doctors are good learners and have always just got on with their own continuing medical education and professional development – that is what being a professional means.

Clair du Boulay

du Boulay C. From CME to CPD: getting better at getting better? Individual learning portfolios may bridge gap between learning and accountability. *BMJ.* 2000; 320(7232): 393–4.

A 21st century NHS [National Health Service] doctor needs 21st century, mature learning skills to actively keep abreast of the pace of change.

Harry El-Sayeh

El-Sayeh HG. A problem with problem-based learning. *BMJ.* 2004 July 30. Available at: www.bmj.com/content/329/7457/92/reply#bmj_el_69225?sid=3ccbd2b2-6802-483a-8a14-9c933f373379 (accessed 1 August 2011).

Like the gap between evidence and practice, there is a gap too between continuing medical education and professional and practice development.

Glyn Jones Elwyn

Elwyn GJ. Professional and practice development plans for primary care teams: life after the postgraduate education allowance. *BMJ.* 1998; 316(7145): 1619–20.

It has long been clear that most physicians receive the majority of continuing medical education (CME) from peer-reviewed medical journals, which is in contrast to how they receive the bulk of their accredited and documented CME necessary for relicensing.

Timothy Fagan

Fagan TC. "User-friendly" CME in the Archives of Internal Medicine. *Arch Intern Med.* 1999; 159: 648.

Shifting the continuing medical education experience from dimly lit halls, with lectures delivered with numerous, complex Powerpoint slides, to practice based learning and improvement will require a large cultural change in the continuing medical education world.

Suzanne Fletcher

Fletcher S. Continuing medical education: pharma and CME: view from the US. *BMJ.* 2008; 337: a1023.

It has been my rule to renew my textbooks every five years, and on each renewal I am continually impressed by my own ignorance.

John Good

Good J. Medical education. *BMJ.* 1920; 2(3112): 295–6.

In the UK around half of continuing medical education is industry funded, but the climate is changing as doctors move to setting their own learning agendas.

Mark Gould

Gould M. Continuing medical education: end of the free lunch? *BMJ.* 2008; 337: a1399.

Little evidence exists that formal continuing medical education – that is, attendance at traditional courses and conferences – has a significant effect on performance or competence.

TM Hayes

Hayes TM. Continuing medical education: a personal view. *BMJ.* 1995; 310(6985): 994–6.

To recapitulate the basic requirements, a doctor should be knowledgeable, capable of assigning priorities, skilful, dedicated, trustworthy, available, flexible, a good listener, a good teacher, a good leader, a good health promoter, and a life long student and researcher.

Astrid Nøklebye Heiberg

Heiberg AN. The doctor in the twenty first century. *BMJ (Clin Res Ed).* 1987; 295(6613): 1602–3.

A doctor's desire to be more competent in the delivery of health care is the most important motivating factor for continuous learning and change.

Hans Asbjørn Holm

Holm HA. Continuing medical education: quality issues in continuing medical education. *BMJ.* 1998; 316(7131): 621.

If we take into account the pivotal role that reading has in a doctor's continuous learning then reading should be generously honoured, allowing doctors to meet at least half of any set annual standard of credit points by reporting their reading and its perceived influence on their practice.

Hans Asbjørn Holm

Holm HA. Should doctors get CME points for reading? Yes: relaxing documentation doesn't imply relaxing accountability. *BMJ.* 2000; 320: 394.

If those in positions of leadership in medicine really do wish to give evidence of self improvement without government intervention, the time to act is now.

John Hubbard

Hubbard JP. Self-education and self-assessment as a new method for continuing medical education. *AMA Arch Surg.* 1971; 103(3): 422–4.

At least we can foretell that new doctors will need to be flexible enough to discard old ideas and absorb new, will need intensely open minds and a far greater capacity for continued learning and relearning than we have needed.

FM Hull

Hull FM. Personal view. *BMJ (Clin Res Ed).* 1984; 288(6435): 1993.

We are what we learn just as we are what we eat.

Alex Jamieson

Jamieson A. E-learning: theories of learning and conversations with e-learners. *Work Based Learn Prim Care.* 2004; 2(1): 62–71(10).

More and more, with medicine undergoing significant and continuous change, medical training programs will need to develop "stem-cell" physicians into differentiated practitioners capable of providing the highest-quality care, conducting cutting-edge research, being life-long learners, and teaching others to do the same.

Michael Johns

Johns MME. The time has come to reform graduate medical education. *JAMA.* 2001; 286(9): 1075–6.

The kind of doctor that I want is one who, when he's not examining me, is home studying medicine.

George Kaufman

Attributed.

For many people, moving from CME [continuing medical education] to CPD [continuous professional development] involves a culture change and requires a set of skills and knowledge about learning that many do not have and may not realise they do not have.

Diane Kelly

Kelly D. The need for needs assessment in continuing medical education. *BMJ.* 2004 May 11. Available at: www.bmj.com/content/328/7446/999?tab=responses (accessed 10 February 2012).

There is a lack of clarity over the purpose of appraisal, revalidation and continuing professional development (CPD) and the connections between each.

Diane Kelly

Kelly D. Perceptions of Scottish appraisers and continuing professional development advisers on general practitioner appraisal, continuing professional development and revalidation. *Educ Prim Care.* 2007; 18: 697–703.

Let me ask a question that might be unpopular with general practitioners (GPs) and the general practice postgraduate educational establishment: Is there a need to make continuing professional development (CPD) – both the process for individuals and the organisations responsible for it – more accountable?

Mayur Lakhani

Lakhani M. Guest editorial: clinical governance and continuing professional development: a question of accountability. *Educ Prim Care.* 2002; 13: 323–5.

Formal learning and academic research, including journals and books, do influence practice and may lead to change – but not in a simple linear way.

John Launer

Launer J. Reflective practice. *Work Based Learn Prim Care.* 2003; 1(1): 56–8(3).

If we assume at every step of our decision making process that we are likely to be ill informed, the possibilities for continuing education are virtually infinite.

Graeme Mackenzie

Mackenzie G. Little less than a revolution required. *BMJ.* 2008 August 31. Available at: www.bmj.com/content/337/bmj.a119/reply#bmj_el_201263?sid=f02266c3-e46f-42f6-95b0-40740e183fa9 (accessed 1 August 2011).

Effective CME [continuing medical education] requires learning needs assessment and GPs have previously been criticised for not being able accurately to assess their own needs.

Sheona MacLeod

MacLeod S. How GPs learn. *Educ Prim Care.* 2009; 20: 271–7.

Learning after certification, CME [continuing medical education], is the longest phase of their educational journey, and perhaps the most important.

Sheona MacLeod

MacLeod S. How GPs learn. *Educ Prim Care.* 2009; 20: 271–7.

The education of most people ends upon graduation; that of the physician means a lifetime of incessant study.

Karl FH Marx

Bulletin of the New York Academy of Medicine. 1929; 5: 156.

The glory of medicine is that it is constantly moving forward, that there is always more to learn.

William Mayo

National Education Association: addresses and proceedings. 1928; 66: 163.

In my opinion the 'reflective practitioner' is at the heart of work based learning. Such a practitioner has the motivation to learn, seeks opportunities to turn 'knowing-in-action' to 'reflection-in-action' and then onwards to 'reflection-on-action'.

Richard McDonough

McDonough R. The reflective practitioner: the essence of work based learning? *Work Based Learn Prim Care.* 2004; 2(4): 373–6(4).

Professional development, sometimes referred to as continuous professional development (CPD), is the systematic maintenance, improvement and broadening of the knowledge, skills and personal qualities necessary for the execution of professional duties throughout one's working life.

Michelle McLean

McLean M. How to professionalise your practice as a health professions educator. *Med Teach.* 2010; 32(12): 953–5.

Teaching communication skills should be included at all levels of medical education and, even more importantly, should be a mandatory element of the medical school curriculum and programmes of continuing medical education.

Siegfried Meryn

Meryn S. Improving doctor-patient communication: not an option, but a necessity. *BMJ.* 1998; 316(7149): 1922–30.

There is no doubt that the majority of clinicians are interested teachers. After all medicine is a continuous learning process for all doctors.

Abdullah Mohammed

Mohammed A. Universities and NHS trusts need to work together to improve undergraduate teaching. *BMJ.* 2005 January 19. Available at: www.bmj.com/content/330/7483/153.1/reply#bmj_el_93383?sid=1e069fc1-8837-4789-925c-3c1714669644 (accessed 1 August 2011).

Although more than half of continuing education is sponsored by drug and device makers, good evidence about the effects of sponsorship is sparse.

Ray Moynihan

Moynihan R. Sponsorship of medical education: is the relationship between pharma and medical education on the rocks? *BMJ.* 2008; 337: a925.

The building of a portfolio takes time and is never finished, as we learn throughout life.

Lesley Moore

Moore LJ. Professional portfolios: a powerful vehicle for reflective exercises and recording work based learning. *Work Based Learn Prim Care.* 2006; 4(1): 25–35(11).

Although medical students might think that the process of learning how to be a physician ends when they finish medical school, those who have been in practice know that, in fact, the learning process never stops.

Marc Nelson

Nelson MS. The physician as learner: linking research to practice. *JAMA.* 1995; 274(9): 775.

If educational efforts appear divorced from the needs and interests of the learner, they are unlikely to make any lasting impact.

Neil Nusbaum

Nusbaum NJ. Continuing professional development and core curricula: a view from the USA. *Educ Prim Care.* 2008; 19: 248–57.

To maintain mental freshness and plasticity requires incessant vigilance; too often, like the dial's hand, it steals from its figure with no pace perceived except by one's friends, and they never refer to it.

William Osler

Osler W. An address on the importance of post-graduate study: delivered at the opening of the museums of the Medical Graduates College and Polyclinic, July 4th, 1900. *BMJ.* 1900; 2(2063): 73–5.

And this is well, perhaps, if you will remember that, having in the old phrase commenced Bachelor of Medicine, you have only reached a point from which you can begin a lifelong process of education.

William Osler

Osler W. An address on the master-word in medicine: delivered to medical students on the occasion of the opening of the new laboratories of the Medical Faculty of the University of Toronto, October 1st, 1903. *BMJ.* 1903; 2(2236): 1196–200.

We doctors do not "take stock" often enough and are very apt to carry on our shelves stale or out of print books.

William Osler

Osler W. On the educational value of the medical society. In: Osler W. *Aequanimitas, With Other Addresses to Medical students, Nurses and Practitioners of Medicine.* London; 1904.

One of the key problems in developing learning is how to recognise and accredit learning undertaken in the workplace.

Nigel Oswald

Oswald N. Agenda for change: agenda for learning change. *Educ Prim Care.* 2005; 16: 644–7.

The tradition of graduating from a training programme and obtaining a licence for life seems naive in this era when the quality of care we provide is so dependent on our efforts to keep up to date.

John Parboosingh

Parboosingh J. Revalidation for doctors: should reflect doctors' performance and continuing professional development. *BMJ.* 1998; 317(7166): 1094–5.

We must move away from linking professional licensing to the accumulation of educational credits in whatever guise.

John Parboosingh

Parboosingh J. Educator with a vision. *BMJ.* 1999; 319(7203): 146.

The key is the relation of continuing education to standards of practice – the integration of learning, and teaching with audit, so that continuing education becomes the means and the measure of improvement in the quality of medical care.

James Parkhouse

Parkhouse J. Stars and stripes: for ever? *BMJ (Clin Res Ed).* 1983; 286(6368): 825–6.

A doctor who finished his education twenty-five years ago and has learned nothing since is a public menace.

George Pickering

Pickering G. Postgraduate education and society: the lesson from medicine. *BMJ.* 1969; 3(5667): 375–8.

Continuing medical education has become so heavily dependent on support from drug and medical device companies that the ethical underpinnings and the reputation of the medical profession may be compromised.

Alfredo Pisacane

Pisacane A. Rethinking continuing medical education. *BMJ.* 2008; 337: a973.

CME [continuing medical education] must expand beyond traditional 'content driven' education and help clinicians function as part of an outcomes-based system of care.

David Price

Price D. Continuing medical education, quality improvement, and organizational change: implications of recent theories for twenty-first-century CME. *Med Teach.* 2005; 27(3): 259–68.

When we can all admit what we do not know, what we cannot do, and that sometimes we are wrong, maybe we will be half way there. Taking the element of chance out of our continuing education and development is another way of ensuring that we are aiming in the right direction.

Fiona Rae

Rae F. Continuing professional development. *BMJ.* 2000 March 2. Available at: www.bmj.com/content/320/7232/393/reply#bmj_el_6876?sid=7f1b5b2e-7b0c-43f6-8a46-f45951808b4f (accessed 1 August 2011).

The "pot filling" approach to medical education in this country has produced generations of medical graduates poorly equipped for the self directed study and performance review that characterises successful continuing medical education outside the formal environment of clinical school.

Geraint Rees

Rees G. Improving preregistration training. *BMJ.* 1992; 304(6832): 981.

Continuing medical education [CME] need not be as expensive as it now is, and physicians attending CME programs ought to be willing and able to pay something for their continuing education.

Arnold Relman

Relman AS. Industry support of medical education. *JAMA.* 2008; 300(9): 1071–3.

Ultimately, educators hope to show improvements in outcomes for patients.

John Roberts

Continuing medical education: news. *BMJ.* 1993; 306: 7.

The advance of medical science is so rapid that without knowing it – and he seldom does – a man easily becomes a medical Rip Van Winkle.

Humphry Rolleston

Rolleston H. The aims and methods of graduate study. *BMJ.* 1920; 1(3081): 77–9.

Medical education is a continuum.

Peter Rubin

Rubin P. Medical education is a continuum. *BMJ.* 2006 September 6. Available at: www.bmj.com/content/333/7566/459/reply#bmj_el_141142?sid=20523c27-2e0d-443d-a7db-86e43c2767d3 (accessed 1 August 2011).

Continuous professional development activities of practicing surgeons should be integrated with the core competency of practice-based learning and improvement (PBLI), which involves a cycle of 4 steps – identifying areas for improvement, engaging in learning, applying new knowledge and skills to practice, and checking for improvement.

Ajit Sachdeva

Sachdeva AK. The new paradigm of continuing education in surgery. *Arch Surg.* 2005; 140: 264–9.

One method of personalised continuing medical education is portfolio based learning, in which the individual learner collects experiential evidence.

Sidha Sambandan

Sambandan S. Continuing medical education: competence and performance are measurable but do not equate with practice. *BMJ.* 1995; 311(7001): 393.

It is important to remember that on-line opportunities also require protected time to develop collective learning but this is often not recognised as being 'proper work' since it occurs at a time and place that is convenient to the participant rather than at a fixed time and place.

John Sandars

Sandars J. Knowledge management: something old, something new! *Work Based Learn Prim Care.* 2004; 2(1): 9–17(9).

There is increasing impetus to use reflective practice as a method of learning for continuing professional development. This concept has become an integral part of personal development plans, and is enshrined as a requirement for the future revalidation of healthcare professionals.

John Sandars

Sandars J. Transformative learning: the challenge for reflective practice. *Work Based Learn Prim Care.* 2006; 4(1): 6–10(5).

A clear message from the available evidence that can guide the provision of CME [continuing medical education] in a new system is that the learner must actively participate in the educational process and that this requires the support of a facilitator.

John Sandars

Sandars J. Continuing medical education across Europe. *BMJ.* 2010; 341: c5214.

All healthcare professionals need to keep their knowledge, skills and attitudes updated to ensure that they can provide high-quality healthcare.

John Sandars

Sandars J. Cost effective continuing professional development. In: Walsh K, editor. *Cost Effectiveness in Medical Education.* Oxford: Radcliffe Publishing; 2010. pp22–9.

Measuring the cost effectiveness of CPD [continuing professional development] will be a major challenge since identifying the true costs of educational interventions and deciding on the appropriate expected benefits that are relevant to all stakeholders is not easy.

John Sandars

Sandars J. Cost effective continuing professional development. In: Walsh K, editor. *Cost Effectiveness in Medical Education.* Oxford: Radcliffe Publishing; 2010. pp22–9.

At a time when Britain is facing serious shortages in the medical workforce, it would be foolish as well as unjust to give anything less than adequate support to individuals genuinely trying to remedy deficiencies in their performance.

Gabriel Scally

Scally G. Tackling deficient doctors: mentoring and appraisal may stave off calls for reaccreditation. *BMJ.* 1997; 314(7094): 1568.

The amount of information needed to maintain clinical currency exceeds the capacity of the lecture, and for many types of learning need, lectures are the wrong method of education.

Michael Scotti Jr

Scotti M Jr. Continuing medical education: actually learning rather than simply listening; reply. *JAMA.* 1996; 275(21): 1638.

Continuing medical education activities occur in artificial learning environments and possibly have little impact on physician performance because they are removed from the health care setting.

Terrence Shaneyfelt

Shaneyfelt TM. Building bridges to quality. *JAMA*. 2001; 286(20): 2600–1.

Recording a doctor's activity in continuing medical education is almost useless because it is possible to attend many educational sessions, score well on tests of knowledge, and be incompetent.

Richard Smith

Smith R. Should GMC leaders be put to the sword? No, doctors must work together. *BMJ*. 2000; 321(7253): 61.

But education does not happen to end with registration, or qualification, with the obtaining of a commission, a diploma, or a degree, and there is no professional life in which this truth can be seen more clearly than in the medical life, in relation to which it is stark staleness to say that education never ceases and that the longer we practise our calling the more we have the opportunity of learning, of testing that learning, and of obtaining its rewards.

Samuel Squire Sprigge

Squire Sprigge S. An address on prizes and performances: delivered at the opening of the medical session at St. George's Hospital, on October 1st. *BMJ*. 1910; 2(2597): 1024–7.

Continuing medical education has become so heavily dependent on support from pharmaceutical and medical device companies that the medical profession may have lost control over its own continuing education.

Robert Steinbrook

Steinbrook R. Financial support of continuing medical education. *JAMA*. 2008; 299(9): 1060–2.

The art of medicine was to be properly learned only from its practice and its exercise.

Thomas Sydenham

Dedicatory epistle, from *Medical Observations.*

How, in the face of all the clerical work he must perform, can a G.P. remain a student?

Malcolm Tate

Tate M. Medical education and the G.P. *BMJ*. 1948; 2(4566): 110–11.

The advantage of work based learning is that it is practical and involves colleagues with whom we interact every day.

Jill Thistlethwaite

Thistlethwaite J. Work based learning in primary care: remembering my past. *Work Based Learn Prim Care*. 2003; 1(1): 59–61(3).

Study leave provision is under ever greater financial pressure, to the point now where many doctors find it very difficult to get approval for funding to attend even one conference a year.

Martin Toal

Toal M. Case not proven. *BMJ*. 2006 July 26. Available at: www.bmj.com/content/333/7560/161/reply#bmj_el_138111?sid=20523c27-2e0d-443d-a7db-86e43c2767d3 (accessed 1 August 2011).

Continuing medical education doesn't just mean keeping up to date with one's own speciality interests. It has to be extended into the wider aspects of continuing professional development, including computer literacy, ethics, appraisal, management, and evidence based medicine.

Peter Toghill

Toghill P. Continuing medical education: where next? Doctors must manage their own education. *BMJ.* 1998; 316(7133): 721–2.

The culture of the education system, now largely shaped by performance in examinations and emphasis on factual content, must be changed to one which values self directed learners and problem solvers.

Angela Towle

Towle A. Continuing medical education: changes in health care and continuing medical education for the 21st century. *BMJ.* 1998; 316(7127): 301–4.

The choice of CME [continuing medical education] objectives should be based on a continuous analysis of quality of care indicators which serve also for verifying the impact of educational activities.

Alberto Tozzi

Tozzi AE. Dreaming of new educational models. *BMJ.* 2008 August 19. Available at: www.bmj.com/content/337/bmj. a973/reply#bmj_el_200850?sid=a15ec792-dfe3-4ba7-b8d0-a79c5a5cccab (accessed 1 August 2011).

In terms of the purpose of revalidation there were three over-riding themes: securing public trust, promoting continuing professional development, and detecting poor performance, with recognition that the purpose might be multifaceted.

Tim van Zwanenberg

van Zwanenberg T. Revalidation: the purpose needs to be clear. *BMJ.* 2004; 328(7441): 684–6.

Medical education is not completed at the medical school: it is only begun.

William Welch

Bulletin of the Harvard Medical School Association. 1892; 3: 55.

The explosion in the amount of medical knowledge available has mandated that medicine is today a learning profession.

Richard Wilbur

Wilbur RS. Continuing medical education: past, present, and future. *JAMA.* 1987; 258(24): 3555–6.

We are working toward eliminating industry support from all of our CME [continuing medical education].

Stephen Willis

Kuehn BM. Successes, challenges emerge from efforts to shift away from industry-funded CME. *JAMA.* 2010; 304(7): 729–31.

Continuing education should be less reliant on presentations and lectures and more focused on practice based learning.

Robert Woollard

Woollard RF. Continuing medical education in the 21st century. *BMJ.* 2008; 337: a119.

Traditional lecture based continuing education is largely ineffective in changing the performance of health professionals and in improving patient care.

Robert Woollard

Woollard RF. Continuing medical education in the 21st century. *BMJ.* 2008; 337: a119.

7. REVALIDATION

We in the health professions have only begun to emerge from the strikingly arrogant posture of asserting that our licences are awarded for life and that we can be fully entrusted to pursue whatever continuing learning we choose, without the need for external monitoring.

Hilliard Jason

Many less well motivated, or isolated, or overworked doctors probably do not actively continue their medical education after qualifying and practise a standard of medicine little changed from that they learnt at medical school.

Michael Brudenell

Brudenell M. Recertification of specialists. *BMJ.* 1989; 298(6671): 455.

Maintenance of certification – the very term draws an extraordinary variety of reactions from surgeons: confusion, bewilderment, resignation, fear, hostility, boredom, and a desperate desire that it just go away.

Jo Buyske

Buyske J. Maintenance of certification: for the protection of the public and the good of the specialty. *Arch Surg.* 2009; 144(2): 101–3.

Being a professional is about self regulation and developing a specific knowledge and ethical base.

Kenneth Calman

Smith R. Education and debate health profile: challenging doctors; an interview with England's chief medical officer. *BMJ.* 1994; 308(6938): 1221–4.

From the start, the aim of revalidation has been to enable doctors to show that they are up to date and fit to practise, and to encourage improvement through meaningful reflection based on evidence drawn from practice.

Graeme Catto

Catto G. GMC and the future of revalidation: building on the GMC's achievements. *BMJ.* 2005; 330(7501): 1205–7.

In a truly knowledge based health service, knowledge must be dispersed throughout the system, along with the clinical responsibility for using that knowledge in practice. The method should be to strengthen education rather than regulation.

Bruce Charlton

Charlton BG. Towards a knowledge based health service may lead to more red tape. *BMJ.* 1994; 309(6956): 740.

We should tackle the doctors at fault rather than tangling all doctors in more red tape and introducing a system of pseudoscience by diktat.

Bruce Charlton

Charlton BG. Towards a knowledge based health service may lead to more red tape. *BMJ.* 1994; 309(6956): 740.

As a profession, we are unsure what to do for the best in order to demonstrate fitness to practise. We sense that something must be done, but are wary of doing something counterproductive.

Maurice Conlon

Conlon M. Revalidation: the long and winding road. *BMJ*. 2006 February 1. Available at: www.bmj.com/content/332/7535/230/reply#bmj_el_127254?sid=20523c27-2e0d-443d-a7db-86e43c2767d3 (accessed 1 August 2011).

Will we be able to achieve a balance between sufficient regulation as a safety net without strangling the internal professional drive to do well by each person we meet?

Peter Davies

Davies PG. Internal or external motivations. *BMJ*. 2006 February 5. Available at: www.bmj.com/content/332/7535/230/reply#bmj_el_127254?sid=20523c27-2e0d-443d-a7db-86e43c2767d3 (accessed 1 August 2011).

Setting up a revalidation process that provides a sensitive method of picking out poorly performing doctors early, while simultaneously providing the stimulus for improvement for the majority, will be a challenge.

Clair du Boulay

du Boulay C. Revalidation for doctors in the United Kingdom: the end or the beginning? The process should celebrate what we do well while showing that we are accountable. *BMJ*. 2000; 320(7248): 1490.

Given the evidence-based environment of medicine today, physician leaders should not be pushing for a greater emphasis on recertification without data to support this process.

F Michael Gloth III

Gloth III FM. Credentialing, recertification, and public accountability. *JAMA*. 2006; 296(13): 1587–8.

I was taught, and still believe, that self-regulation is a hallmark of any profession. Professionals are best placed to decide if a member of the profession is fit to practise, not fit to practise, or if limits should be placed upon his or her practice.

Peter Gooderham

Gooderham P. Threat to the profession. *BMJ*. 2006 July 26. Available at: www.bmj.com/content/333/7560/161/reply#bmj_el_138111?sid=20523c27-2e0d-443d-a7db-86e43c2767d3 (accessed 1 August 2011).

Annual appraisal can be used as a tool to promote quality of care for patients and also to support doctors, but at present many GPs see it as more of a threat than an opportunity.

Stephen Hayes

Hayes S. Appraisal-helpful only if done well. *BMJ*. 2000 November 12. Available at: www.bmj.com/content/321/7270/1220.1/reply#bmj_el_11220?sid=7f1b5b2e-7b0c-43f6-8a46-f45951808b4f (accessed 1 August 2011).

Dysfunctional doctors should be helped back to practise wherever appropriate.

Donald Irvine

Irvine D. The performance of doctors: II. Maintaining good practice, protecting patients from poor performance. *BMJ*. 1997; 314(7094): 1613–15.

Revalidation is an essential part of professionalism directed at meeting patients' expectations of good care.

Donald Irvine

Irvine D. GMC and the future of revalidation: patients, professionalism, and revalidation. *BMJ*. 2005; 330(7502): 1265–8.

We in the health professions have only begun to emerge from the strikingly arrogant posture of asserting that our licences are awarded for life and that we can be fully entrusted to pursue whatever continuing learning we choose, without the need for external monitoring.

Hilliard Jason

Jason H. Continuing education: where does it begin? *Med Teach.* 1979; 1(6): 277–9.

The purpose of professionally led regulation is to ensure that the public can put their trust in registered doctors.

John Jenkins

Jenkins J. Good medical practice. *BMJ.* 2006 February 6. Available at: www.bmj.com/content/332/7535/230/reply#bmj_el_127254?sid=20523c27-2e0d-443d-a7db-86e43c2767d3 (accessed 1 August 2011).

It, therefore, is very clear that a diploma from the College of Surgeons does not confer on the holders the exclusive right of practising surgery, but only of calling themselves members of the Royal College of Surgeons.

George King

King G. On the present condition of the medical profession. *Prov Med Surg J.* 1846; s1–10(12): 138–9.

Obtaining important and useful information about doctors' performance is possible but it is technically difficult and time consuming.

Gary Lafferty

Lafferty G. Patient satisfaction surveys: as reliable as DIY neurosurgery. *BMJ.* 2001 April 3. Available at: www.bmj.com/content/322/7289/792.1/reply#bmj_el_13789?sid=bfae656f-d7d3-4ae5-abb6-1b0e432b89b5 (accessed 1 August 2011).

Revalidation is an essential tool to protect patients from the minority of poorly performing doctors.

Mayur Lakhani

Lakhani M. GMC and the future of revalidation: a way forward. *BMJ.* 2005; 330(7503): 1326–8.

The profession cannot but rejoice in the present laudable effort on the part of many to raise its general standard, and to render it more homogeneous in its character.

Percy Leslie

Leslie P. Out-door practice as a means of medical education. *BMJ.* 1868; 2(413): 582–3.

The focus should be on education rather than on re-licensing. However, if re-licensing is a means to the desired end (education) then so be it.

Sanjiv Lewin

Lewin S. Focus on re-licensing towards a need to provide relevant education! *BMJ.* 2005 April 18. Available at: www.bmj.com/content/330/7494/748.6/reply#bmj_el_104221?sid=1e069fc1-8837-4789-925c-3c1714669644 (accessed 1 August 2011).

Professions have long been recognized to consist of 3 essential characteristics: expert knowledge (as distinguished from a practical skill), self-regulation, and a fiduciary responsibility to place the needs of the client ahead of the self-interest of the practitioner.

Kenneth Ludmerer

Ludmerer KM. Instilling professionalism in medical education. *JAMA.* 1999; 282(9): 881–2.

No review of the subject of training for the practice of medicine can be anything but a waste of time which does not pay regard to the relation of medical practice to the public and to the conditions under which it is conducted and regulated.

Keith Waldegrave Monsarrat

Monsarrat KW. Educational number, session 1935–6: some comments on medical training and practice and their regulation. *BMJ.* 1935; 2(3895): 365–8.

Doctors who have successively waged financial campaigns, devised new strategies to cope with bureaucratic requirements, entered the world of teaching and training – all of which require clever and co-operative teamwork – struggle to integrate the collective practice resources into their appraisals.

Mary Nichols

Nichols M. GP appraisal: how much material do GP appraisers want? *Work Based Learn Prim Care.* 2004; 2(1): 75–8(4).

It is important for the appraiser to establish rapport with the appraisee, to determine his or her ideas, concerns and expectations, to negotiate on the basis of shared understanding and to reach an appraisee-centred outcome.

Mary Nichols

Nichols M. What do appraisers think about during appraisals? *Work Based Learn Prim Care.* 2004; 2(4): 386–9(4).

Appraisees demonstrate a wide range of preferences for the meeting location – it is impossible to predict who will favour where. Let them choose.

Mary Nichols

Nichols M. Practical tips for appraisers. *Work Based Learn Prim Care.* 2005; 3(2): 173–7(5).

Appraisers' work is interesting, challenging and satisfying. It can also be lonely and demanding, and require considerable powers of personal organisation.

Mary Nichols

Nichols M. Stresses on appraisers: Part 1 – process issues. *Work Based Learn Prim Care.* 2005; 3(3): 272–80(9).

The appraiser may well know best, but if the appraisee does not 'own' his or her PDP [personal development planning], the chances of it being fulfilled will be reduced significantly.

Mary Nichols

Nichols M. The role of the appraiser in personal development planning. *Work Based Learn Prim Care.* 2005; 3(1): 61–5(5).

Doctors are the envy of other professions. In poll after poll, the public say that they trust and are more satisfied with doctors, ahead of clergymen, judges, professors and the police.

Olusola Oni

Oni OOA. The regulation of the medical profession: ruminations of an ordinary doctor. *BMJ.* 2005 June 13. Available at: www.bmj.com/content/330/7504/1385/reply#bmj_el_109444?sid=1e069fc1-8837-4789-925c-3c1714669644 (accessed 2 October 2011).

Certification of doctors in this country is hopelessly inconsistent. Hospitals, doctors and patients deserve a far more structured and consistent certification process from the royal colleges. Only when we have proper certification in place, can we address re-certification and revalidation with all the merits it offers.

Jeremy Rawlins

Rawlins JM. Consistent certification before revalidation. *BMJ.* 2006 August 28. Available at: www.bmj.com/content/333/7565/439/reply#bmj_el_141424?sid=20523c27-2e0d-443d-a7db-86e43c2767d3 (accessed 1 August 2011).

Monopoly over medical knowledge lies at the heart of any meaningful discussion of professional regulation.

Marilynn Rosenthal

Rosenthal MM. Regulating medical work. *BMJ.* 1997; 314(7094): 1633.

Doctors in Britain have been insufficiently regulated for too long.

Richard Smith

Smith R. Regulation of doctors and the Bristol inquiry: both need to be credible to both the public and doctors. *BMJ.* 1998; 317(7172): 1539–40.

If we are to be 'revalidated' it must be by the equitable, workable and least expensive process which is clearly an examination. Discussion can take place about the form of the examination, but examination it must be.

William Stevenson

Stevenson W. Revalidation by examination. *BMJ.* 2000 November 12. Available at: www.bmj.com/content/321/7270/1220.1/reply#bmj_el_11220?sid=7f1b5b2e-7b0c-43f6-8a46-f45951808b4f (accessed 2 October 2011).

All this emphasis on re-validation implies that the initial validation of doctors is satisfactory. In fact it is quite a shambles. Each University with a medical school issues its own medical qualification, and there is no effective mechanism for moderating standards.

Richard Wakeford

Wakeford R. Response to responses. *BMJ.* 2000 November 16. Available at: www.bmj.com/content/321/7270/1220.1/reply#bmj_el_11220?sid=7f1b5b2e-7b0c-43f6-8a46-f45951808b4f (accessed 5 October 2011).

8. ASSESSMENT

> Truth is no more at issue in an examination than thirst at a wine-tasting or fashion at a striptease.
>
> **Alan Bennett**

MCQs [multiple-choice questions] test well in the cognitive domain, at least at the lower taxonomic levels, and are the most reliable, reproducible and internally consistent method we have of testing recall of factual knowledge.

John Anderson

Anderson J. For multiple choice questions. *Med Teach.* 1979; 1(1): 37–42.

If our aim is to test a knowledge of medicine rather than knowledge of the English language and its intricacies and the ability to remember accurately complicated instructions, there is little doubt that the multiple true/false and one-from-five types of question are to be preferred in that they are 'purer' and contain much less 'background noise'.

John Anderson
Anderson J. The MCQ controversy: a review. *Med Teach.* 1981; 3(4): 150–6.

Not only do educational assessments influence student learning, but the content of teaching will inevitably influence both learning and the assessment methods used – an academic vicious circle that is all too often pitched at a low taxonomic level.

John Anderson
Anderson J. Testing students' competence. *Med Teach.* 1982; 4(2): 44–6.

But whilst guessing may not be a good strategy in medicine, reasoning and weighing up probabilities to reach the correct answer are to be commended.

John Anderson
Anderson J. *Medical Teacher* 25th Anniversary Series multiple-choice questions revisited. *Med Teach.* 2004; 26(2): 110–13.

A European licensing examination is the only fair way to assess and therefore recruit doctors across and into Europe by achieving standardization, consensus and the effective pooling of resources.

Julian Archer
Archer JC. European licensing examinations: the only way forward. *Med Teach.* 2009; 31(3): 215–16.

Mere examining corporations which have done practically nothing for medical education, and are chiefly engaged in extracting fees from students, should be allowed to retire into obscurity.

James Barr
Barr J. President's address, delivered at the Eightieth Annual Meeting of the British Medical Association. *BMJ.* 1912; 2(2691): 157–63.

Truth is no more at issue in an examination than thirst at a wine-tasting or fashion at a striptease.

Alan Bennett
The History Boys. 2004.

The only parties capable of examining are experienced teachers, who, in consequence of their annually reviewing their special subjects, must be cognisant of details.

John Hughes Bennett
Bennett JH. Professor Bennett on medical education. *BMJ.* 1864; 1(180): 649.

Some students have a dread of MCQs [multiple-choice questions]. Though they believe themselves capable of writing an essay or facing an oral, they freeze before an MCQ paper like a mouse before a snake.

Leonard Biran
Biran LA. Hints for students (and examiners) on answering MCQ questions of the multiple true/false type. *Med Teach.* 1986; 8(1): 41–8.

Separating good from poor performance reliably is the essential function of any examination. But how good is good enough and how poor is unacceptable?

Peter Burrows

Burrows P. Simulated surgery for the assessment of consulting skills. In: Jackson N, Jamieson A, Khan A, editors. *Assessment in Medical Education and Training: a practical guide.* Oxford: Radcliffe Publishing; 2007. pp97–108.

Away with the cant of "Measures, not men!" – the idle supposition that it is the harness and not the horses that draw the chariot along. No Sir, if the comparison must be made, if the distinction must be taken, men are everything, measures comparatively nothing.

George Canning

Speech against the Addington Ministry. 1801.

Trainers' assessments of their trainees are not always reliable owing to the "halo effect" and their variation from trainer to trainer.

Tim Carney

Carney T. A national standard for entry into general practice. *BMJ.* 1992; 305(6867): 1449–50.

I find it hypocritical to criticise junior doctors for being motivated by examinations, when throughout stages I and II of medical education these are the sine qua non for progression and employment.

PD Cartwright

Cartwright PD. Medical education. *BMJ (Clin Res Ed).* 1984; 288(6434): 1911–12.

Few reliable measures of teaching excellence currently exist, and those that do rely heavily on subjective assessments by superiors, peers, and students or exclusive modes of recognition such as awards that carry scant attraction for clinicians.

Yap-Seng Chong

Chong YS. Academic medicine: time for reinvention. *BMJ.* 2004; 328(7430): 45–6.

For some years, examination by written papers has been substituted, and practised as with apparent success in all the medical classes. This method has the advantage of testing all who undergo the trial with far less consumption of their time; but it cannot be practised so often as some reformers would have it, who forget, or may not know, that the labour and consumption of time in examining the written papers of a large class is enormous, and a most ungrateful task.

Robert Christison

Christison R. President's address, delivered at the Forty-Third Annual Meeting of the British Medical Association. *BMJ.* 1875; 2(762): 155–63.

Now this is the age of examinations, and for qualifications in the various departments of art and science the questions to be answered are sometimes so numerous, recondite, and complex that the kind and degree of preparation necessary to answer them are becoming incompatible with true education, genuine study, and thorough work.

Andrew Clark

Clark A. An address on medical education and the duty of the community with regard to it. *BMJ.* 1888; 2(1449): 747–50.

The mere process of cramming conducted by a clever coach may sharpen some of the lower intellectual powers; but it will sap the strength of the higher ones, and, whilst it may carry a student triumphantly through some difficult examination, which may have been made the end of his studies, it will place him in after years at a terrible disadvantage in dealing with the difficult problem of life and work.

Andrew Clark

Clark A. An address on medical education and the duty of the community with regard to it. *BMJ.* 1888; 2(1449): 747–50.

The tendency of the University examinations is to fill the minds of the men with isolated bits of scientific knowledge, very useful for the purpose of answering questions at examination, but not very useful for the higher purpose of thoroughly disciplining the faculties, and for thoroughly furnishing the candidate with that sort of practical knowledge which is essential to the due discharge of his duties in life.

Andrew Clark

Barnes R. The relations of the graduates and convocation of the University of London to the proposed reform of the university. *BMJ.* 1890; 1(1518): 267–8.

In order to build up a picture of an individual doctor's performance, it is helpful to make multiple 'snapshot' assessments of different real clinical problems encountered in the workplace.

Robert Clarke

Clarke R. Foundation programme assessments in general practice. *Educ Prim Care.* 2006; 17: 291–300.

It should be remembered that the OSCE [objective structured clinical examination] was devised to enable the observation and assessment of clinical skills under controlled conditions, and that this is its forte.

Rufus Clarke

Clarke RM. Criterion-referencing: the baby and the bathwater. *BMJ.* 2009 February 24. Available at: www.bmj.com/content/338/bmj.b690/reply#bmj_el_209927?sid=c01598e6-7fa7-4552-bbff-d3bc10847fd9 (accessed 5 October 2011).

Rumours are abroad that the standard is to be reduced, and that the failures in July will be converted into successes in October.

W Bruce Clarke

Clarke WB. The conjoint board examinations. *BMJ.* 1885; 2(1296): 853.

Learning that takes place in the course of the quotidian but of which the learners themselves have little or no cognisance does not lend itself easily to three crucial educational actions: capture (namely, its relatively formalised acknowledgement and systematisation), measurement (that is to say, the assessment of the outcomes of learning and the impact of its application in practice) and accreditation (wherein a learner might obtain some form of externally validated credential).

Mark Cole

Cole M. The practice of developing practice: facilitating the capture and use of informal learning in the workplace. *Work Based Learn Prim Care.* 2004; 2(1): 1–5(5).

Students approach the final two years of training worn out by non-stop testing and with an overt wish to pass exams rather than learn and understand the subjects offered.

John Collier

Collier J. Personal view: medical education as abuse. *BMJ.* 1989; 299(6712): 1408–9.

Examinations are formidable even to the best prepared for the greatest fool may ask more than the wisest man can answer.

Charles Caleb Colton

Lacon. 1820–22. vol. I. p170.

If the General Medical Council administered a national licensing examination and the schools' results were published the schools would be more purposeful and concerned.

Philip Cooles

Cooles P. Medical education. *BMJ.* 1993; 306: 66.

Registrars in general practice are in favour of assessment that is valid, reliable, and equitable and welcome any procedure that will improve their training.

Will Coppola

Coppola W. Proposals may damage one of finest examples of postgraduate medical education. *BMJ.* 1995; 311(7019): 1573.

Perhaps the most important step of an assessment plan is to articulate the knowledge, skills, and attitudes that students are expected to learn.

Scott Cottrell

Cottrell S. A matter of explanation: assessment, scholarship of teaching and their disconnect with theoretical development. *Med Teach.* 2006; 28(4): 305–8.

Examinations are the only effective way to make the average student take a subject seriously.

Desmond Curran

Curran D. The place of psychology and psychiatry in medical education. *BMJ.* 1955; 2(4938): 515–18.

During the past decade the field of clinical assessment has demonstrated a clear move away from dependence on pencil and paper tests and the multiple-choice format as measures of predicting clinical competence to assessing what physicians do in the real world of practice.

W Dale Dauphinee

Dauphinee WD. Assessing clinical performance: where do we stand and what might we expect? *JAMA.* 1995; 274(9): 741–3.

A prerequisite for any qualifying examination is that the examiner is, and is seen to be, at a higher level of competence in the area being examined than the examinee: if the examiner is only seen as primus inter pares what reliance can be placed on his or her assessment?

DR Davies

Davies DR. Recertification of specialists. *BMJ.* 1989; 298(6676): 832.

Content validity is generally viewed as a crucial component of any assessment.

Hilton Dixon

Dixon H. Candidates' views of the MRCGP examination and its effects upon approaches to learning: a questionnaire study in the Northern Deanery. *Educ Prim Care.* 2003; 14: 146–57.

Consideration should be given to inductees undergoing a form of assessment at the end of the induction period. This could improve the learning process.

Fergus Donaghy

Donaghy F. Induction of foundation programme doctors entering general practice. *Educ Prim Care.* 2008; 19: 382–8.

The term face validity is sloppy at best and fraudulent and misleading at worst.
Steven Downing

Available at: http://psg-faimer-2008.wikispaces.com/file/view/July+ml+web+project+report+final+feroze.pdf (accessed 10 Feb 2012).

To one who can look back over thirty or forty years, no fact in medical education bulks more largely than the increasing importance of our examination system. Formerly examinations were meant to eliminate the useless; now they dominate the teaching.
John Duncan

Duncan J. An address delivered at the opening of the section of surgery, at the Annual Meeting of the British Medical Association at Edinburgh, July, 1898. *BMJ.* 1898; 2(1961): 299–300.

Examinations are now passed by most students at the first attempt but are criticised by some for testing the wrong qualities, by others for using wrong methods and by many for encouraging unfortunate habits of learning.
John Ellis

Ellis J. Editorial: 2. The present state of medical education in Britain. *Med Teach.* 1987; 9(3): 243–6.

While there is certainly a benchmark requirement for foundation doctor skills and knowledge base, if the individual medical schools cannot be trusted to deliver this then it undermines the system and I agree that focus could be in danger of changing from producing doctors with a well-rounded medical education to producing clones that can pass the national exam.
Jane Foster

Foster JAH. Idealism: evidence based selection. *BMJ.* 2008 August 28. Available at: www.bmj.com/content/337/bmj. a1279/reply#bmj_el_201185?sid=b74f0c68-fddb-4ccf-81b2-5e2a3899315c (accessed 5 October 2011).

No one opinion do I hold more strongly than this, that our youth, not medical only, but of all kinds, having been for many years past over-examined, are now year by year being more and more over-taught; one of the most urgent needs of medical education seems to me to be, not a multiplication, but a simplification, of medical studies. And, if a wider scope is to be given to physiology, something must be given up to afford the necessary room.
Michael Foster

Foster M. Forty-Eighth Annual Meeting of the British Medical Association, held in Cambridge, August 1880: address in physiology. *BMJ.* 1880; 2(1025): 285–9.

A video-based assessment is close to assessing what a candidate actually does and provided attention is paid to certain aspects, the assessment has a high utility.
Adrian Freeman

Freeman A. Video assessment. In: Jackson N, Jamieson A, Khan A, editors. *Assessment in Medical Education and Training: a practical guide.* Oxford: Radcliffe Publishing; 2007. pp109–13.

Video creates a permanent valid record of performance that can be assessed with reliability.
Adrian Freeman

Freeman A. Video assessment. In: Jackson N, Jamieson A, Khan A, editors. *Assessment in Medical Education and Training: a practical guide.* Oxford: Radcliffe Publishing; 2007. pp109–13.

Exclusive reliance on formal needs assessment could render education an instrumental and narrow process rather than a creative, professional one.

Janet Grant

Grant J. Learning needs assessment: assessing the need. *BMJ.* 2002; 324(7330): 156.

Learning needs assessment can be undertaken for many reasons, so its purpose should be defined and should determine the method used and the use made of findings.

Janet Grant

Grant J. Learning needs assessment: assessing the need. *BMJ.* 2002; 324(7330): 156.

While the OSCE [objective structured clinical examination] may test specific skills, it does not evaluate the comprehensive understanding of the candidate.

Piyush Gupta

Gupta P. Long case vs. OSCE: is there a need for comparison? *BMJ.* 2002 April 1. Available at: www.bmj.com/content/324/7340/748/reply#bmj_el_20889?sid=d5e693ea-0765-423d-ac1d-1c98624d8fdf (accessed 5 October 2011).

Examining in psychiatry is probably less objective than in most specialties since the subject requires a relatively smaller proportion of factual knowledge for clinical practice, and many topics, including psychiatric research, remain open to interpretation.

Alyson Hall

Hall A. Autumn books: for the MRCPsych candidate. *BMJ (Clin Res Ed).* 1984; 289(6452): 1127.

The evidence is that where there is a system of centralized examinations, innovation in assessment is hindered.

Ronald Harden

Harden RM. Five myths and the case against a European or national licensing examination. *Med Teach.* 2009; 31(3): 217–20.

Undergraduate assessments should help focus learning during the course, in identification of individual's [*sic*] strengths and weaknesses (and provide opportunities for the latter to be improved), and ultimately give the public the confidence in the quality and performance of its doctors.

Kamila Hawthorne

Hawthorne K. Assessment in the undergraduate curriculum. In: Jackson N, Jamieson A, Khan A, editors. *Assessment in Medical Education and Training: a practical guide.* Oxford: Radcliffe Publishing; 2007. pp27–40.

While there is a sound educational argument for the drive to raise standards, care must be taken to ensure that educational organisations such as colleges are not seen to be the regulators, that assessment methods are valid, reliable, educational and affordable, and that experienced general practitioners are assisted to remain current.

Richard Hays

Hays R. Improving general practice standards: a lesson from Australia. *Education for General Practice.* 2001; 12(2): 132–4.

Clinical teachers often feel uncomfortable when they are asked to assess the learners in their care.

Richard Hays

Hays R. Determining whether or not learners have achieved the desired standard. In: Hays R. *Teaching and Learning in Clinical Settings.* Oxford: Radcliffe Publishing; 2006. pp79–96.

While it is tempting to think that inappropriate knowledge, skills and attitudes will eventually be detected and dealt with by someone, the reality is that learners with persistent deficiencies can get to final assessments before they are officially noted.

Richard Hays

Hays R. Assessing learning in primary care. *Educ Prim Care*. 2009; 20: 4–7.

Examination, like fire, is a good servant but a bad master.

Thomas Huxley

Starling EH. Medical education in England: the overloaded curriculum and the incubus of the examination system. *BMJ*. 1918; 2(3010): 258–9.

Computer-based assessment (CBA) has an established role in high-stakes licensing examinations worldwide.

Bill Irish

Irish B. The potential use of computer-based assessment for knowledge testing of general practice registrars. *Educ Prim Care*. 2006; 17: 24–31.

There are many established practical and pedagogic advantages to CBA [computer-based assessment] over conventional paper-based assessments.

Bill Irish

Irish B. The potential use of computer-based assessment for knowledge testing of general practice registrars. *Educ Prim Care*. 2006; 17: 24–31.

In educational terms, assessment may be considered as a means of supporting learning rather than just to indicate current or past achievement.

Neil Jackson

Jackson N. Assessment and work based learning in primary care. *Work Based Learn Prim Care*. 2003; 1(2): 89–92(4).

Summative assessment is defined as a means of recording the overall achievement at an endpoint (or given point in time) in a systematic way; it may be applied at the end of a phase of learning or performance.

Neil Jackson

Jackson N. Assessment and work based learning in primary care. *Work Based Learn Prim Care*. 2003; 1(2): 89–92(4).

The point is that there are no quick and easy assessment tools – they all require time and effort.

Brian Jolly

Jolly BC. The long case is mortal. *BMJ*. 2008 June 2. Available at: www.bmj.com/content/336/7655/1250/reply#bmj_el_196478?sid=90b7a8a2-7af4-4018-b137-261049bb6944 (accessed 5 October 2011).

There are many examples of well-written stems for problem-solving MCQs [multiple-choice questions] that are totally destroyed by obvious clues and defects in the choice of distractors.

Bahman Joorabchi

Joorabchi B. How to . . .: construct problem-solving MCQs. *Med Teach*. 1981; 3(1): 9–13.

The establishment of a uniform standard of education by means of conjoint examination is a proposition calculated to obtain, at its first suggestion, the support of all; but, on closer investigation, it will be found that the objections to it are manifold and insuperable.

George Kidd

Kidd GH. An address on medical education. *BMJ.* 1882; 1(1108): 146–8.

The MEQ [modified essay question] is, in effect, an account of a series of events in the evolution of a case study, narrated as they occurred.

James Knox

Knox JDE. Use modified essay questions. *Med Teach.* 1980; 2(1): 20–4.

Revalidation should be regarded as a form of summative assessment and conform to established academic criteria for assessment.

Mayur Lakhani

Lakhani M. GMC and the future of revalidation: a way forward. *BMJ.* 2005; 330(7503): 1326–8.

As recertification moves toward an evaluation of practice, there is a call for competence evaluations that will also examine practice performance.

Donald Langsley

Langsley DG. Medical competence and performance assessment: a new era. *JAMA.* 1991; 266(7): 977–80.

Historically, the competence of physicians has been based on peer review of their performance.

Donald Langsley

Langsley DG. Medical competence and performance assessment: a new era. *JAMA.* 1991; 266(7): 977–80.

Exams measure ability in passing exams, not necessarily anything else.

Gordon Lehany

Lehany GP. Failure to validate outcome measures. *BMJ.* 2002 July 4. Available at: www.bmj.com/content/324/7353/1554/reply#bmj_el_23411?sid=d5e693ea-0765-423d-ac1d-1c98624d8fdf (accessed 5 October 2011).

In undergraduate and postgraduate examinations there is little to equal the scrutiny that is given to a multiple choice question.

David Lowe

Lowe D. How to do it: set a multiple choice question (MCQ) examination. *BMJ.* 1991; 302(6779): 780–2.

Writing multiple choice questions is a laboriously acquired art, and it is much easier to advise how not to write them than to give a simple way of writing them.

David Lowe

Lowe D. How to do it: set a multiple choice question (MCQ) examination. *BMJ.* 1991; 302(6779): 780–2.

What students preparing for the medical profession want is a knowledge of principles and methods, not of details, which are only useful to them for absurd examinations, conducted by specialists who know nothing, and care nothing, about the requirements of medical education.

Benjamin Lowne

Lowne BT. The preliminary scientific examination of the University of London. *BMJ.* 1885; 1(1263): 567.

No single examination format will guarantee acceptability, feasibility, validity, and reliability, but care in identifying the strengths and weaknesses of each approach and clear objectives for the assessment should help staff select a useful range of tests.

Stella Lowry

Lowry S. Medical education: assessment of students. *BMJ.* 1993; 306(6869): 51–4.

Student assessment is often described as "the tail that wags the dog" of medical education. It is seen as the single strongest determinant of what students actually learn (as opposed to what they are taught) and is considered to be uniquely powerful as a tool for manipulating the whole education process.

Stella Lowry

Lowry S. Medical education: assessment of students. *BMJ.* 1993; 306(6869): 51–4.

The only sensible way to ensure that minimum standards are met is to define them and fail any student who does not reach them.

Stella Lowry

Lowry S. Medical education: assessment of students. *BMJ.* 1993; 306(6869): 51–4.

The complexity of assessing a single component of competence has resulted in attempts at multifaceted assessment.

Nick Lyons

Lyons N. Clinical competence: a review of methods used to assess competence and proposals for a realistic future strategy. *Educ Prim Care.* 2002; 13: 326–35.

The literature on assessment of clinical competence of medical practitioners agrees on but one thing: it is difficult.

Nick Lyons

Lyons N. Clinical competence: a review of methods used to assess competence and proposals for a realistic future strategy. *Educ Prim Care.* 2002; 13: 326–35.

From having been many years an examiner myself, I am quite satisfied, that a mere verbal examination furnishes no evidence of the candidate's real or practical knowledge.

James Macartney

Macartney J. On medical reform and the remodelling the profession. *Prov Med Surg J.* 1841; s1–1(17): 282–5.

Individual knowledge assessment is useful but it is easy to have good knowledge and be a bad doctor. General practice is about making multiple decisions, under pressure and trying to do no harm.

Graeme Mackenzie

Mackenzie GM. Team certification is perhaps more important for general practice. *BMJ.* 2006 September 1. Available at: www./content/333/7565/439/reply#bmj_el_141424?sid=20523c27-2e0d-443d-a7db-86e43c2767d3 (accessed 5 October 2011).

The notion of how well a newly qualified doctor should be able to perform constitutes minimum competence.

Peter Maguire

Maguire P. Assessing clinical competence. *BMJ.* 1989; 298(6665): 4–5.

While the idea that communication is an essential aspect of medicine is not new, communication skills teaching and assessment have recently become more visible in medical education.

Gregory Makoul

Makoul G. Communication skills education in medical school and beyond. *JAMA.* 2003; 289(1): 93.

WPBA [workplace-based assessment] provides a unique opportunity in the licensing tripos to achieve comprehensive competency coverage; it addresses the blueprint gaps and tests important attitudinal areas that other components do not.

Jane Mamelok

Mamelok J. Workplace-based assessment (WPBA) portfolios in licensing for general practice specialty training. *Educ Prim Care.* 2009; 20: 139–42.

The notions of self-regulation, self-assessment and self-monitoring are fundamental to meeting societal and professional expectations.

Karen Mann

Mann KV. Reflection: understanding its influence on practice. *Med Educ.* 2008; 42(5): 449–51.

With a few noble exceptions, the examinations are in the book-science; and of hospital practice, all that is asked is some general statement of having "attended", which is quite formal.

Samuel Martyn

Martyn S. Medical education. *BMJ.* 1864; 1(165): 247.

There is a wealth of evidence that extended matching questions are the fairest format but MCQs [multiple-choice questions] should always be combined with practical assessments, as written testing emphasizes learning from written sources.

Paul McCoubrie

McCroubrie P. Improving the fairness of multiple-choice questions: a literature review. *Med Teach.* 2004; 26(8): 709–12.

Assessment of problem-solving skills is best done by placing an individual in a problematical situation and observing his performance.

Christine McGuire

McGuire CH. Assessment of problem-solving skills, 1. *Med Teach.* 1980; 2(2): 74–9.

Common national assessment systems provide the equity inherent in common standards.

Donald Melnick

Melnick DE. Licensing examinations in North America: is external audit valuable? *Med Teach.* 2009; 31(3): 212–14.

Assessment drives learning.

George Miller

Miller G. The assessment of clinical skills/competence/performance. *Acad Med.* 1990; 65(9): S63–7.

Few consultants (by their own admission) that have taught me over the years (let alone registrars and so on) have a breath of knowledge that would enable them to manage anything and everything that a long case examination tosses up haphazardly like a bad Greek salad.

Thomas More

More T. Medicine the profession: a heart of darkness? *BMJ.* 2000 August 15. Available at: www.bmj.com/content/321/7258/398/reply#bmj_el_9244?sid=7f1b5b2e-7b0c-43f6-8a46-f45951808b4f (accessed 5 October 2011).

Striking the best balance between validity and reliability is never easy.

Roger Neighbour

Neighbour R. Reflections on the ethics of assessment. *Educ Prim Care.* 2003; 14: 406–10.

Assess before you teach, if you need to.
Assess after you teach, if you need to.
Assess while you teach, because you need to.

Roger Neighbour

Neighbour R. *The Inner Apprentice.* Oxford: Radcliffe Publishing; 2004.

With the disadvantages of vivas so clearly evident, it does seem surprising that more medical schools have not adopted the structured approach which has been shown to have such a high level of validity and reliability.

David Newble

Newble DI. How to conduct a clinical viva voce examination. *Med Teach.* 1983; 5(4): 157.

A national examination would ruin the current diversity in assessment of medical education and, because assessment has been shown to drive learning, would probably ruin the diversity in education.

Ian Noble

Noble IS. Are national qualifying examinations a fair way to rank medical students? No. *BMJ.* 2008; 337: a1279.

Three aspects of doctors' performance can be assessed – patients' outcomes, process of care, and volume of practice.

John Norcini

Norcini JJ. ABC of learning and teaching in medicine: work based assessment. *BMJ.* 2003; 326(7392): 753–5.

In my view there has been insufficient attention to the interface between our understanding of clinical expertise and the application of this knowledge to improve instruction and assessment.

Geoff Norman

Norman G. Research in medical education: three decades of progress. *BMJ.* 2002; 324(7353): 1560–2.

Although portfolios have been used in summative assessment, occasionally in very high stakes situations, the evidence of reliability and validity is quite sparse.

Geoff Norman

Norman G. Are learning portfolios worth the effort? No. *BMJ.* 2008; 337: 1136.

To link the assessment of medical competence with methods of education is as difficult as measuring the quality of medical care, but that is not an adequate reason for accepting that current systems of medical education are satisfactory.

Kenneth Parry

Parry KM. Postgraduate education in Australia and the United Kingdom compared. *BMJ*. 1981; 282(6257): 52–5.

I for one would rather have my appendix removed by someone who had passed a criterion-referenced assessment of their competence for the procedure than someone who was slightly less incompetent than the failing 30%.

Phil Parslow

Parslow PM. Norm vs criterion referencing. *BMJ*. 2009 February 25. Available at: www.bmj.com/content/338/bmj.b690/reply#bmj_el_209927?sid=c01598e6-7fa7-4552-bbff-d3bc10847fd9 (accessed 5 October 2011).

Exams are fine but they do not indicate competence. Newly qualified drivers in a formal assessment know far more about the Highway Code than drivers who have driven for years. Yet the mature driver is the better driver. A fact known to insurance companies but which cannot be proven in an exam.

Kevin Pearce

Pearce K. Tests only test for what can be tested. *BMJ*. 2006 August 26. Available at: www.bmj.com/content/333/7565/439/reply#bmj_el_141424?sid=20523c27-2e0d-443d-a7db-86e43c2767d3 (accessed 5 October 2011).

For all experience teaches us that the great bulk of students, with a compulsory examination before them, concentrate their vision on that alone, and refuse to look beyond it; so that teaching schools and universities must then teach down to this minimum, and not teach up to their maximum, if they are to preserve their students from mere crammers.

Lyon Playfair

Playfair L. Extract of an address on universities in their relation to professional education. *BMJ*. 1873; 1(633): 165–6.

Criterion referencing works when assessment reflects the curriculum.

Kevin Quinn

Quinn K. Criterion and curriculum. *BMJ*. 2009 February 26. Available at: www.bmj.com/content/338/bmj.b690/reply#bmj_el_209927?sid=c01598e6-7fa7-4552-bbff-d3bc10847fd9 (accessed 5 October 2011).

Norm referencing does not drive excellence whereas criterion referencing will, and remains the best standard for patient safety and care.

Kevin Quinn

Quinn K. Criterion and curriculum. *BMJ*. 2009 February 26. Available at: www.bmj.com/content/338/bmj.b690/reply#bmj_el_209927?sid=c01598e6-7fa7-4552-bbff-d3bc10847fd9 (accessed 5 October 2011).

In an examination those who do not wish to know ask questions of those who cannot tell.

Walter Alexander Raleigh

Some thoughts on examinations, from *Laughter from a Cloud*. 1923.

Faculty development programmes should incorporate the teaching, observing and assessing of history-taking skills and hypotheses generating based on the patient's history.

Subha Ramani

Ramani S. Promoting the art of history taking. *Med Teach*. 2004; 26(4): 374–6.

All doctors have to take so many examinations that they are experts in the subject.
Philip Rhodes
Rhodes P. Examinations. *BMJ (Clin Res Ed)*. 1983; 286(6372): 1202–3.

One of the other problems with both long case examinations and OSCEs [objective structured clinical examinations] is that they are high-pressure examination situations in which nearly everything you do is being watched. This is obviously not like everyday clinical medicine.
Daniel Sado
Sado DM. The long case versus objective structured clinical examinations. *BMJ*. 2002 March 31. Available at: www.bmj.com/content/324/7340/748/reply#bmj_el_20889?sid=d5e693ea-0765-423d-ac1d-1c98624d8fdf (accessed 5 October 2011).

Cheaters do not necessarily need to be subjected to full blown public humiliation but should perhaps be made to take a repeat exam before qualifying at least. If this means repeating a year of medical school, then so be it.
Sumita Saha
Saha S. Cheating at medical school. *BMJ*. 2000 November 23. Available at: www.bmj.com/content/321/7258/398/reply#bmj_el_9244?sid=7f1b5b2e-7b0c-43f6-8a46-f45951808b4f (accessed 5 October 2011).

I have heard doctors say time and time again how some of the best doctors they know and went through medical school with actually scraped through all their exams!
David Samuel
Samuel DG. Variety of medical courses remains the tonic for healthy medical education. *BMJ*. 2008 February 18. Available at: www.bmj.com/content/336/7640/347.1/reply#bmj_el_190644?sid=31284f95-3d82-4668-a4d3-12f808c21b4a (accessed 5 October 2011).

While a national examination would appeal to those wishing to ensure that the core components of the medial education have been understood and achieved by every medical student, irrespective of medical school, the introduction of such a system would merely make students "learn the exam".
David Samuel
Samuel DG. Loss of diversity and autonomy with national exam. *BMJ*. 2008 September 11. Available at: www.bmj.com/content/337/bmj.a1279/reply#bmj_el_201757?sid=b74f0c68-fddb-4ccf-81b2-5e2a3899315c (accessed 5 October 2011).

Above all, recollect that you are not here merely to learn how to pass certain examinations, although that is a duty which has to be kept in mind. Most of you will have in these few years of study your only opportunity of obtaining systematic instruction in scientific principles.
Robert Saundby
Saundby R. An address on modern universities: delivered at the opening of the medical school of University College, Cardiff. *BMJ*. 1898; 2(1971): 1034–8.

It is not clear to me why having a centralised assessment at graduation for medical students is in any way incompatible with a liberal education. We do, and should, encourage students to participate in music, sports, drama and many other activities which we do not attempt to assess.

Michael Schachter

Schachter M. National medical exams. *BMJ.* 2005 October 9. Available at: www.bmj.com/content/331/7520/791/reply#bmj_el_118714?sid=cb764c2a-ad1a-4f84-a8c4-88b3568c267c (accessed 5 October 2011).

There is a widely-spread misconception that subjective tests are by definition unreliable.

Lambert Schuwirth

Schuwirth LWT. Professional development in undergraduate medical curricula from an assessment point of view. *Med Educ.* 2002; 36(4): 312–13.

Although the ability to assess your own deficiencies is considered essential for lifelong learners, most people are not very good at it.

Lambert Schuwirth

Schuwirth L. What the educators are saying. *BMJ.* 2005; 331(7513): 392.

I am certainly not an opponent to the use of CBA [computer-based assessment], but I value a clear and open discussion about its added values before implementing it.

Lambert Schuwirth

Schuwirth L. The use of computer-based assessment. *Med Teach.* 2008; 30(7): 651.

It is indeed disappointing that the system of evaluation of medical graduates in the developed world ignores the art of physical examination.

Vishal Sharma

Sharma V. Clinical skills in developing world: more developed than the West. *BMJ.* 2009 December 18. Available at: www.bmj.com/content/339/bmj.b5448/reply#bmj_el_228489?sid=31b7420e-2cd9-4337-8329-2f40df508216 (accessed 5 October 2011).

Students enter university full of enthusiasm and have their curiosity washed out by multiple choice examinations.

David Shaw.

Dillner L. GMC says it will watch curriculum reforms. *BMJ.* 1994; 308(6925): 361.

It is clear that all too often the examination methods presently employed are of little or no educational value, and may even serve to reduce the educational value of the medical course.

Michael Simpson

Simpson MA. Student research. *BMJ.* 1968; 3(5621): 802.

For a reliable measure of clinical skills, performance has to be sampled across a range of patient problems.

Sydney Smee

Smee S. ABC of learning and teaching in medicine: skill based assessment. *BMJ.* 2003; 326(7391): 703–6.

Case-based discussion (CBD) is a fundamental way we like to learn and a method we have subsequently applied to teaching.

Chris Smith

Smith C. Question design for assessment by case-based discussion (CBD): 'your starter for 10.' *Educ Prim Care.* 2008; 19: 416–32.

Is there not something amiss about contemporary medical education when frequent examinations stifle the intellectual meanderings so essential for an expanded mind?

Daniel Sokol

Sokol DK. Ethics Man: a perforated education. *BMJ.* 2007; 335(7631): 1186.

Incessant assessment at medical school risks the loss of the skills of reflection, deliberation, and communication among tomorrow's doctors.

Daniel Sokol

Sokol DK. Ethics Man: of interviews and examination machines. *BMJ.* 2010; 341: 6899.

At present the course of preparation, as it is miscalled, has but little relation to the examinations to be undergone; and the intervention of the grinder with his practical knowledge of the peculiar views and requirements of the examining bodies, is, to the ordinary intellect, absolutely necessary.

Joseph Stephens

Stephens J. Medical education and medical parasites. *BMJ.* 1864; 1(178): 596–7.

Examinations are times of assessment; any teaching involved during exams and any conviviality on the part of the examiners are added extras, not central to the object of the exercise.

Alex Stewart

Stewart A. What makes a good doctor? *BMJ.* 1998 December 4. Available at: www.bmj.com/content/317/7168/1329.1/reply#bmj_el_1365?sid=35c7ac25-b25d-43e6-9bc0-a5da27e4e533 (accessed 5 October 2011).

The criteria for evaluating student performance should be derived from the framework of expectations that has been established.

Howard Stone

Stone HL. Return to 'basics' in medical education: a commentary. *Med Teach.* 1982; 4(3): 102–3.

A nationally agreed licensing system could unify standards, be regularly assessed and address deficiencies in graduating medical students, making them "fit for purpose" and should be embraced.

Alasdair Strachan

Strachan A. National standards for medical student competencies. *BMJ.* 2005 October 20. Available at: www.bmj.com/content/331/7520/791/reply#bmj_el_119704?sid=cb764c2a-ad1a-4f84-a8c4-88b3568c267c (accessed 5 October 2011).

Formative assessment tools in the workplace facilitate reflection and professional development, enabling the bringing out into the open of those deficiencies that the individual may not have been aware of, or would rather have kept hidden.

Tim Swanwick

Swanwick T. Work based assessment in general practice: three dimensions and three challenges. *Work Based Learn Prim Care.* 2003; 1(2): 99–108(10).

Oral examinations raise specific and knotty problems, not only of validity and reliability, but also of generalisability across contexts.

Tim Swanwick

Swanwick T. Preparing for the MRCGP examination: an issue for trainers and the profession, not just the registrar. *Educ Prim Care.* 2002; 13: 13–17.

Traditionally, medical assessment focused on ritualistic endpoint summative assessments conducted far away from the place of work.

Tim Swanwick

Swanwick T. Work based assessment in general practice: three dimensions and three challenges. *Work Based Learn Prim Care.* 2003; 1(2): 99–108(10).

With any authentic assessment instrument we soon bump up against pragmatic considerations, and in operating a large-scale performance assessment there will always be a trade-off between what is practical and what is valid.

Tim Swanwick

Swanwick T. The video component of the MRCGP examination: threats to validity. *Educ Prim Care.* 2004; 15: 311–27.

When I first became a trainer in 1976 I was not very good. Not because I didn't know much educational theory, which I didn't, but mainly because I was not clear enough about what I did know that might be useful to my marginally more insecure registrar.

Peter Tate

Tate P. Assessment: is it good or bad for training? *Educ Prim Care.* 2002; 13: 306–8.

Requesting patients to agree explicitly whenever a trainee is involved in their care would eventually ruin learning, teaching, and assessment in clinical practice.

Edith ter Braak

ter Braak E. Patients need not give consent in all clinical education. *BMJ.* 2006; 33(7540): 549.

The ultimate goal of optimising competency based training and assessment in medical education is the delivery of the best possible doctors and specialists in the best interest of current and future patients.

Edith ter Braak

ter Braak E. Patients consenting to participate in clinical education: a paradox? *BMJ.* 2006 February 21. Available at: www.bmj.com/content/332/7538/431.1/reply#bmj_el_128619?sid=20523c27-2e0d-443d-a7db-86e43c2767d3 (accessed 5 October 2011).

If we accept that assessment drives change, then to improve consultation skills, the fundamental skills on which our work is based, do we need to be assessed in situ?

Jill Thistlethwaite

Thistlethwaite J. GP assessment: if assessment drives learning, what happens after qualification? *Work Based Learn Prim Care.* 2004; 2(1): 82–4(3).

In 1800 a man could practise as a doctor without passing an examination of any kind. Indeed one itinerant practitioner is reported to have assumed the title of assistant surgeon on the ground that he had served an apprenticeship to the crutchmaker of a hospital.

Frederick Treves

Treves F. Address in surgery. *BMJ.* 1900; 2(2066): 284–9.

As it is the principal responsibility of a medical school to produce competent physicians and not to rank order them, it is more reasonable to compare student achievement to an external standard of performance or criterion.

Jeffrey Turnball

Turnball JM. What is . . . normative versus criterion-referenced assessment. *Med Teach*. 1989; 11(2): 145–50.

We need to assess in a real context, with all the intricacies of that.

Cees van der Vleuten

Pritchard L. Accidental hero. *Med Educ*. 2005; 39(8): 761–2.

By setting assessments at the end of undergraduate or postgraduate training programmes we can at least measure all our graduates against the same ruler and assure the public for some minimal level of competence.

Cees van der Vleuten

van der Vleuten CPM. National, European licensing examinations or none at all? *Med Teach*. 2009; 31(3): 189–91.

My personal opinion is that it is better to prevent malpractices before, during and after the examinations by taking every possible precaution rather than risking the possibility of penalising even one innocent student based on statistical analysis.

Padmini Venkataramani

Venkataramani P. Malpractices in written medical examinations. *BMJ*. 2005 May 11. Available at: www.bmj.com/content/330/7499/1064/reply#bmj_el_106435?sid=1e069fc1-8837-4789-925c-3c1714669644 (accessed 5 October 2011).

Assessment is a statement to the trainees of what is important.

David Wall

Wall D. Assessment, appraisal and evaluation issues. In: Chambers R, Wall D, editors. *Teaching Made Easy: a manual for health professionals*. Oxford: Radcliffe Medical Press; 2000. pp105–29.

To assess incompetence will have punitive implications; to promote competence is to pursue a positive virtue.

Tony Waterston

Waterston T. Incompetence in medical practice. *BMJ*. 1986; 292(6535): 1600.

For my own part, I regard the unbridled licence so unwisely accorded to the present system of education by examination as a monstrous evil; since, instead of educated gentlemen, it tends to produce mere examination-passing machines, as well stuffed with pedantic learning to gratify the unreasonable demands of insatiable examiners, as Michaelmas geese with piquant seasoning, to suit the depraved tastes of confirmed gourmands.

W Roger Williams

Williams WR. Medical education. *BMJ*. 1882; 2: 966.

In order to clarify the use of different methods of combining scores we desperately need more studies linked to future student performance.

Ian Wilson

Wilson I. Combining assessment scores: a variable feast. *Med Teach*. 2008; 30(4): 428–30.

It would seem sensible that a final clinical examination examine the clinical skills of a student in a manner which reflects reality on hospital wards.

Alan Woodall

Woodall A. Clinical examinations should allow students access to reference materials. *BMJ.* 2000 August 11. Available at: www.bmj.com/content/321/7258/398/reply#bmj_el_9244?sid=7f1b5b2e-7b0c-43f6-8a46-f45951808b4f (accessed 15 October 2011).

There are but few men who can pass the said examinations without a great amount of cramming and coaching (*vide* the advertisements in the press); and I think that the time spent in this way could be used to greater advantage in the wards and laboratories of a large hospital.

JP zum Busch

Zum Busch JP. A German view of English medical education. *BMJ.* 1898; 1(1936): 405.

9. FEEDBACK

> Bullying, intimidation, and humiliation are essential in maintaining all hierarchies, but I still can't find the evidence that they are any good for producing doctors.
>
> **John Collier**

It takes two for bullying to happen: someone with the intention to hurt, humiliate, intimidate, undermine or even destroy another person, and someone who allows it to happen.

Kristin Becker

Becker K. Bullying: how to help both sides. *BMJ.* 2001 December 11. Available at: www.bmj.com/content/323/7324/1314.1/reply#bmj_el_18066?sid=bfae656f-d7d3-4ae5-abb6-1b0e432b89b5 (accessed 15 October 2011).

Feedback should be sensitive, timely, face-to-face, and regular.

Ronald Berk

Berk RA. Using the 360° multisource feedback model to evaluate teaching and professionalism. *Med Teach.* 2009; 31(12): 1073–80.

Training in formative assessment is an essential component of any preparatory programme for teachers since both the assessment of educational need and the giving of feedback requires specific skills.

Robert Clarke

Clarke R. Preparing teachers for work-based teaching and assessing. In: Jackson N, Jamieson A, Khan A, editors. *Assessment in Medical Education and Training: a practical guide.* Oxford: Radcliffe Publishing; 2007. pp86–96.

Bullying, intimidation, and humiliation are essential in maintaining all hierarchies, but I still can't find the evidence that they are any good for producing doctors.

John Collier

Collier J. Personal view: medical education as abuse. *BMJ.* 1989; 299(6712): 1408–9.

Might I suggest that if examinations are to fulfil any purpose their aims need to be clearly stated and students need to be given regular feedback sessions, particularly on clinical skills and taking histories, so that they may improve their performance.

John Collier

Collier J. The national curriculum and medical education. *BMJ.* 1989; 298(6673): 602.

Most medical schools have many examinations but do not provide comprehensive feedback on performance so that an examination becomes a moving goalpost at which students can aim only roughly.

John Collier

Collier J. The national curriculum and medical education. *BMJ.* 1989; 298(6673): 602.

We need to measure what we need to measure rather than what is easy to measure, and feedback is an important mechanism in the pursuit of consequential validity.

Hilton Dixon

Dixon H. Candidates' views of the MRCGP examination and its effects upon approaches to learning: a questionnaire study in the Northern Deanery. *Educ Prim Care.* 2003; 14: 146–57.

Destructive criticism is adverse criticism motivated not by a desire for the best but by such motives as aggression or self-aggrandisement or self-protection on the part of the critic.

Raanan Gillon

Gillon R. The function of criticism. *BMJ.* 1981; 283(6307): 1633–9.

Just as many learning opportunities are wasted if they are not accompanied by feedback from an observer, so too are they wasted if the learner cannot reflect honestly on his or her performance.

Jill Gordon

Gordon J. ABC of learning and teaching in medicine: one to one teaching and feedback. *BMJ.* 2003; 326(7388): 543–5.

Learners value feedback highly, and valid feedback is based on observation.

Jill Gordon

Gordon J. ABC of learning and teaching in medicine: one to one teaching and feedback. *BMJ.* 2003; 326(7388): 543–5.

What is needed is not just a handful of allocated or even fully trained mentors but an overall paradigm shift to a culture of coaching, with role models, positive constructive feedback, and good staff management principles.

Sonia Hutton-Taylor

Hutton-Taylor S. Cultivating a coaching culture. *BMJ.* 1999; 318(Suppl.): S2–7188.

The concept of a continuum of student learning with progressive enhancement of knowledge, skills, and attitudes based upon instruction, including self-instruction, and experience, complemented by timely, relevant feedback must be understood and supported by clinical teachers.

Robert Maudsley

Maudsley RF. Effective in-training evaluation. *Med Teach.* 1989; 11(3–4): 285–90.

Many of the feedback models published are designed to protect the learner's self-esteem and motivation.

Elizabeth Molloy

Molloy EK. The feedforward mechanism: a way forward in clinical learning? *Med Educ.* 2010; 44(12): 1157–9.

Students are very desirous of having their problems appreciated by the teaching staff and teaching staff are equally desirous of having feedback (reactions from the students) to enable them to respond.

John Morris

Morris JG. Questionnaires in medical education. *Med Teach.* 1987; 9(4): 395–402.

An important aspect of the role of an e-tutor is giving feedback in order to motivate the learner.

Maura Murphy

Murphy M. Becoming an e-tutor. In: Sandars J, editor. *E-learning for GP Educators.* Oxford: Radcliffe Publishing; 2006. pp81–7.

The difficulty that physicians face in coping with criticism, even with feedback of a very constructive nature, may derive from the rigorous mind-set formation undergone during their training, including both internship and residency experiences.

Lawrence O'Brien

O'Brien LJ. Eradicate neglect, abuse, & the commercial viewpoint. *BMJ.* 2003 October 31. Available at: www. bmj.com/content/327/7422/1001/reply#bmj_el_39485?sid=7f27ee1c-bc1e-486c-bc82-03a5164885cc (accessed 15 October 2011).

All feedback is useful feedback: discuss.

Ed Peile

Peile E. Multi-method research; multi-source feedback: pauci-impact data. *Educ Prim Care.* 2010; 21: 139–40.

The existing evidence supports the identification of feedback as the central component of formative assessment.

Alison Rushton

Rushton A. Formative assessment: a key to deep learning? *Med Teach.* 2005; 27(6): 509–13.

Videotape reviews are almost never as 'painful' as students and residents first think.

Yvonne Steinert

Steinert Y. Twelve tips for using videotape reviews for feedback on clinical performance. *Med Teach.* 1993; 15(2–3): 131–9.

Let's be honest, harassment and belittlement are merely impotent linguistic representations of the multiplicity of truly complex experiences, each fundamentally connected to a specific context and each inextricably linked to the particularized internal state of the perceiver.

Elliot Tapper

Tapper EB. A dead horse, turned on its head. *BMJ.* 2006 September 20. Available at: www.bmj.com/content/333/7570/682/reply#bmj_el_143313?sid=20523c27-2e0d-443d-a7db-86e43c2767d3 (accessed 15 October 2011).

Correcting a student's mistake in an understanding and constructive tone once is worth (or yields the same results as) berating them for the same mistake a hundred times.

Emiliano Amir Tatar

Personal correspondence, 30 June 2011.

Remember the rules for giving feedback: look at the positives first. So often we forget to do that.

Jill Thistlethwaite

Thistlethwaite J. Work based learning in primary care: remembering my past. *Work Based Learn Prim Care.* 2003; 1(1): 59–61(3).

Simulated patients (SPs) are lay people who learn how to portray patients in a consistent and standardised way. In medical education they help students and doctors develop and practise communication, consultation and clinical skills, giving valuable feedback from the patient's perspective.

Jill Thistlethwaite

Thistlethwaite J. The use of incognito simulated patients in general practice: a feasibility study. *Educ Prim Care.* 2003; 14: 419–25.

One of the problems with videotaping, apart from issues of patient consent, is the lack of the patient voice in the feedback process.

Jill Thistlethwaite

Thistlethwaite J. GP assessment: if assessment drives learning, what happens after qualification? *Work Based Learn Prim Care.* 2004; 2(1): 82–4(3).

For learning to take place, learners need to have their assumptions and ways of thinking challenged. This is much more likely to happen when learners are able to enter into a dialogue with a tutor/facilitator and/or other learners and obtain feedback from them.

Geoff Wong

Wong G. Broadband learning: firing on all cylinders? *BMJ.* 2006 June 19. Available at: www.bmj.com/content/332/7555/1403/reply#bmj_el_135847?sid=20523c27-2e0d-443d-a7db-86e43c2767d3 (accessed 15 October 2011).

The negative impact that bullying and harassment have on the wellbeing of students and doctors, overall morale in the medical workforce, and recruitment and retention in the profession demand our continuing efforts to resolve these problems.

Diana Wood

Wood DF. Bullying and harassment in medical schools. *BMJ.* 2006; 333(7570): 664–5.

10. EVALUATION

> No country has produced so many excellent analyses of the present defects of medical education as has Britain, and no country has done less to implement them.
>
> **George Pickering**

One of the most serious impediments to change in medical education is the illusive concept of international standards.

Raja Bandaranyake

Bandaranyake RC. Implementing change in medical education in developing countries. *Med Teach.* 1989; 11(1): 39–45.

The framework of clinical governance allows clinicians to organise their continuing learning and to assemble evidence to review their learning needs and to demonstrate their quality.

Jonathan Burton

Burton J. Work based learning and clinical governance. In: Burton J, Jackson N, editors. *Work Based Learning in Primary Care.* Oxford: Radcliffe Medical Press; 2003. pp119–27.

Educationalists may bemoan the difficulties in evaluating education but the challenges are not unique to education and we can learn much from the extensive research and methodological advances in healthcare evaluation.

Melanie Calvert

Calvert M. Research into cost-effectiveness in medical education. In: Walsh K, editor. *Cost Effectiveness in Medical Education.* Oxford: Radcliffe Publishing; 2010. pp121–9.

But in terms of the question 'how many portfolios is enough?', then the answer is 'one'. The key to effective personal and practice development must lie in quality, not quantity.

Maggie Challis

Challis M. Portfolios: how many is enough? *Educ Prim Care.* 2001; 12: 258–63.

In an ideal world, all practitioners within healthcare strive to improve and are expected to improve their services in a way that places the needs of service users firmly at the centre of the process.

Linda Chapman

Chapman L. Practice development: advancing practice through work based learning. *Work Based Learn Prim Care.* 2004; 2(1): 90–6(7).

In many cases, the continued production of doctors probably depends more on the quality of students that enter medical training than the quality of the teaching they receive.

Yap-Seng Chong

Chong YS. Medical education especially needs help. *BMJ.* 2003 November 2. Available at: www.bmj.com/content/327/7422/1001/reply#bmj_el_39485?sid=7f27ee1c-bc1e-486c-bc82-03a5164885cc (accessed 15 October 2011).

Adequate representation among students and faculty of the diversity in our society is indispensable for quality medical education.

Jordan Cohen

Cohen JJ. The consequences of premature abandonment of affirmative action in medical school admissions. *JAMA.* 2003; 289(9): 1143–9.

The maintenance of a high quality portfolio of learning requires that the learner records not merely that they attended an event but what they learned from it, and how they plan to apply that learning in practice.

Mark Cole

Cole M. The practice of developing practice: facilitating the capture and use of informal learning in the workplace. *Work Based Learn Prim Care.* 2004; 2(1): 1–5(5).

The observations about the informal nature of much of the learning undertaken by health-care practitioners only become problematical when the issue of capture, measurement and accreditation is raised.

Mark Cole

Cole M. Capture and measurement of work based and informal learning: a discussion of the issues in relation to contemporary healthcare practice. *Work Based Learn Prim Care.* 2004; 2(2): 118–25(8).

The most important step in planning your evaluation is to identify for whom the information is intended.

David Cook

Cook DA. Twelve tips for evaluating educational programs. *Med Teach.* 2010; 32(4): 296–301.

Recertification and maintenance of competencies in the US is being introduced only after stepwise evaluation and validation of the assessment methods.

W Dale Dauphinee

Dauphinee WD. GMC and the future of revalidation: self regulation must be made to work. *BMJ.* 2005; 330(7504): 1385–7.

It is obvious that without a mission or goal or set of objectives, it is quite impossible to conduct an orderly planning of the course, or to develop an evaluation system which accurately measures the effectiveness of the program.

Lawrence Fisher

Fisher LA. What can be done about curriculum. *Arch Dermatol.* 1966; 93(5): 536–8.

The point of theory-based evaluation is to test the theory by seeing if (a) the theory is being implemented and (b) if the predicted outcomes then follow. The theory, in other words, helps you to select from the cacophony of life, some variables that you may need to measure to try to make sense of the events.

Carol Fitz-Gibbon

Fitz-Gibbon C. Re: Trials are needed in educational research. *BMJ.* 2002 January 22. Available at: www.bmj.com/content/324/7330/126/reply#bmj_el_18878?sid=d5e693ea-0765-423d-ac1d-1c98624d8fdf (accessed 15 October 2011).

Nowadays, to appraise a man by his coat needs special sartorial training, and is at the best perilous.

Michael Foster

Foster M. An address on university work in relation to medicine: delivered at the opening of Mason University College, Birmingham. *BMJ.* 1898; 2(1971): 1028–34.

No one is more aware than I am of the bad influence which has been exerted upon medical education by the competition which has existed amongst certain of the medical licensing boards of the country, and no one wishes more ardently than I do for a legislative measure which shall place some control upon certain of these bodies.

Arthur Gamgee

Gamgee A. The Owens College Medical School. *BMJ.* 1879; 2(970): 191–2.

At a time when the standard of the medical qualifications granted by even the least efficient of the licensing medical corporations, is being greatly raised, it is expedient that a new university, about to confer medical degrees, should disavow any intention to seek popularity by conferring titles upon any but the most honourable terms.

Arthur Gamgee

Gamgee A. Introductory address on the progress of the Owens College. *BMJ*. 1883; 2(1188): 665–8.

A plethora of evaluation models have been developed that can assist the evaluator in choosing the optimum method for their particular evaluation.

John Goldie

Goldie J. Cost-effective educational evaluation. In: Walsh K, editor. *Cost Effectiveness in Medical Education*. Oxford: Radcliffe Publishing; 2010. pp101–11.

The question for medical educators considering whether to evaluate is not whether they can afford the cost of evaluation, but can they afford not to?

John Goldie

Goldie J. Cost-effective educational evaluation. In: Walsh K, editor. *Cost Effectiveness in Medical Education*. Oxford: Radcliffe Publishing; 2010. pp101–11.

As with the practice of medicine, the best hope for understanding the quality of current educational techniques and for evaluating proposed new approaches is by conducting and disseminating research based on sound principles.

Robert Golub

Golub RM. Medical education theme issue 2009: call for papers. *JAMA*. 2009; 301(9): 972.

The pursuit of excellence is a training in itself and need not necessarily be vocational.

JC Griffiths

Griffiths JC. The problem of bottlenecks. *BMJ*. 1981; 282(6280): 1976.

I submit that it is more important to maintain the quality of medical education than the present number of students.

Anne Grüneberg

Grüneberg A. University budgets and medical education. *BMJ (Clin Res Ed)*. 1981; 282(6280): 1987–8.

The profession have a right to demand uniformity of qualification in each of its ranks throughout the United Kingdom.

Charles Hastings

Hastings C. Medical legislation. *Assoc Med J*. 1856; s3–4(162): 111–12.

If approached by the education institution that places students in the practice, teaching practices should engage actively with the QA [quality assurance] process in order to improve its value to the practice, the education institution and the learners who attend the placements.

Richard Hays

Hays RB. Preparing the practice for an education QA visit. *Educ Prim Care*. 2009; 20: 425–8.

Whenever a real answer is sought on effectiveness of educational programme a careful examination of the goals and evidence of accomplishment of the process and outcome are required.

PT Jayawickramarajah

Jayawickramarajah PT. How to evaluate educational programmes in the health professions. *Med Teach.* 1992; 14(2–3): 159–66.

There is no one method for meeting educational needs: needs are different, people are different; some may appreciate one educational method, others heartily dislike it.

Robert Jones

Jones RV. Partners in practice: getting better; education and the primary health care team. *BMJ.* 1992; 305(6852): 506–8.

Uniform standards of education have been fatal to intellectual progress wherever they have been tried.

George Kidd

Kidd GH. An address on medical education. *BMJ.* 1882; 1(1101): 146–8.

The adoption of innovative medical curricula requires an equally innovative evaluative method to first describe and then to analyse its impact on traditional medical education.

Peter Leggat

Leggat PA. Traditional and innovative approaches to medical education in Australia and the move to graduate schools. *Med Teach.* 1997; 19(2): 93–4.

Perhaps it is time to reflect as to whether there is convincing long term follow up data on the validity of the long case. It may be that we are merely making the same mistake with ever increasing confidence.

David Lucey

Lucey D. Long case penalises the individual. *BMJ.* 2002 April 5. Available at: www.bmj.com/content/324/7340/748/reply#bmj_el_20889?sid=d5e693ea-0765-423d-ac1d-1c98624d8fdf (accessed 14 September 2011).

The irony really is the notion that people go into the public sector to be mediocre . . . no, in the main, they have mediocrity thrust upon them.

Chris Manning

Manning C. The carrot in the UK is now the removal of the stick. *BMJ.* 2002 April 14. Available at: www.bmj.com/content/324/7341/838/reply#bmj_el_21113?sid=d5e693ea-0765-423d-ac1d-1c98624d8fdf (accessed 14 August 2011).

Quality is a personal responsibility: it's never being satisfied with the way you do things.

Ernest McAlpine Armstrong

Smith R. A BMA secretary for quality: interview by Richard Smith. *BMJ.* 1993; 306(6888): 1328–30.

For any educational process to improve, it has to be subject to periodic external review.

Lalitha Mendis

Mendis L. Infrastructure and not the training is at fault. *BMJ.* 2004 April 8. Available at: www.bmj.com/content/328/7443/779/reply#bmj_el_56070?sid=3f545f3a-8b62-4679-979a-2c0b244a4cd7 (accessed 15 October 2011).

But, in all questions that relate to medical education, I am strongly of opinion that no man can give a really sound and valuable judgment upon them who is not actively engaged at the moment in teaching.

William Mitchell Banks

Mitchell Banks W. The five years' curriculum. *BMJ.* 1892; 2(1663): 1082–3.

There is a risk with evaluation of healthcare teaching practice that the essential elements are hardest to define and measure.

Kay Mohanna

Mohanna K. Evaluating teaching sessions: is your teaching style effective? In: Mohanna K, Chambers R, Wall D. *Your Teaching Style: a practical guide to understanding, developing and improving.* Oxford: Radcliffe Publishing; 2008. pp89–101.

He never showed signs of a lively imagination, nor of a quick intelligence you find in some; but these were qualities which led me to forsee that his judgement would be strong, a quality essential to the exercise of our art . . . Eventually after much hard slog, he succeeded in graduating with glory; and I can say without vanity that in his two years on the benches, no candidate has made more noise than he in the disputes of our school. He has made himself formidable, and no thesis can be advanced without his arguing the opposite case to its ultimate extreme.

Molière

Le Malade Imaginaire.

One of the objectives of audit is to get clinical staff to consider the justification for the interventions that make up their clinical practice. The link between medical audit and medical education and training is crucial for this and for the development of approaches to audit.

Fiona Moss

Moss F. From audit to quality and beyond: authors' reply. *BMJ.* 1991; 303(6806): 852–3.

Good quality medical education should produce doctors who are capable of obtaining succinct and accurate histories and performing appropriate examinations.

Mark Moss

Moss M. Diagnosis of deep "vein" thrombosis. *BMJ.* 2004 October 20. Available at: www.bmj.com/content/329/ 7470/821/reply#bmj_el_79792?sid=3f545f3a-8b62-4679-979a-2c0b244a4cd7 (accessed 15 October 2011).

Quality education is more than a 'flash in the pan': it is about sustained development of practice over time.

Ed Peile

Peile E. Three-dimensional training. *Educ Prim Care.* 2010; 21(2): 67.

No country has produced so many excellent analyses of the present defects of medical education as has Britain, and no country has done less to implement them.

George Pickering

Pickering G. The purpose of medical education. *BMJ.* 1956; 2(4985): 113–16.

What if increased hours of direct patient care during internship yields more competent senior residents and having more of these experienced senior residents on duty at night (a casualty of the duty hours regulations) improves care more than intern fatigue compromises it?

Louis Rice

Rice LB. Evidence-based evaluation of physician work hour regulations. *JAMA.* 2009; 301(5): 484.

A greatly improved educational programme for house officers will require more than commitment and effort from NHS [National Health Service] and academic staff: it will also need protected time, enshrined in contracts.

Peter Richards

Richards P. Educational improvement of the preregistration period of general clinical training: Council of Deans of United Kingdom Medical Schools and Faculties. *BMJ.* 1992; 304(6827): 625–7.

Trainers are a much valued resource and we need to ensure their continued participation by recognising how much effort they put in to achieve such high-quality sessions and listening to their concerns about group size, continuity and other pressures they are under.

Carolyn Rigby

Rigby C. Half-day release in vocational GP training: a case study of redesign based on qualitative evaluation. *Educ Prim Care.* 2010; 21: 354–9.

Prejudice should play no part in assessing standards of medical education.

Alexander Ross

Ross APJ. St George's University School of Medicine, Grenada: benefit or liability? *BMJ.* 1982; 285: 437.

In my judgment, gentlemen, there are two objects which are of quite paramount interest to all who wish to improve our medical education: first, to insist upon a very high standard of efficiency and public spirit in all the examining boards of the country; secondly, to insist upon a very great simplification, if not an almost entire extinction, of that ponderous code of detailed regulations under which now we either groan or sleep.

John Simon

Simon J. Address on medical education and the examining boards. *BMJ.* 1868; 1(369): 65–7.

Each medical school should develop and implement guidelines for ethics in clinical teaching, evaluate their impact, and share the findings of these evaluations.

Peter Singer

Singer PA. Intimate examinations and other ethical challenges in medical education: medical schools should develop effective guidelines and implement them. *BMJ.* 2003; 326(7380): 62–3.

Learning contracts can be a useful learning and evaluation tool within a clinical setting provided the supervisor shafts their role from one of imparter of knowledge to facilitator of learning.

Patricia Solomon

Solomon P. Learning contracts in clinical education: evaluation by clinical supervisors. *Med Teach.* 1992; 14(2–3): 205–10.

There hasn't been one medical school that has failed since the publication of the Flexner Report. I think that this is an interesting fact, that either demonstrates medical schools are so wonderful, or the situation is so critical that nobody wants to examine it.

Eugene Stead

Stead EA. Wisdom from a medical elder. *CMAJ.* 2004; 171(12): 1465–6.

The trouble is that the GMC's [General Medical Council's] only sanction is like a nuclear deterrent – it can close a medical school, but it is never going to do that.

Angela Towle

Dillner L. GMC says it will watch curriculum reforms. *BMJ.* 1994; 308(6925): 361.

Just as examinations define students' academic success, so the academic success of university staff is defined by excellence outside education: higher status is mainly attained through outstanding research or excellence in clinical work rather than educational achievements.

Cees van der Vleuten

van der Vleuten C. Improving medical education. *BMJ.* 1993; 306(6873): 284–5.

Evaluation measures the teaching. It is not the same as assessment, which measures what the learner has learned.

David Wall

Wall D. Assessment, appraisal and evaluation issues. In: Chambers R, Wall D, editors. *Teaching Made Easy: a manual for health professionals.* Oxford: Radcliffe Medical Press; 2000. pp105–29.

A major fault in our present medical education is the lack of cohesion between those responsible for welding the individual parts of the finished machine.

Beckwith Whitehouse

Whitehouse B. The British tradition and the new outlook. *BMJ.* 1942; 2(4264): 357–9.

When enthusiasm is discouraged, effort is unrewarded, and imaginations are unfired what can we expect but a "let's just get by" mentality?

John Woodhouse

Woodhouse J. Disillusion in medicine. *BMJ.* 1991; 303(6796): 246.

11. MEDICAL EDUCATION RESEARCH

> One truism in educational research is that few self evident truths are true.
> **Geoff Norman**

It is well acknowledged that RCTs [randomised controlled trials] are rarely if ever relevant in educational research.

Julian Archer

Archer J. Medical education research: reasons to be cheerful. *BMJ.* 2007; 335(7617): 414–15.

As clinicians, committed to using evidence and research to guide our practice and support clinical governance, we should not stray from the same approach to our educational practice and educational governance.

Paul Bradley

Bradley P. Evidence and research: clinical and educational parallels. *BMJ.* 2009 March 3. Available at: www.bmj.com/content/338/bmj.b690/reply#bmj_el_209927?sid=c01598e6-7fa7-4552-bbff-d3bc10847fd9 (accessed 15 October 2011).

Much of the research in medical education has been focused on undergraduates, but it is clear that practical training and competency assessment in the workplace also needs to be effective.

Melanie Calvert

Calvert M. Research into cost-effectiveness in medical education. In: Walsh K, editor. *Cost Effectiveness in Medical Education.* Oxford: Radcliffe Publishing; 2010. pp121–9.

It's true, that by blundering about, we stumbled on gold, but the fact remains that we were looking for gold.

Francis Crick

What Mad Pursuit. 1988.

Considering that academicians who devote themselves primarily to medical education have a decreased likelihood of promotion are not reimbursed for teaching time, there is insufficient funding especially to perform high-quality medical education research, which is particularly difficult to conduct, and that they have increased risk for medical liability, can there be any wonder why would-be professors do not profess?

Catherine DeAngelis

DeAngelis CD. Professors not professing. *JAMA.* 2004; 292(9): 1060–1.

It is unlikely that there will ever be a randomized controlled trial to compare the care provided by certified vs noncertified physicians, as it would be difficult to get patients to participate in such a project.

Gary Freed

Freed GL. Credentialing, recertification, and public accountability: reply. *JAMA.* 2006; 296(13): 1588.

There is a pressing need for more research into effectively treating wounded healers at local levels, and strategies that work and evaluate new techniques for teaching the wounded healer.

Lisa Graves

Graves L. Teaching the wounded healer. *Med Teach.* 2008; 30(2): 217–19.

There is almost as much unknown about the nature of a systematic review that seeks to provide best evidence for decisions about effectiveness in healthcare education as there is about many of the teaching and learning processes that we all participate in as healthcare educators.

Marilyn Hammick

Hammick M. A BEME review: a little illumination. *Med Teach.* 2005; 27(1): 1–3.

But why think. Why not trie the expt.

John Hunter

John Hunter to Edward Jenner. Correspondence, 2 August 1775.

Rigorously designed research into the effectiveness of education is needed to attract research funding, to provide generalisable results, and to elevate the profile of educational research within the medical profession.

Linda Hutchinson

Hutchinson L. Evaluating and researching the effectiveness of educational interventions. *BMJ*. 1999; 318(7193): 1267–9.

Although the Delphi method removes the risk that the outcome will be heavily dominated by a single expert, one of the main difficulties with the method is that the membership of the consultation and steering groups will have a significant effect on the outcome of the process.

Neil Johnson

Johnson N. Developing a national person specification for entry to general practice training. *Educ Prim Care*. 2002; 13: 21–7.

There is a need for medical academics whose main contribution to scholarship is in the field of education rather than research.

Sam Leinster

Leinster S. Reviving academic medicine in Britain. *BMJ*. 2000 March 8. Available at: www.bmj.com/content/320/7235/591/reply#bmj_el_6941?sid=7f1b5b2e-7b0c-43f6-8a46-f45951808b4f (accessed 15 October 2011).

Physician educators who are in general trained in the 'natural science' or 'positivist' model of research are reluctant to accept any investigation with results that fail to demonstrate the following four criteria; they must be clear, unambiguous, observable, and distinguishable.

David Lloyd

Lloyd DA. Can medical education be researched? *Med Teach*. 1991; 13(2): 145–8.

Those who are just entering upon, as well as those who are proceeding with, their studies, will do well to be upon their guard against some of the subtle theories upon which they may chance to stumble, and to receive with caution those theories which attempt to explain everything; there are many things which are essentially above our reach, and when we cannot exalt our capacities to the comprehension of them, it is better to say so, than endeavour to bring them down to the level of our capacities.

James Long

Long J. Introductory lecture delivered at the Liverpool Royal Institution: October 1, 1841. *Prov Med Surg J*. 1841; s1–3(54): 23–9.

There are many inherent difficulties in conducting high-quality educational research. Perhaps the most immediate of these is a lack of money and time.

Stephen Lurie

Lurie SJ. Raising the passing grade for studies of medical education. *JAMA*. 2003; 290(9): 1210–12.

The arguments for and against different methods of teaching medical students how to be a doctor has been raging for decades and will continue to run and run. A study that provides firm evidence of the superiority of one method over another will, I wager, never be done.

Paul McCoubrie

McCoubrie P. The PBL debate is a distraction. *BMJ*. 2004 July 21. Available at: www.bmj.com/content/329/7457/92/reply#bmj_el_67922?sid=3f545f3a-8b62-4679-979a-2c0b244a4cd7 (accessed 15 October 2011).

Case studies are powerful tools for understanding human experience and learning from it.

Anne McKee

McKee A. Getting to know case study research: a brief introduction. *Work Based Learn Prim Care.* 2004; 2(1): 6–8(3).

Whatever form it takes, a good case study supports learning and, by implication, informs decision making and practice.

Anne McKee

McKee A. Getting to know case study research: a brief introduction. *Work Based Learn Prim Care.* 2004; 2(1): 6–8(3).

It is very difficult to discuss problems in medical education without rattling a few skeletons.

George Miller

Miller GE. Problems of medical education. *Arch Dermatol.* 1965; 91(4): 292–7.

Why do clear thinking clinicians and researchers sometimes apply illogical thought to education?

Jill Morrison

Morrison J. *Med Educ.* 2000; 34(6): 490–1.

One truism in educational research is that few self evident truths are true.

Geoff Norman

Norman G. The long case versus objective structured clinical examinations: the long case is a bit better, if time is equal. *BMJ.* 2002; 324(7340): 748–9.

Perhaps the most important evidence of progress in the discipline is that we are now more likely than before to demand evidence to guide educational decision making.

Geoff Norman

Norman G. Research in medical education: three decades of progress. *BMJ.* 2002; 324(7353): 1560–2.

Conservatism and old fogeyism are totally different things; the motto of the one is, Prove all things, and hold fast that which is good; of the other, Prove nothing, but hold fast that which is old.

William Osler

Osler W. An address on the importance of post-graduate study: delivered at the opening of the museums of the Medical Graduates College and Polyclinic, July 4th, 1900. *BMJ.* 1900; 2(2063): 73–5.

While basic scientists work in a bedrock of established fact and dominant paradigms, bedsprings might be a more appropriate metaphor for the environment of the researcher into learning.

Nigel Oswald

Oswald N. Commentary: the next steps for research in learning. *Educ Prim Care.* 2005; 16: 432–3.

There is a growing body of research indicating that medical students' empathy and moral development are often stunted during medical school.

Reidar Pedersen

Pedersen R. Empathy development in medical education: a critical review. *Med Teach.* 2010; 32(7): 593–600.

Some debates in medical education can appear to the outsider to have an almost religious fervour to them, which may be off putting.

Stewart Petersen

Petersen S. Time for evidence based medical education: tomorrow's doctors need informed educators not amateur tutors. *BMJ.* 1999; 318(7193): 1223–4.

Much research about medical education proceeds devoid of theory.

David Prideaux

Prideaux D. Researching the outcomes of educational interventions: a matter of design: RCTs have important limitations in evaluating educational interventions. *BMJ.* 2002; 324(7330): 126–7.

Impact or outcome research may provide external sponsors with the information they need, but, if rigorously conducted, it will also provide generalisable findings for the wider medical education community.

David Prideaux

Prideaux D. Promises and delivery: a research imperative for new approaches to medical education. *BMJ.* 2004; 329(461): 331–2.

In the first place the trend of modern medical education and training is distinctly of a progressively more and more scientific character, and aims at preparing the student so that he may be able in the future to carry on research with real advantage to himself and to others.

Frederick Roberts

Roberts FT. The Harveian oration: delivered before the Royal College of Physicians of London, June 21st, 1905. *BMJ.* 1905; 1(2321): 1369–70.

Research and self-honest observation over decades have revealed that many of the experiences of medical school may overwhelm and exhaust rather than inspire and instruct students.

Laura Weiss Roberts

Roberts LW. Understanding depression and distress among medical students. *JAMA.* 2010; 304(11): 1231–3.

I have now seen a good many years of student life, and have watched the results of a good many educational experiments, and as the result of the experience, the advice I offer you is to attend all the practical classes you can.

William Rutherford

Rutherford W. An address on the value of practical studies. *BMJ.* 1888; 1(1428): 1002–4.

Though questionnaires are rarely phrased in Phoenician, they often use words foreign to their intended audience.

Michael Simpson

Simpson MA. How to . . . design and use a questionnaire in evaluation and educational research. *Med Teach.* 1984; 6(4): 122–7.

Doctors use some two million pieces of information to manage patients, but little research has been done on the information needs that arise while treating patients.

Richard Smith

Smith R. What clinical information do doctors need? *BMJ.* 1996; 313(7064): 1062–8.

I believe that research should inform teaching, or else one just delivers old knowledge, freshly packaged.

Michael Snaith

Snaith M. Is medical school for students, teachers or researchers. *BMJ.* 2002 May 27. Available at: www.bmj.com/content/324/7335/437/reply#bmj_el_19996?sid=d5e693ea-0765-423d-ac1d-1c98624d8fdf (accessed 15 October 2011).

The open and relatively tolerant Dutch culture, slightly scared from traditions and regulations, makes a fertile soil for investigation, experimentation and improvement of medical education, in a way that might have surprised Boerhaave – but he would have liked it, had he lived now instead of in the Golden Age?

Olle ten Cate

ten Cate O. Medical education in the Netherlands. *Med Teach.* 2007; 29(8): 752–7.

It is good to philosophise about education and its role, but pragmatically educationalists have to test what their input is achieving.

Jill Thistlethwaite

Thistlethwaite J. Reflection on 'Reflections on the ethics of assessment'. *Educ Prim Care.* 2004; 15: 125.

Educational interventions are remarkably similar to health treatments in that when they work their effect sizes tend to be small.

Carole Torgerson

Torgerson C. Trials are needed in educational research. *BMJ.* 2002 January 21. Available at: www.bmj.com/content/324/7330/126/reply#bmj_el_18878?sid=d5e693ea-0765-423d-ac1d-1c98624d8fdf (accessed 15 October 2011).

Fewer RCTs have been undertaken in medical education than is optimal.

Carole Torgerson

Torgerson CJ. Educational research and randomised trials. *Med Educ.* 2002; 36(11): 1002–3.

The argument that a randomised controlled trial will not control for the myriad of factors associated with an educational intervention is misleading.

Carole Torgerson

Torgerson CJ. Researching outcomes of educational interventions. *BMJ.* 2002; 324(7346): 1155.

If a research project is not worth doing at all, it is not worth doing properly.

Unknown

Research in medical education is thriving.

Cees van der Vleuten

van der Vleuten CPM. Research in medical education: doctoral dissertation reports. *Med Teach.* 2010; 32(4): 288–9.

Basic research is what I am doing when I don't know what I am doing.

Wernher von Braun

Attributed.

A second task involved in the rebuilding of medicine is to ensure, as and when the human resources are available, that those who hold key positions in centres of medical education and research shall be men interested not only in research and routine teaching but also in general ideas.

Francis Walshe

Walshe FMR. The integration of medicine. *BMJ.* 1945; 1(4403): 723–7.

The whole theory of modern education is radically unsound. Fortunately, in England, at any rate, education produces no effect whatsoever.

Oscar Wilde

The Importance of Being Earnest. 1895.

In a world into which fifty million children are born each year we ought to have better guides to education than the speculations of Plato and Dewey.

Leslie Witts

Witts LJ. Traditional tutorial wisdom. *BMJ.* 1960; 1(5185): 1550, 1551.

Educational interventions (of whatever type) are complex; as such, they cannot be reduced into simple "black-box" interventions and pooled into a quantitative analysis without introducing important problems.

Geoff Wong

Wong G. Internet-based education for health professionals. *JAMA.* 2009; 301(6): 598–9.

Learning

12. PROBLEM-BASED LEARNING

> Discussion clarifies thinking.
>
> **John McMichael**

The one consistency about PBL [problem-based learning] is that student and faculty satisfaction appears to be greater.

Mark Albanese

Albanese M. Life is tough for curriculum researchers. *Med Educ.* 2009; 43(3): 199–201.

Problem-based learning (PBL) serves as an educational method to foster self-directed learning, integration across disciplines, small-group learning and decision-making strategies.

Samy Azer

Azer SA. Becoming a student in a PBL course: twelve tips for successful group discussion. *Med Teach.* 2004; 26(1): 12–15.

When students are aware about their roles in PBL [problem-based learning] tutorials and what they need to do, they usually perform better and group dynamics are maintained.

Samy Azer

Azer SA. Challenges facing PBL tutors: 12 tips for successful group facilitation. *Med Teach.* 2005; 27(8): 676–81.

A trigger is the starting point of problem-based learning (PBL) cases.

Samy Azer

Azer SA. Twelve tips for creating trigger images for problem-based learning cases. *Med Teach.* 2007; 29(2–3): 93–7.

Enthusiasts for PBL [problem-based learning] talk of a commitment to life long learning as if earlier generations have not had that.

John Belstead

Belstead JS. PBL in the clinical environment. *BMJ.* 2006 February 14. Available at: www.bmj.com/content/332/7537/365.1/reply#bmj_el_128164?sid=20523c27-2e0d-443d-a7db-86e43c2767d3 (accessed 15 October 2011).

Identifying material for a course of problem based learning requires teachers to analyse their discipline for the critical elements that are essential to medical practice.

John Bligh

Bligh J. Problem based, small group learning. *BMJ.* 1995; 311(7001): 342–3.

Problem based learning is an educational method that uses problems as the starting point for student learning.

John Bligh

Bligh J. Problem based, small group learning. *BMJ*. 1995; 311(7001): 342–3.

Questioning is one of the most widely used skills of medical teaching.

George Brown

Brown G. Self assessment. *Med Teach*. 1983; 5(1): 27–9.

The facilitator of a learning group has to be especially skilled in group dynamics, as learning groups are often run for those who have already achieved a great deal in their own fields and want to develop themselves and their ideas further.

Ruth Chambers

Chambers R. Delivering relevant teaching well. In: Chambers R, Wall D, editors. *Teaching Made Easy: a manual for health professionals*. Oxford: Radcliffe Medical Press; 2000. pp77–104.

The exploration of knowledge, learning through curiosity, the critical evaluation of evidence and a capacity for self-education are all fostered in small-group interactions.

Joy Crosby

Crosby J. Learning in small groups. *Med Teach*. 1996; 18(3): 189–202.

Whilst there is certainly a role for problem based learning in the medical curriculum, traditional methods of teaching cannot be dismissed, particularly as the majority of medical students are school leavers, with little experience of problem based learning.

Shreelata Datta

Datta ST. New methods of teaching need to be assessed before being accepted *BMJ*. 2004 July 23. Available at: www.bmj.com/content/329/7457/92/reply#bmj_el_68324?sid=3f545f3a-8b62-4679-979a-2c0b244a4cd7 (accessed 15 October 2011).

The most outstanding, complicating and time consuming factor in case based problem-solving tests is the element of interaction.

Erik de Graff

de Graff E. Simulation of initial medical problem-solving: a test for the assessment of medical problem-solving. *Med Teach*. 1988; 10(1): 49–55.

Problem-based learning is grounded in the belief that learning is most effective when students are actively involved and learn in the context in which that knowledge is to be used.

Grahame Feletti

Feletti G. The disaster simulation: a problem-based learning or assessment experience for primary care professionals. *Med Teach*. 1995; 17(1): 39–45.

I think PBL [problem-based learning] has become a catchy marketing pitch to draw attention away from the real issue of quality in medical education.

Hartley Flege

Flege H. Just acting? *BMJ*. 2004 July 27. Available at: www.bmj.com/content/329/7457/92/reply#bmj_el_68776?sid=3f545f3a-8b62-4679-979a-2c0b244a4cd7 (accessed 15 October 2011).

The teacher should facilitate students' learning by asking questions requiring problem solving skills rather than simple recall of facts.

Jean-Jacques Guilbert

Guilbert JJ. What is a medical teacher's job? *Med Teach*. 1979; 1(1): 21–3.

Trying to link PBL [problem-based learning] to one educational theory is too simplistic.

Hossam Hamdy

Hamdy H. The fuzzy world of problem based learning. *Med Teach*. 2008; 30(8): 739–41.

The OSCE [objective structured clinical examination] approach is reductive as it hinders the development of higher order consultation skills such as patient centredness and in particular the integration of clinical problem solving.

Adrian Hastings

Hastings A. Let us return to reality. *BMJ*. 2006 September 20. Available at: www.bmj.com/content/333/7567/546/reply#bmj_el_142183?sid=20523c27-2e0d-443d-a7db-86e43c2767d3 (accessed 18 October 2011).

Inquiry learning is more effective than deductive methods in helping students gain understanding and works well when learners have prior knowledge.

Kevork Hopayian

Hopayian K. Using mock studies to teach evidence-based practice: description of workshops and evaluation of GP trainees' experiences. *Educ Prim Care*. 2008; 19: 321.

Most attempts at longitudinal, controlled intervention studies in PBL [problem-based learning] have been overtaken by events.

Brian Jolly

Jolly B. Jigsaws and the march of time. *Med Educ*. 2007: 41(6): 535–6.

In a programmed lecture a single teacher can transform an amphitheatre into a small-group tutorial.

Bahman Joorabchi

Joorabchi B. How to: construct and use a problem-based programmed lecture. *Med Teach*. 1982; 4(1): 6–9.

Problem-based learning, self-directed learning, task-based learning and situated learning to name but four are in essence terminological constructs describing aspects of learning unproven by any useful clinical outcome measure yet enthusiastically employed based upon their enjoyment by those involved.

Darren Kilroy

Kilroy DA. Turning aspiration into action in medical education. *BMJ*. 2006 September 11. Available at: www.bmj.com/content/333/7567/544/reply#bmj_el_142089?sid=20523c27-2e0d-443d-a7db-86e43c2767d3 (accessed 15 October 2011).

I remember very little about benzene rings, but the critical thinking and problem-solving skills of organic chemistry formed the foundation of my medical training.

Daniel Kramer

Kramer DB. Changing premedical requirements. *JAMA*. 2007; 297(1): 37.

Students who have been exposed to teachers using the problem-based approach in their secondary education might be more adaptive to this type of learning. If this is the case, close liaison of medical schools with secondary schools is important.

Wai-Ching Leung

Leung WC. Teaching time required and students' past experience should be considered too. *BMJ*. 1999 March 8. Available at: www.bmj.com/content/318/7184/657.1/reply#bmj_el_2623?sid=3b793041-95a4-4870-a5d9-9fc0c51e668f (accessed 15 October 2011).

Problem based learning has the potential to liberate students from unimaginative didactic teaching in which facts, that are relatively useless in the long term, are passed on as pearls of wisdom for students to forget once they have regurgitated them in their finals.

Jennifer Majoor

Majoor J. The challenges of problem based teaching. *BMJ*. 1999 March 24. Available at: www.bmj.com/content/318/7184/657.1/reply#bmj_el_2623?sid=3b793041-95a4-4870-a5d9-9fc0c51e668f (accessed 15 October 2011).

Tutors can gain much from facilitating adult learning, but must move away from authoritarianism and dispensing facts.

Gillian Maudsley

Maudsley G. Roles and responsibilities of the problem based learning tutor in the undergraduate medical curriculum. *BMJ*. 1999; 318(7184): 657–61.

Undergraduate medical curriculums that use problem based learning rather than a traditional approach need a different type of medical educator.

Gillian Maudsley

Maudsley G. Roles and responsibilities of the problem based learning tutor in the undergraduate medical curriculum. *BMJ*. 1999; 318(7184): 657–61.

PBL [problem-based learning] is not about sacrificing the basic sciences.

Jean McKendree

McKendree J. What PBL is and isn't. *BMJ*. 2004 October 7. Available at: www.bmj.com/content/329/7457/92/reply#bmj_el_66800?sid=3f545f3a-8b62-4679-979a-2c0b244a4cd7 (accessed 15 October 2011).

While there are many methods under the umbrella term PBL, most approaches include being specific about the ultimate outcomes that are expected to be achieved. What is not specified is a single path for achieving that outcome.

Jean McKendree

McKendree J. What PBL is and isn't. *BMJ*. 2004 October 7. Available at: www.bmj.com/content/329/7457/92/reply#bmj_el_66800?sid=3f545f3a-8b62-4679-979a-2c0b244a4cd7 (accessed 15 October 2011).

Any curriculum, whether PBL, systems or specialty based, should cover an agreed core of knowledge, skills and attitudes and there should be no presumption that adopting PBL precludes students from learning facts, any more than there should be the presumption that students on non-PBL courses are unable to think for themselves.

Hamish McKenzie

McKenzie H. PBL is not the whole story. *BMJ*. 2004 July 27. Available at: www.bmj.com/content/329/7457/92/reply#bmj_el_68717?sid=3f545f3a-8b62-4679-979a-2c0b244a4cd7 (accessed 15 October 2011).

Whatever the pedagogic approach, PBL or otherwise, the single most important factor that shapes the undergraduate educational experience is the quality with which that approach is implemented.

Hamish McKenzie

McKenzie H. PBL is not the whole story. *BMJ.* 2004 July 27. Available at: www.bmj.com/content/329/7457/92/reply#bmj_el_68717?sid=3f545f3a-8b62-4679-979a-2c0b244a4cd7 (accessed 15 October 2011).

To ensure responsibility for all components of the PBL programme, a medical education unit with full-time dedicated and experienced staff should be functional at implementation.

Michelle McLean

McLean M. Sustaining problem-based learning reform: advice in hindsight! *Med Teach.* 2004; 26(8): 726–8.

Discussion clarifies thinking.

John McMichael

McMichael J. Adult education: for the academic clinical teacher. *BMJ.* 1955; 2(4938): 510–11.

The use of small groups to encourage active participation and deep learning as well as learning group skills and the ability to express and defend new ideas is well established in medical education.

Honor Merriman

Merriman H. Clinical governance for primary care teams: how useful is a learning set for individuals from different teams? *Educ Prim Care.* 2003; 14: 189–201.

When self-directed learning in PBL [problem-based learning] is conceived as a goal, the small group is crucial to its achievement because it is in the small group that students learn to find their way and take responsibility for their own learning in medicine, an arena that is new for them.

Barbara Miflin

Miflin B. Small groups and problem-based learning: are we singing from the same hymn sheet? *Med Teach.* 2004; 26(5): 444–50.

Although PBL is an example of student centred learning, it is not necessarily the same as student directed learning.

Jill Morrison

Morrison JM. Evidence base for PBL in UK medical schools. *BMJ.* 2004 July 15. Available at: www.bmj.com/content/329/7457/92/reply#bmj_el_67271?sid=3f545f3a-8b62-4679-979a-2c0b244a4cd7 (accessed 15 October 2011).

In PBL, the factual knowledge covered by students can be tightly structured by Faculty by means of carefully written "problems", supporting activities, such as clinical and laboratory sessions, and appropriate assessments.

Jill Morrison

Morrison JM. Evidence base for PBL in UK medical schools. *BMJ.* 2004 July 15. Available at: www.bmj.com/content/329/7457/92/reply#bmj_el_67271?sid=3f545f3a-8b62-4679-979a-2c0b244a4cd7 (accessed 15 October 2011).

Another challenge for the proponents of adult learning theory might be to explain why it has been so difficult to demonstrate significant differences in learning outcomes of students from problem-based medical schools compared to conventional medical schools.

David Newble

Newble D. Are our assumptions about experienced adult learners in medicine warranted. *BMJ.* 2002 July 30. Available at: www.bmj.com/content/325/7357/200/reply#bmj_el_24253?sid=d5e693ea-0765-423d-ac1d-1c98624d8fdf (accessed 15 October 2011).

I think it might be fruitful to start viewing PBL as a term used to denote a family of teaching approaches that share some common principles and to encourage descriptions of each individual approach on a series of consistent common dimensions.

Mark Newman

Newman MJ. PBL type teaching approaches: rigorous evidence still required. *BMJ.* 2008 May 7. Available at: www.bmj.com/content/336/7651/971/reply#bmj_el_194977?sid=a15ec792-dfe3-4ba7-b8d0-a79c5a5cccab (accessed 15 October 2011).

Our experience of introducing problem based learning mirrors that of others, with initial apprehension being slowly overcome.

Paul O'Neill

O'Neill PA. Problem based learning at medical school . . . and has been introduced successfully in Manchester. *BMJ.* 1995; 311(7020): 1643.

Learners' engagement with, and participation in, educational learning activities is widely accepted to enhance their learning.

Ed Peile

Peile E. Interactivity and case learning. *BMJ.* 2006; 332(7551): 1201.

Problem based learning, an educational intervention characterised by small group and self directed learning, is one of medical education's more recent success stories, at least in terms of its ubiquity.

David Prideaux

Prideaux D. Researching the outcomes of educational interventions: a matter of design: RCTs have important limitations in evaluating educational interventions. *BMJ.* 2002; 324: 126.

What is important in doctors' practice is what doctors do and not what they know. Medical knowledge needs to be transferred to clinical practice. PBL is a better means of transferring knowledge to practice than didactic teaching.

Brian Rambihar

Rambihar BV. What doctors do is more important than what doctors know. *BMJ.* 2004 July 13. Available at: www.bmj.com/content/329/7457/92/reply#bmj_el_126491?sid=20523c27-2e0d-443d-a7db-86e43c2767d3 (accessed 15 October 2011).

Remember that the only foolish question is the one you thought of but failed to pose.

George Romanes

Romanes G. Students are an essential part of the education of their institutions. *BMJ.* 2004 January 20. Available at: www.bmj.com/content/327/7429/1430/reply#bmj_el_44809?sid=7f27ee1c-bc1e-486c-bc82-03a5164885cc (accessed 15 October 2011).

Although active participation and interaction are essential to a successful workshop, the participants must also feel that they have learned something.

Yvonne Steinert

Steinert Y. Twelve tips for conducting effective workshops. *Med Teach.* 1992; 14(2–3): 127–31.

One of the strengths of small-group teaching is the opportunity for students to become actively involved in the process of learning.

Yvonne Steinert

Steinert Y. Twelve tips for effective small-group teaching in the health professions. *Med Teach.* 1996; 18(3): 203–7.

Tell me and I'll forget. Show me and I may not remember. Involve me and I'll understand.

Unknown

In problem based learning (PBL) students use "triggers" from the problem case or scenario to define their own learning objectives.

Diana Wood

Wood DF. ABC of learning and teaching in medicine: problem based learning. *BMJ.* 2003; 326: 328–30.

13. SIMULATION

> The huge benefit of simulation is that it shifts the steep and dangerous part of the learning curve away from patients.
>
> **Ian Curran**

Whilst the use of VR [virtual reality] simulation in surgical training is something that should be supported, it should not be seen as a possible replacement for traditional training techniques.

Gareth Bashir

Bashir G. Technology and medicine: the evolution of virtual reality simulation in laparoscopic training. *Med Teach.* 2010; 32(7): 558–61.

Game-based learning invites opportunities for richly immersive learning activities, but is expensive to implement, and time consuming to develop.

Michael Begg

Begg M. Leveraging game-informed healthcare education. *Med Teach.* 2008; 30(2): 155–8.

Organising a session of the simulated surgery is a complex business requiring advance planning, booking of personnel, preparation of paperwork, arranging the rotation, timing the consultations and recording the marks.

Peter Burrows

Burrows P. Simulated surgery for the assessment of consulting skills. In: Jackson N, Jamieson A, Khan A, editors. *Assessment in Medical Education and Training: a practical guide.* Oxford: Radcliffe Publishing; 2007. pp97–108.

The huge benefit of simulation is that it shifts the steep and dangerous part of the learning curve away from patients.

Ian Curran

Reynolds T, Kong ML. Shifting the learning curve. *BMJ.* 2010; 341: c6260.

One of the important things a simulated patient can do is to give 'feedback' at the end of a teaching session and this is where the simulated patient can come out of role completely.

Margaret Davies

Davies M. The way ahead: teaching with simulated patients. *Med Teach.* 1989; 11(3–4): 315–20.

The actor-patient has evolved over the past several years from a purely passive live mannequin, upon whom the techniques of physical examination may be demonstrated before a large audience, to an active participant in the educational process.

Roger Duvoisin

Duvoisin RC. Simulated patients (programmed patients): the development and use of a new technique in medical education. *Arch Neurol.* 1972; 26(6): 555.

An area that is attracting a lot of attention in education circles is that of 'serious gaming', the application of video game principles and techniques to instructional design.

Rachel Ellaway

Ellaway R. eMedical teacher. *Med Teach.* 2007; 29(9–10): 1001–2.

We would like simulation to be embedded in the fabric of how we do health care.

David Gaba

Volker R. Medical simulation gets real. *JAMA.* 2009; 302(20): 2190–2.

Respecting these the old adage which declares that a barber learns his trade by practising on fools does not apply.

Jonathan Hutchinson

Hutchinson J. Address in surgery. *BMJ.* 1895; 2(1805): 273–7.

Simulation offers an environment in which learners can train until they reach specified levels of competency and in which "permission to fail" can be built into the learning process without jeopardizing patient safety.

Roger Kneebone

Kneebone RL. Practice, rehearsal, and performance: an approach for simulation-based surgical and procedure training. *JAMA.* 2009; 302(12): 1336–8.

Repeated practice is essential to gain expertise.

Roger Kneebone

Kneebone RL. Practice, rehearsal, and performance: an approach for simulation-based surgical and procedure training. *JAMA.* 2009; 302(12): 1336–8.

As clinicians and educators we need to decide what it is that is most important for people to learn and use simulation to construct environments that allow people to learn those things.

Roger Kneebone

Reynolds T, Kong ML. Shifting the learning curve. *BMJ.* 2010; 341: c6260.

By teaching in a wider range of settings and making more use of simulated situations we can allow students to explore aspects of medicine that are crucially important but difficult to cover in a traditional teaching hospital.

Stella Lowry

Lowry S. Trends in health care and their effects on medical education. *BMJ.* 1993; 306: 255–8.

On any plane flight I am comforted in the knowledge that the pilots are regularly subjected to simulator exercises and medical checks to establish fitness.

Chris Manning

Manning C. Revaluation and the plaudit cycle. *BMJ.* 1999 October 30. Available at: www.bmj.com/content/319/7218/1180/reply#bmj_el_11171?sid=7f1b5b2e-7b0c-43f6-8a46-f45951808b4f (accessed 15 October 2011).

Performance ratings based on simulation will be more reliable, not only because they are based on a better sample of student responses, but also because detailed criteria for judging performance can be specified in advance and examiners can be trained to apply these criteria consistently.

Christine McGuire

McGuire CH. Assessment of problem-solving skills, 2. *Med Teach.* 1980; 2(3): 118–22.

Simulations . . . provide opportunities for participants to deal with the consequences of their actions, an element of instruction that is often lacking in other forms of education.

Max Miller

Miller MD. Simulations in medical education: a review. *Med Teach.* 1987; 9(1): 35–41.

It is a constant cry that medical students want responsibility, but in the same way and for the same reasons as airline pilots learn much of their skills on simulators, we cannot grant students real responsibility for clinical decisions until they have demonstrated their ability to cope with them.

Max Rendall

Rendall M. Controversy: Pomr; the case in favour. *Med Teach.* 1979; 1(3): 147–50.

Debriefing allows for discharge of emotion and capturing the learning.

Faith Stafford

Stafford F. The significance of de-roling and debriefing in training medical students using simulation to train medical students. *Med Educ.* 2005; 39(11): 1083–5.

By participating in a role-play, medical students or residents can discover their own feelings about a particular situation and gain insight into the patient's presenting problems or life situation.

Yvonne Steinert

Steinert Y. Twelve tips for using role-plays in clinical teaching. *Med Teach.* 1993; 15(4): 283–91.

While the use of simulated patients for training and assessment is extremely powerful, work based learning around the consultation is probably best carried out with 'real' patients.

Jill Thistlethwaite

Thistlethwaite J. GP assessment: if assessment drives learning, what happens after qualification? *Work Based Learn Prim Care.* 2004; 2(1): 82–4(3).

Expert patients lie on the continuum between real and simulated patients.

Jill Thistlethwaite

Thistlethwaite J. Learning from patients. *Work Based Learn Prim Care.* 2004; 2(4): 370–2(3).

14. E-LEARNING

> To enhance learning educational media will need to be discursive, adaptive, interactive and reflective.
>
> **Alex Jamieson**

An essential part of e-learning is the opportunity to enter a discussion with colleagues.

David Bossano

Bossano D. A personal experience of using e-learning. In: Sandars J, editor. *E-learning for GP Educators.* Oxford: Radcliffe Publishing; 2006. pp15–18.

Both undergraduate and postgraduate medical education is changing and will need to change further to ensure adequate skills in learning and problem solving, communication, teamwork, information technology, ethics, and the behavioural and social sciences.

Cyril Chantler

Chantler C. Reinventing doctors: will move doctors from this winter of discontent to a position of leadership. *BMJ.* 1998; 317(7174): 1670–1.

Abundant research now reassures us regarding the effectiveness of e-learning in comparison to non-intervention, and the essential equivalence of e-learning in comparison to traditional methods.

David Cook

Cook DA. The failure of e-learning research to inform educational practice, and what we can do about it. *Med Teach.* 2009; 31(2): 158–62.

It is hoped that the next few years will see an accumulation of evidence to guide our use of WBL [web-based learning].

David Cook

Cook DA. Where are we with web-based learning in medical education? *Med Teach.* 2006; 28(7): 594–8.

I recall from my medical school days watching a guinea pig, strategically placed on the professor's desk, die from anaphylactic shock when challenged with an allergen. It is hard to imagine that I could not have learned this equally well by reading about it or watching a computer simulation.

Marjorie Cramer

Cramer M. Use of animals in medical education. *JAMA.* 1991; 266(24): 3421–2.

There can be little doubt that the rapidity and complexity of change in the need for and of health care, advances in science and technology, as well as change in demographic, social, environmental and economic conditions – nationally, regionally and world-wide should make the ability to adapt to change and to participate in change the single most important outcome of continuing medical education.

Charles Engel

Engel CE. Editorial-3: continuing medical education for change? *Med Teach.* 1988; 10(3–4): 269–71.

Reduced funding, rising student numbers, geographical dispersal, and increased competition in a complex global market have put medical schools under pressure to embrace computer assisted learning.

Trisha Greenhalgh

Greenhalgh T. Computer assisted learning in undergraduate medical education. *BMJ.* 2001; 322: 40.

Learners often have access to a rich range of learning resources via computers, and so location is becoming less relevant to learning, but the defining quality of medical education comes from interactions with patients with stories to tell, clinical signs to demonstrate, and episodes of care to share with learners.

Richard Hays

Hays R. Evolving community-based medical education: integrating undergraduate and postgraduate education. *Educ Prim Care.* 2008; 19: 235–40.

In my view it is in our interest as e-learners that those who design e-learning should understand contemporary learning theory, that is to say, they should understand what they are doing.

Alex Jamieson

Jamieson A. E-learning. *Work Based Learn Prim Care.* 2003; 1(2): 137–46(10).

To enhance learning educational media will need to be discursive, adaptive, interactive and reflective.

Alex Jamieson

Jamieson A. Future trends in e-learning. In: Sandars J, editor. *E-learning for GP Educators.* Oxford: Radcliffe Publishing; 2006. pp137–44.

The three main areas to focus on when designing a course on e-learning are: instructional design principles, the educational media and evaluation.

Peter Johnson

Johnson P. Running a short course on e-learning: a GP tutor's perspective. In: Sandars J, editor. *E-learning for GP Educators.* Oxford: Radcliffe Publishing; 2006. pp89–95.

Electronic learning tools offer an exciting potential for improving student learning, either as an aid to or as a replacement for traditional teaching methods.

Klaus-Dietrich Kronke

Kronke KD. Computer-based learning versus practical course in pre-clinical education: acceptance and knowledge retention. *Med Teach.* 2010; 32(5): 408–13.

E-learning holds out the promise of being an affordable and flexible means through which NHS trusts can deliver the education and training critical to their business, despite continuing financial constraints and restrictions in working hours.

Sue Lacey-Bryant

Lacey-Bryant S. E-learning: fulfilling its promise? *Work Based Learn Prim Care.* 2007; 5(2): 111–14(4).

E-learning is an exciting opportunity to drive up standards of patient care by finding innovative ways of supporting GPs in their efforts to keep up to date.

Mayur Lakhani

Lakhani M. Foreword. In: Sandars J, editor. *E-learning for GP Educators.* Oxford: Radcliffe Publishing; 2006. pv.

A major benefit of work based learning degrees is that study times are more flexible than for a standard degree programme and can be tailored to meet the competing needs of work and home life.

Richard McDonough

McDonough R. Accrediting work based learning in primary care for an academic qualification. *Work Based Learn Prim Care.* 2004; 2(3): 214–19(6).

The concept that instructional text is used rather than read has escaped the notice of many authors and publishers.

PJ McLeod

McLeod PJ. How to produce instructional text for a medical audience. *Med Teach.* 1991; 13(2): 135–44.

The idea of blending learning activities is not particularly new but is attracting more attention because a blended approach seems to be an efficient and effective way forward for many institutions wanting to make better use of information and communication technology (ICT) and e-learning.

Gary Motteram

Motteram G. Blended learning. In: Sandars J, editor. *E-learning for GP Educators.* Oxford: Radcliffe Publishing; 2006. pp39–42.

Computer-assisted instruction enhances learning, allowing the student the discretion of content, time, place, and pace of instruction. Information conveyed can take several forms, some better suited to undergraduate medical education, others more applicable to graduate and continuing education.

Thomas Piemme

Piemme TE. Computer-assisted learning and evaluation in medicine. *JAMA.* 1988; 260(3): 367–72.

Medicine consists of science, wisdom, and technology. We teach the science; we ignore the study of human behaviour from which wisdom could derive; and we profess to despise technology though we see it all around us.

Robert Platt

Platt R. Thoughts on teaching medicine. *BMJ.* 1965; 2(5461): 551–2.

The advent of microcomputers has dramatically expanded the possibilities in information dissemination and medical education.

Mike Pringle

Pringle M. Autumn books: video cassette; tool or toy? *BMJ (Clin Res Ed).* 1984; 289(6452): 1127.

The potential for e-learning can only be achieved if an approach is used that concentrates on the education and recognises that the role of technology is to enhance the learning, rather than trying to find educational uses for new technology.

John Sandars

Sandars J. What is e-learning? In Sandars J, editor. *E-learning for GP Educators.* Oxford: Radcliffe Publishing; 2006. pp1–5.

Improving the effectiveness of e-learning in medical education should have a focus on improving the intervention to produce the desired impact, either on changing clinical behaviour or improving patient outcomes.

John Sandars

Sandars J. Cost effective e-learning in medical education. In: Walsh K, editor. *Cost Effectiveness in Medical Education.* Oxford: Radcliffe Publishing; 2010. pp40–7.

It is surprising that there has not been more interest in evaluating the cost effectiveness of e-learning in medical education, especially with its rapid and widespread uptake as an educational approach at both undergraduate and postgraduate levels, including continuing professional development.

John Sandars

Sandars J. Cost effective e-learning in medical education. In: Walsh K, editor. *Cost Effectiveness in Medical Education.* Oxford: Radcliffe Publishing; 2010. pp40–7.

The main benefit of e-learning for both providers and learners is that it can provide consistent quality of content at a time and a place that is convenient to both parties.

John Sandars

Sandars J. Cost effective e-learning in medical education. In: Walsh K, editor. *Cost Effectiveness in Medical Education.* Oxford: Radcliffe Publishing; 2010. pp40–7.

Given the central role of informatics notions in clinical practice, including health care technology, many observers have argued that the discipline ought to be taught to physicians in training, from the preclinical years through graduate medical education and beyond.

Edward Shortliffe

Shortliffe EH. Biomedical informatics in the education of physicians. *JAMA.* 2010; 304(11): 1227–8.

The e-portfolio is micromanaging medical education. It is just doctors spending more time "recording" and less time "doing" education.

Des Spence

Spence D. From the frontline: the errr-portfolio. *BMJ.* 2009; 339: 2863.

New modes of delivery are needed for the current generation of health and social care professionals that fit in with their work commitments and enable them to continue to learn on a lifelong basis – this cannot be effectively achieved by expecting busy professionals to continue to take time off work.

Andrew Thornett

Thornett A. Training in e-learning in health and social care: where do we go from here? *Work Based Learn Prim Care.* 2004; 2(2): 158–9(2).

Education and learning change subtly as a question posed online is quite likely to be answered immediately and it becomes possible for medical learners to reach further for an exchange of opinion or a discussion of aspects of healthcare as the need arises.

Veronica Wilkie

Wilkie V. Online learning in primary care: the importance of e-professionalism. *Educ Prim Care.* 2009; 20: 423–4.

The internet is here to stay, and those who teach, mentor and facilitate the next generation of healthcare workers need to embrace web-based and e-learning, so that the learning styles of those they teach can be used to maximum effect.

Veronica Wilkie

Wilkie V. Online learning in primary care: the importance of e-professionalism. *Educ Prim Care.* 2009; 20: 423–4.

15. INTERPROFESSIONAL EDUCATION

> Oh wad some pow'r the giftie gie us to see oursels as others see us.
>
> **Robert Burns**

I am dying with the help of too many physicians.

Alexander the Great

Attributed.

It is the unwitting deterioration of standards of medical education that we should be trying to avoid in order not to allow the distinction between doctors and nurses to be blurred.

Angshu Bhowmik

Bhowmik A. Blurring of distinctions. *BMJ.* 2005 December 12. Available at: www.bmj.com/content/331/7529/0.7/reply#bmj_el_123652?sid=cb764c2a-ad1a-4f84-a8c4-88b3568c267c (accessed 15 October 2011).

Oh wad some pow'r the giftie gie us to see oursels as others see us.

Robert Burns

Burns R. To a mouse. 1786.

As interprofessional working, and the benefits it can bring, has become more widely recognised across primary and secondary care, the concept of interprofessional education or learning has been developed.

Charles Campion-Smith

Campion-Smith C. Practice team learning in primary care. *Work Based Learn Prim Care.* 2006; 4(4): 301–10(10).

The true value of interprofessional learning is greatest when the learners study a common topic of interest and importance to themselves and the patients they care for. If the learning is effective, they will see how the team as a whole can better understand the needs of the patients or organisation.

Charles Campion-Smith

Campion-Smith C. Practice team learning in primary care. *Work Based Learn Prim Care.* 2006; 4(4): 301–10(10).

When successful, interprofessional team learning in primary care can be a fruitful, effective and economical way of responding to the constant demands for change and practice development.

Charles Campion-Smith

Campion-Smith C. Practice team learning in primary care. *Work Based Learn Prim Care.* 2006; 4(4): 301–10(10).

Learning in teams is best facilitated by the progressive mastery of more and more complex tasks incorporating the best practices of cooperative learning as part of an experiential learning process.

Marcel D'Eon

D'Eon M. A blueprint for interprofessional learning. *Med Teach.* 2004; 26(7): 604–9.

Would it not be more effective to envisage a substantial amount of interprofessional learning taking place in clinical settings, where students are dealing with real life circumstances; where they can see the contributions of the different members of the team; where they can learn to work together and can indeed take over each other's roles where appropriate?

Janet Finch

Finch J. Interprofessional education and teamworking: a view from the education providers. *BMJ.* 2000; 321(7269): 1138–40.

At an undergraduate level, combining education for different health professionals has much to commend it, encouraging the mutual respect needed for their future professional lives.

Andrew Frank

Frank A. Interprofessional education and team working. *BMJ.* 2000 November 8. Available at: www.bmj.com/content/321/7269/1138/reply#bmj_el_11016?sid=7f1b5b2e-7b0c-43f6-8a46-f45951808b4f (accessed 12 September 2011).

If we are to bring relevant groups together to refine and improve the education and the education experience of young doctors-to-be (and presumably other health professionals) it is my impression that we first need to redefine what it is we are trying to produce. What is the desired outcome of all the medical education and the contact with the healthcare setting?

Stan Goldstein

Goldstein S. Outcomes for medical education. *BMJ.* 2000 March 6. Available at: www.bmj.com/content/320/7235/633/reply#bmj_el_6909?sid=7f1b5b2e-7b0c-43f6-8a46-f45951808b4f (accessed 12 September 2011).

One of the advantages of learning in primary care is that multi-professional teamwork is well established and patients are plentiful.

Richard Hays

Hays R. Assessing learning in primary care. *Educ Prim Care.* 2009; 20: 4–7.

Work based learning necessitates effective collegiate relationships across professional boundaries and could therefore be perceived as an opportunity to promote interprofessional working.

Julie Hughes

Hughes J. Advanced practice roles in primary care: a critical discussion of the policy and practice implications. *Work Based Learn Prim Care.* 2005; 3(2): 119–28(10).

Moving some roles to other healthcare professionals will require review of medical students' and doctors' training.

Linda Hutchinson

Hutchinson L. Medical education: challenges of training doctors in the new English NHS. *BMJ.* 2006; 332(7556): 1502–4.

In the dining rooms of teaching hospitals and in the bars at conferences specialist surgeons may be heard forecasting the imminent demise of the general surgeon and his replacement by specialised multidisciplinary teams who will concentrate on one system, or even part of one system.

Miles Irving

Irving M. The general surgeon. *BMJ (Clin Res Ed).* 1986; 292(6522): 741–2.

Work based learning as a model of lifelong learning enables healthcare professionals working as individuals and in teams in the NHS [National Health Service] to participate in regular and systematic educational activity.

Neil Jackson

Jackson N. Work based learning and the retention and development of the NHS workforce. *Work Based Learn Prim Care*. 2003; 1(1): 5–9(5).

Multiprofessional education is a strand of the cultural change considered essential for the modernisation of healthcare services.

Sue Lacey-Bryant

Lacey-Bryant S. E-learning: 'more bang for your buck?' *Work Based Learn Prim Care*. 2006; 4(2): 166–70(5).

The barrier holding back interdisciplinary education is not that doctors, nurses and other clinical staff are unwilling to learn management skills and techniques: many already do. It is that the NHS [National Health Service] has no history of supporting managers without a medical, nursing or therapy background to gain an insight into the clinical area for which they are responsible.

Rachel Lissauer

Lissauer RJ. Don't have a clinical background but . . . *BMJ*. 2003 March 25. Available at: www.bmj.com/content/326/7390/652.2/reply#bmj_el_30870?sid=7f27ee1c-bc1e-486c-bc82-03a5164885cc (accessed 12 September 2011).

Our patients love the nurse, availability is more important than the highest expertise.

Geoffrey Marsh

Handysides S. General practice enriching careers in general practice new roles for general practitioners. *BMJ*. 1994; 308: 513.

In my opinion a medical man in starting on his career – should not only know all a nurse does and a great deal more, but be able to do all that she can do.

Wesley Mills

Mills W. Some considerations bearing on the surgeon, the patient, the student, and the nurse, based largely on the personal experiences of the writer. *BMJ*. 1910; 1: 682.

Collaborative learning needs to be interconnected, and parallels the interconnectedness of collaborative working.

Sue Morrison

Morrison S. A case study of interprofessional learning and working at Marylebone Health Centre. *Work Based Learn Prim Care*. 2006; 4(2): 116–29(14).

The move from continuing medical education for doctors to continuing professional development for the whole primary care team presents new challenges for multidisciplinary learning and performance monitoring.

Mike Pringle

Pringle M. Clinical governance in primary care: participating in clinical governance. *BMJ*. 2000; 321: 737.

The main places of clinical learning are obviously the wards, the outpatients department, laboratories, and operating theatres; your teachers are the patients, nurses, consultants, colleagues and many others.

Philip Rhodes

Rhodes P. Studying for a higher diploma. *BMJ (Clin Res Ed)*. 1983; 286(6363): 461–2.

Medical students are not passive bystanders during their training. They are an integral part of the health care team who admittedly are there to learn but at the same time do contribute.

Michael Ruse

Ruse M. Student experience and view point is necessary. *BMJ.* 2004 January 21. Available at: www.bmj.com/content/327/7428/1362/reply#bmj_el_47671?sid=3f545f3a-8b62-4679-979a-2c0b244a4cd7 (accessed 12 September 2011).

Interprofessional/multiprofessional education is a goal defined professionally and politically and instinctively it feels right. Many of us are trying to find ways to overcome inherent barriers and move in this direction.

Patsy Stark

Stark P. Interprofessional education: how do we know if it improves patient care? *BMJ.* 2001 March 16. Available at: www.bmj.com/content/322/7287/676.2/reply#bmj_el_13310?sid=bfae656f-d7d3-4ae5-abb6-1b0e432b89b5 (accessed 12 September 2011).

If receptionists are recognised as offering health advice, it is important that it is the correct advice. We need to be sure that our receptionists are trained in what they are doing, and work within clear boundaries.

Rebecca Torry

Torry R. Reception staff and health advice. *Work Based Learn Prim Care.* 2005; 3(1): 31–40(10).

Interprofessional education creates the opportunity for learners from different professions to work together during the educational process, to develop a better understanding of related healthcare discipline perspectives and to simulate future professional interactions.

Prathibha Varkey

Varkey P. Practical tips and strategies for designing and implementing interprofessional curricula. *Educ Prim Care.* 2010; 21: 41.

One hopes that effective interprofessional education decreases medical errors, enhances quality of care and promotes patient-centred care and professional satisfaction.

Prathibha Varkey

Varkey P. Practical tips and strategies for designing and implementing interprofessional curricula. *Educ Prim Care.* 2010; 21: 41.

So often the doctors produced by medical schools are not equipped to provide the health services that people need.

Henry Walton

Robb J. Interdisciplinary training needed in medical education. *BMJ.* 1993; 307: 941.

Once students are accepted into medical school, a major element in their training is the process of identity development as a doctor.

Cynthia Whitehead

Whitehead C. The doctor dilemma in interprofessional education and care: how and why will physicians collaborate? *Med Educ.* 2007; 41(10): 1010–16.

Group learning facilitates not only the acquisition of knowledge but also several other desirable attributes, such as communication skills, teamwork, problem solving, independent responsibility for learning, sharing information, and respect for others.

Diana Wood

Wood DF. ABC of learning and teaching in medicine: problem based learning. *BMJ.* 2003; 326: 328–30.

16. LEARNING FROM EXPERIENCE

You can not learn surgery sitting on your ass.

Ward Griffen

All experience is an arch to build upon.

Henry Brooks Adams

The Education of Henry Adams. 1907.

A student must be interested in his subject, and a lot can be done towards this end by a man with many years in practice who is liked and respected and who can make the student interested by drawing on his experiences of people and patients to illustrate and italicize his teaching.

David Alexander

Alexander DF. The G.P.'s clinical training. *BMJ.* 1950; 2(4678): 575.

For the things we have to learn before we can do, we learn by doing.

Aristotle

Nicomachean Ethics.

They be the best physicians, which being learned incline to the traditions of experience, or, being empirics, incline to the methods of learning.

Francis Bacon

Smith WG. Introductory remarks delivered at the opening of the section of pharmacology and therapeutics: at the Annual Meeting of the British Medical Association at Ipswich, July–August, 1900. *BMJ.* 1900; 2(2066): 292–4.

I would not have every ignorant asse to be made a chirurgeon by my booke, for they would do more harm with it than good.

George Bacon

Elliston WA. President's address: delivered at the Sixty-Eighth Annual Meeting of the British Medical Association. *BMJ.* 1900; 2(2066): 273–80.

Go to the pine if you want to learn about the pine.

Matsuo Basho

The Narrow Road to the Deep North. 1966.

Ask any person the question, Based on your personal experience, what quality do you most associate with physicians you consider "good," and what quality do you most associate with physicians you consider "bad?" The top response is: the "good" physician is one who listens; the "bad" physician is one who is inattentive and rushed.

Abraham Bergman

Bergman AB. Learning to listen. *Arch Pediatr Adolesc Med.* 2003; 157: 414–15.

Man can learn nothing except by going from the known to the unknown.
Claude Bernard
An Introduction to the Study of Experimental Medicine. ch. 2.

Reflection can translate and transform an experience into learning, which can then be utilised in the next cycle of experience.
Sue Bryant
Bryant S. Case study: the elderly skier. *Work Based Learn Prim Care.* 2007; 5(1): 36–44(9).

Each contact between patient and their family doctor contributes to an evolving story, and each individual consultation can draw on this prior shared experience. The value of this personal relationship is determined by the communication skills of the family doctor and is in itself therapeutic.
Francesco Carelli
Carelli F. Continuity and the European definition. *BMJ.* 2003 November 25. Available at: www.bmj.com/content/327/7425/1219/reply#bmj_el_41337?sid=7f27ee1c-bc1e-486c-bc82-03a5164885cc (accessed 12 September 2011).

What is all Knowledge too but recorded Experience, and a product of History; of which, therefore, Reasoning and Belief, no less than Action and Passion, are essential materials?
Thomas Carlyle
On History, from *Essays.*

Doctors do not appear to learn from their mistakes; they merely repeat them.
William Casey
Casey WF. Resuscitation needed for the curriculum. *BMJ (Clin Res Ed).* 1985; 291(6493): 484–5.

A workshop is a good format if you want to exchange ideas and experiences in a relatively new area.
Ruth Chambers
Chambers R. Delivering relevant teaching well. In: Chambers R, Wall D, editors. *Teaching Made Easy: a manual for health professionals.* Oxford: Radcliffe Medical Press; 2000. pp77–104.

Numbers of practitioners, no doubt, learn to treat children with accuracy and skill; but this knowledge is acquired after their student days are over, by the experience of actual practice.
WB Cheadle
Cheadle WB. An address delivered at the opening of the section of diseases of children. *BMJ.* 1888; 2(1442): 361–3.

What we call experience is often a dreadful list of ghastly mistakes.
J Chalmers Costa
The Trials and Triumphs of the Surgeon. ch. 1.

Although nature commences with reason and ends in experience it is necessary for us to do the opposite, that is to commence as I said before with experience and from this to proceed to investigate the reason.
Leonardo da Vinci
Movement and weight, from *The Notebooks of Leonardo da Vinci.*

Reflection is a continuous process that enables the practitioner to improve practice by questioning their own actions, seeking the advice of colleagues and learning from the experience of others as well as from more orthodox sources.

Sylvia Debreczeny

Debreczeny S. Developing practice nurses through work based learning. *Work Based Learn Prim Care.* 2003; 1(2): 109–18(10).

The main benefit of work based learning is to recognise the learning opportunities that occur during the working day. Such opportunistic learning could result from chance queries or unusual experiences, which may stimulate coffee room or corridor discussions, but may either not be followed up or remain unrecognised as a learning experience and therefore not consolidated.

Sylvia Debreczeny

Debreczeny S. Developing practice nurses through work based learning. *Work Based Learn Prim Care.* 2003; 1(2): 109–18(10).

Read little, see much, do much.

Baron Guillaume Dupuytren

Attributed.

The years teach much which the days never know.

Ralph Waldo Emerson

Experience, from *Essays: second series.* 1844.

The nature and qualities of the teaching materials that you use can have a substantial effect on the educational experience of your students.

Richard Farrow

Farrow R. ABC of learning and teaching in medicine: creating teaching materials. *BMJ.* 2003; 326(7395): 921–3.

Learning by one's mistakes cannot be considered an ideal form of medical education.

Tim Fenton

Fenton T. Junior hospital doctors' hours of work campaign. *BMJ (Clin Res Ed).* 1985; 291(6490): 285.

Clinicians still seem resistant to dropping unreliable examination procedures from teaching or structured examinations, perhaps because of their medical education, clinical experience, or lack of awareness of existing literature.

Christopher Frank

Frank C. Medical education: evidence based checklists for objective structured clinical examinations. *BMJ.* 2006; 333(7567): 546–8.

Physicians, like beer, are best when they are old.

Thomas Fuller

The Holy State and the Profane State.

Contemporary views of learning posit that people construct knowledge based on previously held beliefs and experiences.

Ben Graffam

Graffam B. Active learning in medical education: strategies for beginning implementation. *Med Teach.* 2007; 29(1): 38–42.

I submit that the teaching of medicine must lie in the hands of those who are actively practising it, and it would be disastrous to have theoretical systems of teaching imposed from outside upon our schools by doctrinaires, wholly divorced from practical experience of medical education.

Ernest Graham Little

Graham Little E. A medical minister of health. *BMJ.* 1925; 2(3387): 1032–3.

From the very commencement the student should set out to witness the progress and effects of sickness and ought to persevere in the daily observation of disease during the whole period of his studies.

Robert Graves

Introductory Lectures. 1850.

Richard Branson has observed that complaints are free market research. Structured reflection will allow individuals to learn from the experience and make any necessary adjustments and move on.

Brenda Greaves

Greaves B. Compliments and complaints. *Work Based Learn Prim Care.* 2003; 1(2): 153–5(3).

You can not learn surgery sitting on your ass.

Ward Griffen

Schein M. *Aphorisms and Quotations for the Surgeon.* Shrewsbury: TFM Publishing; 2003. ch 28, pp68–74.

The intern suffers not only from inexperience, but also from over-experience.

William Stewart Halsted

Bulletin of the Johns Hopkins Hospital. 1904; 15: 267.

We must turn to nature itself, to the observations of the body in health and disease to learn the truth.

Hippocrates

Aphorisms.

Practice – hospital practice – should be the basis of all your studies, the source from which they flow, the test to which they are every day referred.

Timothy Holmes

Holmes T. An address on medical education. *BMJ.* 1885; 2(1293): 681–5.

Some experience of popular lecturing had convinced me that the necessity of making things plain to uninstructed people, was one of the very best means of clearing up the obscure corners in one's own mind.

Thomas Huxley

Man's Place in Nature and Other Anthropological Essays: collected essays. 1894.

Reason, Observation, and Experience – the Holy Trinity of Science.

Robert Ingersoll

The Gods.

To restate the obvious, a good GP may be old or youngish, black or white, man or woman, and so may a bad GP. What matters far more is experience, compassion, and a liking for people, and of these the first is directly related to age.

John Ioannou

Ioannou J. Medical unemployment. *BMJ (Clin Res Ed)*. 1982; 285(6343): 742.

The motto of all the mongoose family is, 'Run and find out'.

Rudyard Kipling

The Jungle Book. 1897.

Medical education has enshrined apprenticeship as one of its critical tools.

Daniel Klass

Klass DJ. Will e-learning improve clinical judgment? *BMJ*. 2004; 328(7499): 1147–8.

The most fitted to teach practical medicine and surgery are those successfully and daily engaged in its practice.

Thomas Lewis

Lewis T. The Huxley lecture on clinical science within the university. *BMJ*. 1935; 1(3873): 631–6.

It takes more than the issuing of educational manifestos – the translation of fossilized notions into carefully worded behavioural objectives – to change the experience of being at a medical school.

Marshall Marinker

Marinker M. The way we teach . . . general practice. *Med Teach*. 1980; 2(2): 63–70.

One of the meanings given to the word "academic" in the Oxford English Dictionary is, "not leading to an answer; impractical." How such a meaning came to be ascribed to a word more understandably associated with the search for answers is beyond the scope of this lecture.

Marshall Marinker

Marinker M. Should general practice be represented in the university medical school? *BMJ*. 1983; 286: 855.

Experience is the great teacher; unfortunately, experience leaves mental scars, and scar tissue contracts.

William Mayo

Mayo WJ. In the time of Henry Jacob Bigelow. *JAMA*. 1921; 77(8): 597–603.

At one time, anyone who joined a health professions faculty taught, irrespective of whether they had been trained or had any experience.

Michelle McLean

McLean M. How to professionalise your practice as a health professions educator. *Med Teach*. 2010; 32(12): 953–5.

A doctor learns chiefly from his own experience. The more information he has about his own working methods and the outcome of his actions, the greater his self knowledge will be.

Ian McWhinney

McWhinney IR. Medical audit in North America. *BMJ*. 1972; 2(5808): 277–9.

Experience isn't history, it's biography. Of the myriad things that happen to us or which we see happen to others only those which are "internalised" – that is, connected up with our other observations and values – constitute experience.

David Metcalfe

Metcalfe D. The chains of education, experience, and culture. *BMJ.* 1992; 305(6844): 33–4.

Most men are to some extent handicapped in the practice of the medical profession by a lack of experiences of the sort which fall to their patients. Development and the highest preparation for action come from the mind that has felt sorrows and pain as well as joy.

Wesley Mills

Mills W. Some considerations bearing on the surgeon, the patient, the student, and the nurse, based largely on the personal experiences of the writer. *BMJ.* 1910; 1: 682.

[A]bove all things, what pleases me in him, and what I am glad to see him follow my example in, is that he is blindly attached to the opinions of the ancients, and that he would never understand nor listen to the reasons and the experiences of the pretended discoveries of our century concerning the circulation of the blood and other opinions of the same stamp.

Molière

Le Malade Imaginaire.

To make yourselves, then, perfectly acquainted with the different diseases to which the body is subject, you must see those diseases yourselves, and your observation must not be a cursory one.

John Morgan

Morgan J. Clinical lectures in course of delivery during the present session, at Guy's Hospital. *Prov Med Surg J.* 1841; s1–2(28): 21–5.

My own work in student learning has shown me that experienced adult learners ultimately approach their study and learning in ways which are no different from those used by students entering directly from school.

David Newble

Newble DI. Don't presume about experienced adult learners in medicine. *BMJ.* 2002; 325(7367): 779.

Except for what he gains by experience, it is safe to say that what the newly qualified general practitioner does not already know he will never know adequately.

Bernard Peck

Peck BJ. The teaching of dermatology to medical students. *BMJ.* 1955; 2(4938): 523–5.

Novices may learn from seeing how experts develop their reasoning, and experts exposed to the thought processes of the less experienced may reflect on their unconscious expertise.

Ed Peile

Peile E. How can experts and novices learn together? *BMJ.* 2004; 329(7471): 902.

The student learns not by being told but by doing.

George Pickering

Pickering G. Postgraduate medical education: the present opportunity and the immediate need. *BMJ.* 1962; 1(5276): 421–5.

The first staggering fact about medical education is that after two and a half years of being taught on the assumption that everyone is the same, the student has to find out for himself that everyone is different, which is really what his experience has taught him since infancy.

Robert Platt

Platt R. Thoughts on teaching medicine. *BMJ*. 1965; 2(5461): 551–2.

He gains wisdom in a happy way, who gains it by another's experience.

Plautus

Mercator.

Never miss the opportunity to serve on a few committees. The experience is invaluable. It will teach you much about your fellow doctors, and you will learn techniques of how to persuade others to your point of view.

Philip Rhodes

Rhodes P. Committees. *BMJ (Clin Res Ed)*. 1983; 286(6377): 1563–4.

One legacy of medical education is overvaluing scientific measurement and undervaluing subjective experiences.

Helen Riess

Riess H. Empathy in medicine: a neurobiological perspective. *JAMA*. 2010; 304(14): 1604–5.

The joining together of individuals, to share knowledge and experiences, has been recognised as an essential part of problem solving and action taking since the earliest history of mankind.

John Sandars

Sandars J. Knowledge management: sharing knowledge. *Work Based Learn Prim Care*. 2004; 2(2): 111–17(7).

Education is when you read the fine print; experience is what you get when you don't.

Pete Seeger

Loose Talk.

What is required is not so much clinical instruction as instruction in the method of conducting a practice – a thing which no hospital can provide.

HM Stanley Turner

Stanley Turner HM. Responsible Experience under Guidance. *BMJ*. 1935; 2(3896): 473–4.

I repeat our hospitals should be more thrown open to students, and they should be encouraged to visit them, and inquire for themselves into the hidden mysteries of disease; by no other means will they attain that quickness of perception and readiness of resource without which no one will ever attain success as a physician or surgeon.

Edward Thompson

Thompson EC. Address on the past, present, and future of medicine. *BMJ*. 1882; 2(1135): 607–12.

No one can acquire skill in chemistry, physiology, or histology without practising experiments and manipulations in the laboratory; and it is equally impossible for students to become skilful physicians or surgeons who have not had actual personal labour in our hospitals.

Edward Thompson

Thompson EC. Address on the past, present, and future of medicine. *BMJ*. 1882; 2(1135): 607–12.

And the lowest form of student life was the dresser, who was frankly a cheap form of labour which he undertook in the wards in return for casual teaching and experience.

Arthur Thomson

Thomson A. History and development of teaching hospitals in England. *BMJ*. 1960; 2(5201): 749–51.

It is simply not possible for a physician, having gained a consultant appointment or its equivalent, to become buried in clinical practice and to rely solely on experience if society is to be provided with a high standard of medical care for the ensuing 25–30 years.

Anthony Toft

News. *BMJ*. 1993; 306: 7.

A young doctor makes a full graveyard.

Unknown

Good surgical judgement comes from experience and experience comes from poor surgical judgement.

Unknown

If you've seen one case of chest pain, you've seen one case of chest pain.

Unknown

No man is a good doctor who has never been sick himself.

Unknown

No one becomes a good doctor before he fills a churchyard.

Unknown

Residents must be relieved of time-consuming, nonmedical chores and internal medicine training must be redefined to provide experiences which are important to gain competence.

Eleanor Wallace

Wallace EZ. Service vs education in internal medicine residency: need for a resolution. *Arch Intern Med*. 1988; 148(6): 1296.

We risk replacing the value of embedded experienced performance with a mentality where 'can sometimes do' is good enough to tick the box.

Val Wass

Wass V. The impact of change in healthcare delivery on medical education. *Educ Prim Care*. 2007; 18: 551–7.

Experience is the name every one gives to their mistakes.

Oscar Wilde

Lady Windermere's Fan. 1892.

Personal experience of the worry and stress of illness in our own families can teach us many things and must help make us better doctors.

Derek Wooff

Wooff D. Personal view. *BMJ*. 1988; 297(6660): 1417.

17. LEARNING FROM PATIENTS

> There are two objects of medical education: To heal the sick, and to advance the science.
>
> **Charles Mayo**

The deficiencies which I think good to note . . . I will enumerate . . . The first is the discontinuance of the ancient and serious diligence of Hippocrates, which used to set down a narrative of the special cases of his patients, and how they proceeded, and how they were judged by recovery or death.

Francis Bacon

The Advancement of Learning. bk II.

Let the young know they will never find a more interesting, more instructive book than the patient himself.

Giorgio Baglivi

Available at: http://medicalstate.tumblr.com/post/6597839959/let-the-young-know-they-will-never-find-a-more
(accessed 10 February 2012).

The enlightened public will look to their medical attendants as guides, philosophers, and friends, both in health and disease.

James Barr

Barr J. President's address, delivered at the Eightieth Annual Meeting of the British Medical Association. BMJ. 1912; 2(2691): 157–63.

I now say to general practitioners: Perfect your own education, you have the means at hand; teach your patients the laws of health, which is the most valuable asset of the nation.

James Barr

Barr J. The future of the medical profession. BMJ. 1918; 2(3012): 318–21.

One: The history is by far the most important part of a patient encounter. Two: Don't believe a word patients say.

Daniel Bercu

Personal correspondence, 28 June 2011.

The ability to listen is arguably the most important clinical skill in medicine.

Abraham Bergman

Bergman AB. Learning to listen. Arch Pediatr Adolesc Med. 2003; 157: 414–15.

The public is not always sagacious, but in the long run, it does somehow contrive to find out who are the skilled lawyers and doctors.

John Shaw Billings

Public Health Reports. 1874–75; 2: 384.

There is certainly a need for medical schools to ensure their graduates emerge 'fit for purpose'; but there are, of course, many purposes to which doctors' skills may be put. The hugely diverse range of careers available to doctors – not to mention the diverse range of problems faced by their patients – can best be served by a similarly diverse palette of educational experience.

Ben Braithwaite

Braithwaite B. Diversity in education is the solution, not the problem. *BMJ.* 2005 October 12. Available at: www. bmj.com/content/331/7520/791/reply#bmj_el_119006?sid=cb764c2a-ad1a-4f84-a8c4-88b3568c267c (accessed 12 September 2011).

Just as duties to patients should be measured against the capacity to deliver these duties, so learning should be undertaken in a way which is sustainable.

Jonathan Burton

Burton J. Work based learning in action: collaborative learning and personal learning. In: Burton J, Jackson N, editors. *Work Based Learning in Primary Care.* Oxford: Radcliffe Medical Press; 2003. pp25–48.

The most important thing to learn is how to listen to your patients. Not just hear them, actually listen to them. If the patient is convinced that you're really listening they'll tell you everything you need, and they'll do anything you ask.

Stephen Carr

Personal correspondence, 1 July 2011.

Education must become more focussed and relevant to the needs of the learner, patients and the NHS [National Health Service] as a whole.

Ruth Chambers

Chambers R. Teaching and education should be relevant to the needs of the learner, patients and the NHS as a whole. In: Chambers R, Wall D, editors. *Teaching Made Easy: a manual for health professionals.* Oxford: Radcliffe Medical Press; 2000. pp1–27.

Like clinical research, medical education may expose patients to risks that are not offset by the prospect of benefits to those individual patients but instead by the prospect of benefits to other individuals.

Winston Chiong

Chiong W. Justifying patient risks associated with medical education. *JAMA.* 2007; 298(9): 1046–8.

In teaching hospitals where out-patients are essentially consultative, the physician should stress the technique of consultation.

Henry Cohen

Cohen H. Methods and men in the teaching of clinical medicine. *BMJ.* 1950; 2(4677): 478–81.

The practice of studying stories provides a means of analysing all manner of narratives, from our own reflective accounts to the (hi)stories that patients and clients provide.

Mark Cole

Cole M. Fictional realities. *Work Based Learn Prim Care.* 2007; 5(2): 80–8(9).

If doctors find it difficult to listen to patients, understand their preferences, and involve them in decisions about their care, they may need training in the competencies for shared decision making.

Angela Coulter

Coulter A. Patients' views of the good doctor: doctors have to earn patients' trust. *BMJ.* 2002; 325(7366): 668–9.

Do patients use professional medical exams to get a second opinion?

John Dearlove

Dearlove JC. Do patients use professional medical exams to get a second opinion? *BMJ.* 2002 March 9. Available at: www.bmj.com/content/324/7334/404/reply#bmj_el_20442?sid=d5e693ea-0765-423d-ac1d-1c98624d8fdf (accessed 12 September 2011).

The attitude of the physician towards the profession in general, and particularly towards the patient, will determine to a large extent a number of aspects of his or her functioning.

Charles de Monchy

de Monchy C. Professional attitudes of doctors and medical teaching. *Med Teach.* 1992; 14(4): 327–31.

The first acts of a graduate are apt to be his precedents through coming years, for there is no era in his life in which self-complacency is so exalted as the time which passes between receiving his diploma with its blue ribbon, and receiving crape and gloves, to wear at the funeral of his first patient.

Daniel Drake

Drake D. *West J Med Surg.* 1844; 2: 354.

A medical school education that trains physicians to provide effective, efficient, patient-centered care to our increasingly multicultural citizenry is a critical step in transforming our health care system.

Michael Drake

Drake MV. The need for diversity in medical education: barriers to be broken. *Arch Ophthalmol.* 2009; 127(10): 1387–8.

The idea that health care actually harms patients has been around for some time, but until now little has been done to educate future doctors about the problem.

Oliver Ellis

Ellis O. Patient safety: putting safety on the curriculum. *BMJ.* 2009; 339: b3725.

I believe it is important to be informed of the nature of the disease in each individual patient, because we are not all formed in the same fashion, but we differ markedly from one another in many respects.

Rufus of Ephesus

On the Interrogation of the Patient.

As patient care is shifted from in-hospital ward care to alternative care, we should consider teaching students in other clinical settings as well.

Martin Finkel

Finkel M. Medical education toward the 21st century. *JAMA.* 1985; 254(15): 2060–1.

The patient may well be safer with a physician who is naturally wise than with one who is artificially learned.

Benjamin Franklin

Poor Richard's Almanack. 1760.

Being pleasant, warm, concerned, and, where appropriate, compassionate on the one hand and being medically and scientifically competent on the other are not mutually exclusive attributes.

Raanan Gillon

Gillon R. Doctors and patients. *BMJ (Clin Res Ed).* 1986; 292(6518): 466–9.

One of the keys to respect for autonomy is good communication, and thus respect for patients' autonomy requires doctors to acquire and maintain skill in communicating with them – not just in telling but also in understanding.

Raanan Gillon

Gillon R. Doctors and patients. *BMJ (Clin Res Ed)*. 1986; 292(6518): 466–9.

It is reasonable to assume that cheaters in medical school will be more likely than others to continue to act dishonestly with patients, colleagues, insurers, and government.

Shimon Glick

Glick SM. Cheating at medical school: schools need a culture that simply makes dishonest behaviour unacceptable. *BMJ*. 2001; 322(7281): 250–1.

When we're looking at applicants who ... want to go into primary care and serve the underserved in rural Wisconsin, we should care a bit less whether they got an A or a B in organic chemistry but we should care a lot more as to what kind of track record of community engagement and community service they have.

Robert Golden

Voelker R. Medical education meets health reform: new models are needed for patient-centered care. *JAMA*. 2010; 304(21): 2349.

By all means, improve medical education, and increase the likelihood that practising doctors are worthy of their licences, but let's not try to pretend that we can ensure that no patient will ever be harmed by a doctor's incompetence.

Neville Goodman

Goodman N. Expediency before principle is common. *BMJ*. 2005 January 6. Available at: www.bmj.com/content/ 330/7481/1/reply#bmj_el_91408?sid=1e069fc1-8837-4789-925c-3c1714669644 (accessed 12 September 2011).

In order to teach the students midwifery St. Swithin's supervised the reproductive activities of the few thousand people who lived in the overcrowded area surrounding the hospital.

Richard Gordon

Doctor in the House.

If the patients truly had a choice, what would they prefer? Doctors who are well trained and knew what they were doing or pleasant social beings who let it all hang out so that the customers could choose whether they wanted tegretol or epilim irrespective of the type of the epilepsy they had. Brave new world?

Jayaprakash Gosalakkal

Gosalakkal JA. Are patients in UK so different from the rest of the Western world? *BMJ*. 2006 June 26. Available at: www.bmj.com/content/332/7556/1502/reply#bmj_el_137505?sid=20523c27-2e0d-443d-a7db-86e43c2767d3 (accessed 12 September 2011).

Reaccreditation is mainly for patients. Like the original licence to practise, it should be an assurance that education has been effective, competencies have been acquired, and patients can consult with confidence.

Denis Pereira Gray

Gray DP. Reaccrediting general practice. *BMJ*. 1992; 305(6852): 488–9.

What is needed now is the development of collaborative patient-educator organizations (across conditions and advocacy groups) that can work with existing medical organizations to ensure that medical education and training fully incorporate the important knowledge patients have about chronic disease and how physicians can help meet their needs.

Stuart Green

Green S. Medical education and chronic disease. *JAMA.* 2004; 292(24): 2974.

Patient care in general and patient-physician communication in particular will not improve until the most clinically adept and highly motivated bedside clinicians return to center stage as the role models for students and residents.

M Andrew Greganti

Greganti MA. Clinical role models: importance of attending faculty: reply. *Arch Intern Med.* 1991; 151(4): 818–21.

The "rambo resident" fills in the void and sets the tone for more junior learners – a technologically focused, clinically immature, and psychosocially barren approach that neglects the patient as a person with "human" needs.

M Andrew Greganti

Greganti MA. Clinical role models: importance of attending faculty: reply. *Arch Intern Med.* 1991; 151(4): 818–21.

GP expertise is in diagnosing undifferentiated problems in a relatively stable patient population over time, thus building up a body of clinical knowledge informed by an understanding of the social context of the patient.

Gail Greig

Greig G. Mutual learning between general practitioners with community hospital beds and consultants in Scotland. *Work Based Learn Prim Care.* 2004; 2(4): 338–51(14).

Never forget that it is not a pneumonia, but a pneumonic man who is your patient.

William Withey Gull

Published Writings, Memoir II.

I have yet to see the solitary spleen in bed 5, or the hip replacement on ward 10; visions of a lonesome organ or a prosthesis abound, but do not materialise.

Ian Guy

Guy I. Curious and curiouser? *BMJ.* 2003 June 17. Available at: www.bmj.com/content/326/7402/1337/reply#bmj_el_33424?sid=7f27ee1c-bc1e-486c-bc82-03a5164885cc (accessed 12 September 2011).

When any additional person joins in a consultation with a patient there is a wonderful opportunity to use them to think out loud.

Helen Halpern

Halpern H. Thinking out loud. *Educ Prim Care.* 2006; 17: 258–64.

Medical education is not without its pains and its anxieties. The realities of disease and death are themselves painful and often shocking.

Denis Hill

Hill D. Acceptance of psychiatry by the medical student. *BMJ.* 1960; 1(5177): 917–18.

The ultimate object of study in medicine is the patient himself, not a piece of him, such as his kidneys or his respiratory system.

Denis Hill

Hill D. Acceptance of psychiatry by the medical student. *BMJ.* 1960; 1(5177): 917–18.

The object of attendance at the routine laboratories is not to train students to be pathologists but to give a powerful stimulus to learning by seeing the practical uses of pathology in relation to patients.

Kenneth Hill

Hill KR. Medical education. *BMJ.* 1962; 2(5308): 854, 855.

I will prescribe regimens for the good of my patients according to my ability and my judgment and never do harm to anyone.

Hippocrates

The Hippocratic Oath.

Some patients, though conscious that their condition is perilous, recover their health simply through their contentment with the goodness of the physician.

Hippocrates

Precepts. VI.

As a trainee doctor you are taught all the time to underestimate symptoms. In general, students are taught to be manly and tough and they tend to feel that patients always overemphasise their symptoms. In the same way doctors underemphasise their own symptoms.

Walter Holland

Court C. British study highlights stigma of sick doctors. *BMJ.* 1994; 309(6954): 561–2.

Once in a while you will have a patient of sense, born with the gift of observation, from whom you may learn something.

Oliver Wendell Holmes

The Young Practitioner, from *Medical Essays.*

Paradoxically, as the eyesight and spine deteriorate, clinical knowledge continues to accrue. Why does the profession not recognise this by negotiating contracts which allow clinicians to withdraw from the most complex, tiring work as they age, to increase their involvement in outpatient consultation, under-graduate and post-graduate teaching, management or other related activities, without financial penalty?

Russell Hopkins

Hopkins R. Consequence of ageing among doctors. *BMJ.* 1998 October 2. Available at: www.bmj.com/content/317/7161/811/reply#bmj_el_817?sid=6a4ef178-62d7-4865-ac37-192d0fd43924 (accessed 12 September 2011).

Primary care staff can draw on the skills of patient-centred practice to achieve effective student learning: these skills are of potential value to the broader teaching community.

Amanda Howe

Howe A. Has a decade made a difference? The contribution of UK primary care to basic medical training in 2004. *Educ Prim Care.* 2005; 16: 10–19.

Medical education has an important role in shifting to a truly patient led culture.

Linda Hutchinson

Hutchinson L. Medical education: challenges of training doctors in the new English NHS. *BMJ*. 2006; 332(7556): 1502–4.

From inability to let well alone; from too much zeal for the new and contempt for what is old; from putting knowledge before wisdom, science before art and cleverness before common sense; from treating patients as cases; and from making the cure of the disease more grievous than the endurance of the same, Good Lord, deliver us.

Robert Hutchison

Favourite prayers: the physician's prayer. *BMJ*. 1998; 317(7174): 1687.

Most patients in most disciplines are managed at home unless they are very seriously ill, and teaching of clinical method must be organised to take account of this and use outpatient, day patient, and domiciliary arenas.

DJ Jolley

Jolley DJ. Bed numbers and good medical education. *BMJ (Clin Res Ed)*. 1986; 292(6535): 1596.

Every medical examination is intimate and soon the medical students begin to appreciate this. Examination of the fundus of the uterus is just as intimate for a gynaecologist as examining the fundus of the eye is to an ophthalmologist.

Nikhil Kaushik

Kaushik NC. What examination is not intimate? *BMJ*. 2003 January 14. Available at: www.bmj.com/content/326/7402/1326.3.full (accessed 11 October 2011).

What will ultimately be of greatest benefit to our patients – and will give to the profession the best hope of stability and a sense of direction as circumstances change – is the maintenance by doctors of the highest standards of medical practice.

Robert Kilpatrick

Kilpatrick R. Profile of the GMC: portrait or caricature? *BMJ*. 1989; 299(6691): 109–12.

It is of course essential that patients' representatives should be included in the development of mechanisms to ensure high standards of ethical practice in medical education.

Peter Lapsley

Lapsley P. Patients in medical education and research. *BMJ*. 2004; 329(7461): 334.

At entry to medical school, were each student to be given a copy of the Universal Declaration of Human Rights and asked to commend its essence to memory, by the time of graduation each article would be linked to recollections of people met and understood, people taken care of as patients and encountered as peers.

Jennifer Leaning

Leaning J. Human rights and medical education: why every medical student should learn the Universal Declaration of Human Rights. *BMJ*. 1997; 315: 1390–1.

If the medical profession wants to remove this curious contradiction of aiming on the one hand to educate ethically and clinically competent doctors 'fit for practice' and at the same time continues to tolerate disrespectful and unprofessional attention towards their future doctors by some colleagues, this requires firstly acknowledgement, personal accountability and redress to enhance rather than undermine the well being of doctors and ultimately patients.

Heidi Lempp

Lempp H. Belittlement and harassment in US medical schools. *BMJ.* 2006 October 9. Available at: www.bmj.com/content/333/7570/682/reply#bmj_el_143313?sid=20523c27-2e0d-443d-a7db-86e43c2767d3 (accessed 12 September 2011).

Another obvious response to the shortage of suitable patients in our traditional teaching hospitals is to move the students out into the community, where the patients and much of the health care are.

Stella Lowry

Lowry S. Trends in health care and their effects on medical education. *BMJ.* 1993; 306(6872): 255–8.

The history of diagnostic logic must be as old as that of medicine itself; the motivation to improve it has probably never been stronger than it was in the mind of the caveman patient as he felt the rasp of the trepan drilling a hole in his skull.

Fergus Macartney

Macartney FJ. Diagnostic logic. *BMJ (Clin Res Ed).* 1987; 295(6609): 1325–31.

There is a wholesome tendency in medical education at the present time to bring back into the picture the patient himself, who during the biochemical and bacteriological period has been supplanted by the experimental animal.

Charles Macfie Campbell

Macfie Campbell C. The general practitioner's approach to his nervous or mental patients. *BMJ.* 1932; 2(3756): 1186–9.

It is at the bedside of the patient that the observer must study disease; there he will see it in its true character, stripped of those false shades by which it is so frequently disguised in books.

Louis Martinet

Exposition of the Various Methods of Examination Used in Medicine: a manual of pathology. 1827.

There are two objects of medical education: To heal the sick, and to advance the science.

Charles Mayo

Collected Papers of the Mayo Clinic and Mayo Foundation. 1926; 18: 1093.

The safest thing for a patient is to be in the hands of a man engaged in teaching medicine. In order to be a teacher of medicine the doctor must always be a student.

Charles Mayo

Proceedings of the Staff Meetings of the Mayo Clinic. 1927; 2: 223.

From 30 years' experience of teaching both school leavers and graduates, patients would be better served by doctors entering medical school after the age of 22.

Peter McCrorie

McCrorie P. Graduate students are more challenging, demanding, and questioning. *BMJ.* 2002; 325(7366): 676.

Clinical teaching is a compromise between providing a service for patients and meeting the needs of students.

Roy Meadow

Meadow SR. The way we teach . . .: paediatrics. *Med Teach.* 1979; 1(5): 237–43.

It is stated vaguely but emphatically that the trend of recent hospital teaching is to send him into practice with the conviction that patients are so many laboratory problems, and with a corresponding evasion of his personal responsibility to study the patient, collect his own observations, and form his own judgements.

Keith Waldegrave Monsarrat

Monsarrat KW. Educational number, session 1935–6: some comments on medical training and practice and their regulation. *BMJ.* 1935; 2(3895): 365–8.

The chief event in the last period of the student's course is his contact with patients. No rules can ensure that he will learn how best to approach problems of human disorder.

Keith Waldegrave Monsarrat

Monsarrat KW. Educational number, session 1935–6: some comments on medical training and practice and their regulation. *BMJ.* 1935; 2(3895): 365–8.

Patients employed in medical education provide consent in the context of extant care they are receiving (not always the case in research).

Kelechi Nnoaham

Nnoaham KE. Education is not research. *BMJ.* 2004 August 12. Available at: www.bmj.com/content/329/7461/332/reply#bmj_el_70695?sid=3f545f3a-8b62-4679-979a-2c0b244a4cd7 (accessed 11 June 2011).

Unfortunately, despite both professional obligation and patients' expectations, the performance of doctors declines over time.

John Norcini

Norcini J. Where next with revalidation? *BMJ.* 2005; 330(7506): 1458–9.

Grading is inevitable in medicine, but just as in boxing or lawn tennis a man's grading is that which he makes for himself, so in medicine a doctor's grading is the position he attains in the eyes of his fellows and his patients. Academic training, degrees, honours, appointments, publications, all these things count, but they count little beside that indefinable quality a man's real worth.

Heneage Ogilvie

Ogilvie H. The granny racket. *BMJ.* 1950; 1(4655): 683–5.

If the licence to practise meant the completion of his education how sad it would be for the doctor, how distressing to his patients!

William Osler

Osler W. An address on the importance of post-graduate study: delivered at the opening of the museums of the Medical Graduates College and Polyclinic, July 4th, 1900. *BMJ.* 1900; 2(2063): 73–5.

But there is another side of the question of books and libraries – man does not live by bread alone, and while getting his medical education and making his calling and election sure by hard work, the young doctor should look about early for an avocation, a pastime, that will take him away from patients, pills and potions.

William Osler

Osler W. Remarks on the medical library in post-graduate work. *BMJ.* 1909; 2(2544): 925–8.

You cannot be a perfect doctor, till you have been a patient.
Stephen Paget
Confessio Medici. ch. 7.

His patients should be his book, they will never mislead him.
Paracelsus
The Book of Tartaric Diseases. ch. 13.

It may be more important to know what kind of person has the disease, than to know what kind of disease he has.
Paracelsus
Tait I. Personal view. BMJ. 1970; 1(5699): 815.

One of the essential qualities of the clinician is an interest in humanity, for the secret of the care of the patient is in caring for the patient.
Francis Peabody
Peabody F. The care of the patient. JAMA. 1927; 88(12): 877–82.

Each learner must be responsible for addressing their own needs in the interests of offering better service to patients, and the emphasis on supporting the recognition of personal learning needs is well placed.
Ed Peile
Peile E. Special needs education for general practitioners. Educ Prim Care. 2010; 21: 283–4.

Evidence that patients are less likely to trust medical practitioners who lack communication skills is mounting. Such skills are also vital in doctor-doctor scenarios and when negotiating a complex career pathway.
Adam Poole
Poole AJ. Communication training: it's all talk. BMJ. 2002 August 15. Available at: www.bmj.com/content/325/7359/297.2/reply#bmj_el_24708?sid=d5e693ea-0765-423d-ac1d-1c98624d8fdf (accessed 1 October 2011).

If the gap between knowledge about how to behave towards patients from diverse backgrounds and the way we actually behave towards them is to be reduced then innovation from the students or the communities themselves is what will take education forwards more than recommendations from the GMC [General Medical Council] or medical educators in medical education units.
Vibhore Prasad
Prasad V. Cultural diversity: whose responsibility? BMJ. 2005 February 21. Available at: www.bmj.com/content/330/7488/403/reply#bmj_el_97322?sid=1e069fc1-8837-4789-925c-3c1714669644 (accessed 1 June 2011).

Now is the time to step into the 21st century with a new medical education system, one that allows for compassionate, appropriate quality care to patients at an affordable cost; one that educates young medical professionals in ways that allow them to develop their professional skills without stripping them of their ideals and humanity; and one that treats patients and physicians as if they are feeling human beings, not just organic objects the system can use in the name of medical education.
Charles Rainey
Rainey CJ. Observations on the human cost of residency training. JAMA. 1997; 277(11): 866.

A medical profession that is being educated by an industry that sells the drugs physicians prescribe and other tools physicians use is abdicating its ethical commitment to serve as the independent fiduciary for its patients.

Arnold Relman

Relman AS. Medical professionalism in a commercialized health care market. *JAMA*. 2007; 298(22): 2668–70.

Talk to any pillar of the medical establishment in Britain and the chances are he will shake his greying head, deplore current standards of medical education, and remind you that in his day students really knew the meaning of hard work and, what is more, were shining examples of Renaissance man; well educated, cultivated, and kind to patients.

Tessa Richards

Richards T. Medical education in India: in poor health. *BMJ*. 1985; 290(6475): 1132–5.

To deliver a patient centered agenda we have to understand both our own and our patient's personalities, and have the skill and confidence to harmonize them.

Geoffrey Robinson

Robinson G. Patient centredness and physician personality. *BMJ*. 2001 March 1. Available at: www.bmj.com/content/322/7284/468/reply#bmj_el_12930?sid=bfae656f-d7d3-4ae5-abb6-1b0e432b89b5 (accessed 22 August 2011).

Service is education and when doctors stop learning from involvement in clinical activity it will prove a retrograde step both for them and particularly the patients under their care.

RH Salter

Salter RH. Stop denigrating service. *BMJ*. 1995; 310(6978): 538.

The skill of learner centred facilitation lies in the ability to know when and how to involve the learner.

Shake Seigel

Seigel S. Patient centred care requires learner centred education. *BMJ*. 2001 March 3. Available at: www.bmj.com/content/322/7284/444/reply#bmj_el_12973?sid=bfae656f-d7d3-4ae5-abb6-1b0e432b89b5 (accessed 12 September 2011).

He will be the physician that should be the patient.

William Shakespeare

Troilus and Cressida.

Marrying an institution's responsibility to the public that its graduates are competent and that the education they receive helps minimize errors in patient care is of the highest importance in medical education today.

James Shumway

Shumway JM. Components of quality: competence, leadership, teamwork, continuing learning and service. *Med Teach*. 2004; 26(5): 397–9.

If doctors lack the capacity to relate well to patients; to gather useful, unambiguous and accurate information; and to impart advice and instructions comprehensibly, memorably and influentially, their ability to reach arcane diagnoses or to propose elegant therapeutic plans will be no more relevant to health care than an appreciation of the tonic variations in Mahler's symphonies or the niceties of macrame.

Michael Simpson

Simpson MA. Teaching communication skills. *Med Teach.* 1984; 6(4): 120–1.

We measure the success of our physician graduates by how effective they are in positively changing the health both of their patients and the community around them.

Lawrence Smith

Mitka M. Report: growth of medical schools brings opportunity to redefine their mission. *JAMA.* 2009; 301(11): 1114–15.

Students need time to reflect on what they are learning, and to make sense of the snapshots of patients' lives that they are privileged to see.

Leslie Southgate

Southgate L. Foreword. In: Hays R. *Teaching and Learning in Clinical Settings.* Oxford: Radcliffe Publishing; 2006. piv.

Clinical teaching – that is, teaching and learning focused on, and usually directly involving, patients and their problems – lies at the heart of medical education.

John Spencer

Spencer J. ABC of learning and teaching in medicine: learning and teaching in the clinical environment. *BMJ.* 2003; 326(7389): 591–4.

Each patient has a fascinating story to tell, collect them in your heart and you will maintain compassion.

Jack Springer

Personal correspondence, 21 June 2011.

Medical arrogance kills patients.

Jack Springer

Personal correspondence, 21 June 2011.

My method [is to] lead my students by hand to the practice of medicine, taking them every day to see patients in the public hospital, that they may hear the patient's symptoms and see their physical findings. Then I question the students as to what they have noted in their patients and about their thoughts and perceptions regarding the causes of the illness and the principles of treatment.

Sylvius

Whitman N. *Creative Medical Teaching.* Salt Lake City: University of Utah School of Medicine; 1990.

The skills needed in the patient-centred approach do not come as an automatic bonus to any qualification, however erudite. They require to be taught. We still know too little about how best to do this. We need to experiment and discover.

Ian Tait

Tait I. Personal view. *BMJ.* 1970; 1(5699): 815.

Real patients teach us a lot if we only have the time to reflect on our interactions. Learning from patients is an important part of work-based learning.

Jill Thistlethwaite

Thistlethwaite J. Learning from patients. *Work Based Learn Prim Care*. 2004; 2(4): 370–2(3).

It is not enough for a student to have the opportunity of following his teacher round the wards of a hospital, a unit in a hundred or a hundred and fifty others, poking his nose over his comrade's shoulder, and standing upon tiptoe to try and get a glance at what is going on at the bedside of the patient, that the desired end is to be attained.

Edward Thompson

Thompson EC. Address on the past, present, and future of medicine. *BMJ*. 1882; 2(1135): 607–12.

There are no free lunches, and if the NHS [National Health Service] pays for general practitioners' continuing education then it has a right to expect evidence that this is likely to improve patient care.

Peter Toon

Toon P. Educating doctors, to improve patient care: a choice between self directed learning and sitting in lectures struggling to stay awake. *BMJ*. 1997; 315(7104): 326.

A doctor who cannot take a good history and a patient who cannot give one are in danger of giving and receiving bad treatment.

Unknown

Better to go without medicine than call in an unskilful physician.

Unknown

Choose your specialist and you choose your disease.

Unknown

Westminster Review. 1906 May 18.

As a patient I would not have confidence in a doctor who had been caught cheating in her final examinations.

Bryan Vernon

Vernon B. Responding to cheating. *BMJ*. 2000 August 15. Available at: www.bmj.com/content/321/7258/398/reply#bmj_el_9244?sid=7f1b5b2e-7b0c-43f6-8a46-f45951808b4f (accessed 12 September 2011).

If by a "practical man" we mean a doctor who is equipped by his training to apply promptly and efficiently such treatment as may be the best for his patient, then, of course, "the practical man" is the best kind of man.

Swale Vincent

Vincent S. Medical research and education. *BMJ*. 1920; 2(3119): 562–5.

Communication has always been a particularly thorny problem for medical education and practice, and genetic counselling offers an even greater challenge.

David Weatherall

Weatherall DJ. The troubled helix: social and psychological implications of the new human genetics. *BMJ*. 1996; 312: 1174.

Educators can begin modelling a patient centred agenda from the very start of medical training, by placing a premium on students' integrity, interpersonal manner, and reflective skills.

Caroline Wellbery

Wellbery C. Personal view: medical education must be more patient centred to be relevant. *BMJ.* 2006; 333(7572): 813.

I now think that the first requirement for teaching patient-centred medicine is for medical teachers to adopt a learner-centred approach towards their students. This does not mean that we should abandon basic clinical method or lower standards but that we should start where students are.

David Whittaker

Whittaker D. Learner-centred teaching in family medicine. *BMJ.* 2006 October 31. Available at: www.bmj.com/content/333/7574/920.5/reply (accessed 12 September 2011).

I want to get a job where I can learn something of general medicine; the neurologists just talk and do nothing.

George Widal

Personal reply to Clovis Vincent.

Poor clinical performance may be the medical issue of greatest concern to the general public and the press, but most doctors realise that clinical performance and welfare of patients often come second to the interests of institutions and loyalty to colleagues.

Peter Wilmshurst

Wilmshurst P. Personal views: devaluing clinical skills. *BMJ.* 2000; 320(7251): 1739.

Themes

18. ARTS AND HUMANITIES

> At the end of their careers, physicians tend to wax poetic about the art of medicine and how it is being lost. (The same art seems to be lost every generation.)
>
> **Ezekiel Emanuel**

Every age hath its book.
Koran 13.

What sculpture is to a block of marble, education is to a human soul.
Joseph Addison
Addison J. *Spectator.* November 1711.

I read Shakespeare and the Bible and I can shoot dice. That's what I call a liberal education.
Tallulah Bankhead
Attributed.

If we dispensed with the year of arts and made our medical curriculum more facile, we might attract more students to our portals, but would we be doing our duty to our profession or to the public?
John Banks
Banks JT. An address on medical reform. *BMJ.* 1883; 1(1155): 294–6.

If at 16 they opt for medicine, by that not ignoble choice they slam the door, at once and for good, on literae humaniores.
Lindsey Batten
Batten LW. Adult medical education: a general practitioner's viewpoint. *BMJ.* 1955; 2(4938): 511–13.

Medicine and medical education must turn away from a traditional tough-minded heroic outlook (gendered male) that upholds autonomy, to embrace a tender-minded, more collaborative and feminine medicine.
Alan Bleakley
Bleakley A. Social comparison, peer learning and democracy in medical education. *Med Teach.* 2010; 32(11): 878–9.

To avoid having the profession of medicine become marginalized, we must continue to seek diversity of education not for the sake of multiculturalism or because of a need for a special division called Medical Humanities, but because we need to restore humanity to our practice.
Michael Bogdasarian
Bogdasarian MA. The medical humanities and medical education. *JAMA.* 2006; 295(9): 997.

Art is meant to disturb, science reassures.
Georges Braque
Le Jour et la nuit: Cahiers 1917–52.

Dr Weiss, at forty, knew that her life had been ruined by literature.
Anita Brookner
A Start in Life. 1981.

In science, read, by preference, the newest works; in literature, the oldest.
Edward Bulwer-Lytton
Caxtoniana: hints on mental culture. 1863.

Some said, John, print it, others said, Not so;
Some said, It might do good, others said, No.
John Bunyan
Apology for his Book.

The languages, especially the dead,
The sciences, and most of all the abstruse,
The arts, at least all such as could be said
To be the most remote from common use,
In all these he was much and deeply read.
Byron
Don Juan.

In the end, any model of "the medical humanities" suffers perhaps most egregiously from an inability to pay for itself within medical centers.
Rafael Campo
Campo R. "The medical humanities," for lack of a better term. *JAMA*. 2005; 294(9): 1009–11.

Perhaps in the effort to devise teaching strategies that address the humanities as they relate to medicine, we will reflect more deeply on our own day-to-day behavior and thus become better models of providing the humanistic care that we aspire to give.
Rafael Campo
Campo R. The medical humanities and medical education: reply. *JAMA*. 2006; 295(9): 997–8.

Medicine is my lawful wife but literature is my mistress. When I am bored with one I spend a night with the other.
Anton Chekhov
Letter to Suvorin, 1888.

The artistic temperament is a disease that afflicts amateurs. It is a disease which arises from men not having sufficient power of expression to utter and get rid of the element of art in their being.
GK Chesterton
Heretics. 1905.

The cultivation of the mind is a kind of food supplied for the soul of man.
Cicero
De Finibus Bonorum et Malorum.

Art for art's sake, with no purpose, for any purpose perverts art. But art achieves a purpose which is not its own.

Benjamin Constant

Diary, 11 February 1804.

To heal and to care has always required more than scientific expertise and technical skill. It requires a rich understanding of human nature, an idealistic engagement with values, and an exposure to the broad panorama of the social sciences and humanities.

Richard Cruess

Cruess RL. Medicine and books: developing professional judgement in health care. *BMJ.* 1998; 316(7135): 947.

Does not contemporary medical education threaten to diminish, even extinguish, the usually significant altruistic aspirations of those involved? And if so, what are we all going to do about that?

Larry Culliford

Culliford L. Time flies. *BMJ.* 1999 August 19. Available at: www.bmj.com/content/319/7207/458.3/reply#bmj_el_4316?sid=3b793041-95a4-4870-a5d9-9fc0c51e668f (accessed 12 September 2011).

It is to be regretted, but I fear it is inevitable, that the study of the old humanities must be curtailed, and must even in some measure disappear from medical education.

James Cuming

Cuming J. Address in medicine. *BMJ.* 1892; 2(1648): 230–6.

Medical education does not need the equivalent of a Billy Graham crusade to exaggerate its sins and offer repentance, salvation, and the cheap disruptive thrills of being born again.

Colin Currie

Currie C. Global village fête. *BMJ.* 1988; 297(6648): 630.

At the end of their careers, physicians tend to wax poetic about the art of medicine and how it is being lost. (The same art seems to be lost every generation.)

Ezekiel Emanuel

Emanuel EJ. Changing premed requirements and the medical curriculum. *JAMA.* 2006; 296(9): 1128–31.

A purely scientific education is inadequate for a profession which deals with so close a relationship between mind and matter, and an education in the arts alone is insufficient for minds compelled to live in a material world.

John Fairlie

Fairlie J. Response. *BMJ.* 2000 January 18. Available at: www.bmj.com/content/319/7219/1216/reply#bmj_el_6262?sid=7f1b5b2e-7b0c-43f6-8a46-f45951808b4f (accessed 2 October 2011).

Medicine is said to be a synthesis of art and science but science generally dominates medical education.

William Foster

Foster W. Should poetry be included in the curriculum for specialty registrars? *Educ Prim Care.* 2007; 18: 712–23.

If anyone wishes to observe the works of nature, he should put his trust not in books of anatomy but in his own eyes.

Galen

Galen on the Usefulness of the Parts of the Body.

Talent develops in quiet places, character in the full current of human life.
Goethe
Torquato Tasso. 1790.

The purpose of art is the lifelong construction of a state of wonder.
Glenn Gould
Gould G. Commencement address, York University, Toronto, 1982.

Historically the training of medical men from the earliest times has had a cultural association, particularly with religion. Thus the witch-doctor (with his psychosomatic associations) and the priests of ancient times (with access to the gods of health) tended to underline the importance of medicine as an art or mystique rather than the application of pure techniques.
Kenneth Hill
Hill KR. Some reflections on medical education and teaching in the developing countries. *BMJ*. 1962; 2(5304): 585–7.

I would argue that our success or failure in teaching empathy and humanism begins with the manner in which teaching itself is done.
Harold Horowitz
Horowitz HW. Hey! I'm a teacher too. *JAMA*. 1998; 280(9): 765.

When I was a boy I wanted to know all about the clouds and the grasses, and why the leaves changed colour in the autumn, I watched the ants, bees, birds, tadpoles, and caddis-worms: I pestered people with questions about what nobody knew or cared anything about.
John Hunter
Sampson Handley W. Makers of John Hunter. *BMJ*. 1939; 1(4076): 313–17.

Blest be the hour wherein I bought this book;
His studies happy that composed the book,
And the man fortunate that sold the book.
Ben Jonson
Every Man Out of His Humour.

Can any medical man pretend to any real celebrity, or to occupy any high position safely, who has not carefully studied the mechanism of the human body, with its multiplied parts and its varied functions?
James Thomas Law
Law JT. Address, delivered at the opening of the present session of Queen's College, Birmingham. *Prov Med Surg J.* 1846; s1–10(41): 485–8.

The book is the greatest interactive medium of all time. You can underline it, write in the margins, fold down a page, skip ahead. And you can take it anywhere.
Michael Lynton
Lynton M. *Daily Telegraph.* August 1996.

The hearts of men are their books; events are their tutors; great actions are their eloquence.
Thomas Macaulay
Essays.

Arts and humanities have a contribution to make both in improving health and in educating doctors.

Jane Macnaughton

Macnaughton J. Arts and humanities in medical education. In: Harrison J, van Zwanenberg T, editors. *GP Tomorrow*. 2nd ed. Oxford: Radcliffe Medical Press; 2002. pp67–77.

Arts may well provide relaxation and replenishment, parallels and lessons about people (sometimes specifically about doctors and patients), but they also afford opportunities for deeper engagement and reflection.

John Middleton

Middleton J. Art for the sake of 'caritas'. *Educ Prim Care*. 2008; 19: 360–3.

Young men ought to come well prepared for the study of Medicine, by having their minds enriched with all the aids they can receive from the languages, the liberal arts.

Montesquieu

A Discourse Upon the Institution of Medical Schools in America.

There is a growing perception of the value of the inclusion of humanities based subjects to enable students of medicine to broaden their understanding of the human condition and thus retain their humanity.

Jane Moore

Moore JR. The humanities in medical education. *BMJ*. 2010 March 31. Available at: www.bmj.com/content/340/bmj. c1590/reply#bmj_el_233764?sid=31b7420e-2cd9-4337-8329-2f40df508216 (accessed 12 September 2011).

I do not for a moment suggest that a doctor is not fit to practise if he is not liberally educated, but only that he will be the better doctor if he is.

Arthur Morgan Jones

Morgan Jones A. Medical progress and medical education. *BMJ*. 1952; 2(4782): 466–9.

While science has undeniably contributed massively to modern medicine, it has mainly nourished the analytical skills of clinicians and not their overtly human face 'at the bedside', while it seems clear that the humanities could contribute most significantly to the latter aspect of medicine.

Peter Morrell

Morrell P. Re: medicine, intelligence, and the humanities. *BMJ*. 2000 June 30. Available at: www.bmj.com/content/320/7247/1483.1/reply#bmj_el_8569?sid=7f1b5b2e-7b0c-43f6-8a46-f45951808b4f (accessed 12 September 2011).

Though reports and commissions over the last 60 years have repeatedly recommended a liberal education for health professionals, it remains regrettably true that training institutions, especially medical schools, have by and large been slow, reluctant, or plainly unwilling to accept proposals to include the study of the humanities in the medical curriculum.

Philip Mosley

Mosley P. Role of the humanities in the education of health professionals. *Med Teach*. 1989; 11(1): 99–101.

There is no doubt that literature broadens ones [*sic*] horizons but when it comes to medical education the fundamentals of safe and knowledgeable practice come first.

Martyn Neil

Neil M. There is no need for a literary component to medical education. *BMJ.* 2005 December 19. Available at: www. bmj.com/content/331/7530/1482/reply#bmj_el_124193?sid=cb764c2a-ad1a-4f84-a8c4-88b3568c267c (accessed 12 September 2011).

It is a defect in our whole education that the artist sense is deliberately repressed; the prizes tend to go to possessors of superior memories rather than to those who can observe and reason best.

John Nixon

Nixon JA. The art and science of medicine in relation to professional training. *BMJ.* 1928; 2(3530): 363–4.

To be instructed in the arts, softens the manners and makes men gentle.

Ovid

Epistolæ Ex Ponto. II. 9. 47.

The art of medicine cannot be inherited, nor can it be copied from books.

Paracelsus

Kline GA. The discovery, elucidation, philosophical testing and formal proof of various exceptions to medical sayings and rules. *CMAJ.* 2004; 171(12): 1491–2.

Learn from the birds what food the thickets yield;
Learn from the beasts the physic of the field;
The arts of building from the bee receive;
Learn of the mole to plough, the worm to weave.

Alexander Pope

Essay on Man.

Good medicine requires humanity, which can be achieved with or without spirituality or a personal belief in a god. Such humanity may be enhanced by our recognition and understanding of diverse belief systems and the importance placed on them and their associated customs and rituals, which impact health and well being.

Vivian Rambihar

Rambihar VS. Chaos: weaving together the threads of art, science, humanity and the humanities. *BMJ.* 2000 June 19. Available at: www.bmj.com/content/320/7247/1483.1/reply#bmj_el_8569?sid=7f1b5b2e-7b0c-43f6-8a46-f45951808b4f (accessed 12 September 2011).

In my own academic career I have heard it argued that there should be included in the curriculum: English literature, logic, moral philosophy, economics, history, mathematics, computer science, and jurisprudence – and, of course, anthropology. Surely an enlightened clinical teacher must be encouraged to draw his understanding and expression from a variety of subjects without feeling that specialists have always to be imported to do a demarcated job.

Ian Richardson

Richardson IM. More anthropology for medical students. *BMJ.* 1981; 282(6260): 314.

The physician ought to know literature, to be able to understand or to explain what he reads.

Saint Isidore of Seville

Etymologiae. IV.

My problem is this: the arts can certainly make us feel happier and give us more resources to draw on when our spirits need to be revived and refreshed. But does an appreciation for poetry or painting make us better doctors?

John Salinsky

Salinsky J. Commentary: art for whose sake? Some thoughts about poetry in the curriculum. *Educ Prim Care.* 2007; 18: 683–4.

Art for art's sake is an empty phrase. Art for the sake of the true, art for the sake of the good and the beautiful, that is the faith I am searching for.

George Sand

Letter to Alexandre Saint-Jean, 1872.

We study the past for its interest and in expectation of enlarging our understanding and increasing our powers of appreciation. Like all worthwhile achievement, appreciation requires practice.

David Smithers

Smithers D. On some medicoliterary alliances. *BMJ (Clin Res Ed).* 1985; 291(6511): 1796–1801.

Comments on the humanities should not be a separate program, or a separate calling, but should be part of the character of all teachers of medical students and thereby of their students.

Howard Spiro

Spiro H. The medical humanities and medical education. *JAMA.* 2006; 295(9): 997.

Gentlemen, in our education, that education which ends only with the grave, let us echo the desire of David that our days may be so numbered that we shall incline our hearts unto Wisdom.

Samuel Squire Sprigge

Squire Sprigge S. An address on prizes and performances: delivered at the opening of the medical session at St. George's Hospital, on October 1st. *BMJ.* 1910; 2(2597): 1024–7.

We know that adults learn best when the subject is seen as real and relevant to their everyday needs and they can then see rapid value for their everyday work.

George Taylor

Taylor G. Why use the arts in medial education? In: Powley E, Higson R. *The Arts in Medical Education: a practical guide.* Oxford: Radcliffe Publishing; 2005. pp1–4.

Science can be learned by anyone, even the mediocre. Art, however, is a gift from heaven.

Armand Trousseau

Attributed.

Everyone must decide how to balance education in science and the humanities, but, whatever the proportion, education must be a discipline as habitual as the 9 o'clock surgery, not something to be fitted in if time permits.

CW Walker

Walker CW. Adult education: for the general practitioner. *BMJ.* 1955; 2(4938): 513–15.

One must have a heart of stone to read the death of Little Nell without laughing.

Oscar Wilde

Leverson A. *Letters to the Sphinx.* 1930.

19. PROFESSIONALISM

> All professions are a conspiracy against the laity.
>
> **George Bernard Shaw**

Physician, heal thyself.

Luke 4.23.

One starting point from which to consider improvements in medical education is the current shortcomings of the profession. High up on any list, I fancy, would be our ignorance of, and often our contempt for, techniques of management, and our lack of understanding of the economic constraints within which we must operate.

Donald Acheson

Acheson D. University, medical school, and community. *BMJ.* 1970; 2(5711): 683–7.

It is of concern that given the high level of investment from the pharmaceutical industry in medical education so little of it has been devoted to training the professional side of the partnership in compliance with industry's own promotional codes of practice.

Peter Aitken

Aitken P. We need to agree on the conflicts and train to manage them. *BMJ.* 2008 March 1. Available at: www.bmj.com/content/336/7642/476/reply#bmj_el_191338?sid=a15ec792-dfe3-4ba7-b8d0-a79c5a5cccab (accessed 12 September 2011).

But, while the field of medical education has been thus extended, and is still extending, the time for acquiring such professional instruction ought to be extended also.

William Aitken

Aitken W. Introductory lecture on the influence of human progress on medical education. *BMJ.* 1872; 1(590): 411–13.

We are all human, and we have been human for much longer than we have been professionals.

Mark Albanese

Albanese M. Three blind mice: might make good reviewers. *Med Educ.* 2006; 40(9): 828–30.

The physician himself, if sick, actually calls in another physician, knowing that he cannot reason correctly if required to judge his own condition while suffering.

Aristotle

De Republica. III. 16.

For some years the serious problem of supplying adequate medical manpower for the needs of the country has exercised professional medical educators, government officials, and many others whose interests are both official and unofficial.

William Bean

Bean WB. Physicians for a growing America: report of the Surgeon General's Consultant Group on Medical Education, Public Health Service Publication No. 709. *Arch Intern Med.* 1961; 108(4): 651–2.

In calmer times, it was assumed that the teacher in a medical school knew how and what to teach, the professor knew how and what to profess, and the physician knew whom to care for and how. Teaching institutes, a term of modern ugliness, tend to have a rancid doctrinaire air of professionalism about them.

William Bean

Bean WB. Report of the Second Institute on Clinical Teaching. *Arch Intern Med.* 1963; 112(2): 286–8.

What, then, seems to me desirable in the actual condition of medicine is to bring the scientific and practical departments of the profession into harmony with one another, and to produce such co-operation among practitioners that their methods of treatment should assume more of a fixed and uniform character.

John Hughes Bennett

Bennett JH. Addresses and papers read at the Thirty-Fourth Annual Meeting of the British Medical Association: the address in medicine. *BMJ.* 1866; 2(294): 179–86.

A doctor needs to be liberally as well as professionally educated.

Douglas Black

Gillon R. The function of criticism. *BMJ (Clin Res Ed).* 1981; 283(6307): 1633–9.

But the profession must not complain, for "Salus populi suprema lex."

James Black

Black J. Dr. Black on medical reform. *Prov Med Surg J.* 1840; s1–1(9): 147–9.

I divided my life into three parts: in the first I learned my profession, in the second I taught it, in the third I enjoy it.

John Bland-Sutton

The Story of a Surgeon.

And it has been sarcastically said, that there is a wide difference between a good physician and a bad one, but a small difference between a good physician and no physician at all; by which it is meant to insinuate, that the mischievous officiousness of art does commonly more than counterbalance any benefit derivable from it.

Gilbert Blane

Elements of Medical Logic. 1819.

Whether we intend it or not, to all intents and purposes we have freed students from responsibility for acquiring knowledge, and this is the origin of the professional incompetence, maladjustment, and irresponsibility which are so often encountered.

V Brzheski

Ryan M. Standards in Soviet medical institutes. *BMJ (Clin Res Ed).* 1985; 290(6467): 530–1.

Professionalism, in part, seems to involve having a balanced understanding of, and respect for, the needs of your patients, your employer, and your profession.

Christopher Bulstrode

Bulstrode C. Educating for professionalism: creating a culture of humanism in medical education. *BMJ.* 2001; 322(7302): 1609.

Most learning groups set out to have wide and inclusive educational objectives, trying to reflect the range of requirements for the professional practice of their members and very often responding to case material brought by members.

Jonathan Burton

Burton J. Learning groups for health professionals: models, benefits and problems. *Work Based Learn Prim Care.* 2003; 1(2): 93–8(6).

The ever-changing nature of knowledge, the changing roles of primary care professionals and the changing expectations of how professionals will perform means that primary care professionals are never fully prepared.

Jonathan Burton

Burton J. Work based learning in action: collaborative learning and personal learning. In: Burton J, Jackson N, editors. *Work Based Learning in Primary Care.* Oxford: Radcliffe Medical Press; 2003. pp25–48.

To be a member of a group whose purpose is to review professional competency is to be exposed to many anxieties, such as showing one's weakness or inadequacy.

Jonathan Burton

Burton J. Learning groups for health professionals: models, benefits and problems. *Work Based Learn Prim Care.* 2003; 1(2): pp93–8(6).

The important psychological trick is not to interpret the criticism of our professions or even our own self-criticism as an assault on our self or professional image. To be self-critical and to acknowledge the validity of the criticisms of others are the first steps towards making changes in the way we do things.

Jonathan Burton

Burton J. The way we live now: some thoughts on history from recent TV programmes, websites, journals and newspapers. *Work Based Learn Prim Care.* 2004; 2(1): 102–5(4).

Work based learning should be subject to the same rigour as other forms of professional development which are all, of course, concerned with improving the care of patients.

Jonathan Burton

Burton J. Understanding and promoting work based learning in primary care. *Work Based Learn Prim Care.* 2004; 2(3): 199–201(3).

I think that we have undervalued the professionalism of doctors.

Kenneth Calman

Smith R. Education and debate health profile: challenging doctors; an interview with England's chief medical officer. *BMJ.* 1994; 308(6938): 1221.

Professionalism is central to sustaining the public's trust in the medical profession; it is the essence of the doctor-patient relationship.

Jordan Cohen

Cohen JJ. Professionalism in medical education, an American perspective: from evidence to accountability. *Med Educ.* 2006; 40(7): 607–17.

While all practitioners are required to keep up to date with the unfolding nature of their area of practice, it is in practice that they apply that knowledge, polish their skills, hone their professional capacities and hence develop expertise.

Mark Cole

Cole M. The practice of developing practice: facilitating the capture and use of informal learning in the workplace. *Work Based Learn Prim Care.* 2004; 2(1): 1–5(5).

All 'fictions' – whether they be our own recollection and retelling of particular events or artistic creations, such as novels – provide the reflective and reflexive practitioner with material through which to develop personally and professionally.

Mark Cole

Cole M. Fictional realities. *Work Based Learn Prim Care.* 2007; 5(2): 80–8(9).

But some time during the nineteenth century – perhaps after surgery turned from amputation to repair – a medical degree descended like a small halo, and ever since the ordinary citizen has secretly resented it or been dazzled by it.

Alistair Cooke

Cooke A. The doctor in society. *BMJ (Clin Res Ed).* 1981; 283(6307): 1652–5.

The real challenges are how to produce expert professionals in a shorter time, with poor infrastructure, in a culture that emphasises competency rather than expertise.

Nicola Cooper

Cooper NA. Training doctors in the new English NHS: political correctness or evidence based education? *BMJ.* 2006; 333(7558): 99.

Professional status is . . . an implied contract to serve society over and beyond all specific duty to client and employer in consideration of the privileges and protection society extends to the profession.

Ralf Dahrendorf

Smith R. Profile of the GMC: the day of judgment comes closer. *BMJ.* 1989; 298(6682): 1241–4.

Although we are still fairly ignorant about the way professional attitudes and skills develop in doctors in the United Kingdom, there is sufficient evidence to suggest caution in equating confidence with competence in the early years of training.

Sue Dowling

Dowling S. Junior doctors' confidence in their skill in minor surgery. *BMJ.* 1991; 302(6784): 1083.

At its best, medical education can make students feel good about themselves and what they are learning, as well as preparing them for good professional practice.

Len Doyal

Doyal L. Closing the gap between professional teaching and practice: a policy can help protect students from being asked to behave unethically. *BMJ.* 2001; 322(7288): 685–6.

Telling stories is more than just entertaining, it is a fundamentally powerful way for professionals from different backgrounds or contexts to share and understand one another's practice, meanings and cultures.

Rachel Ellaway

Ellaway R. eMedical teacher. *Med Teach.* 2008; 30(1): 112–13.

The notion of a professional incorporates a specialized skill, acquired via training, the exercise of judgement, the acceptance of a duty to the occupation and to a client above self-interest, and some level of autonomy.
Peter Ellis
Ellis P. Have changes in the context of doctors' work altered the concept of the professional in medicine? *Med Teach.* 2004; 26(6): 529–33.

Although as a profession we must always seek to reduce errors and improve our performance, I believe that it is time for us to re-examine our own unrealistic omnipotent fantasies. It is also time for society at large to acknowledge that life is finite, and that it is unreasonable always to expect a positive outcome to ill health.
Brian Fine
Fine BP. Unrealistic expectations of doctors and patients. *BMJ.* 2002 April 21. Available at: www.bmj.com/content/324/7341/838/reply#bmj_el_21113?sid=d5e693ea-0765-423d-ac1d-1c98624d8fdf (accessed 12 September 2011).

That salutary and lucrative profession.
Edward Gibbon
The History of the Decline and Fall of the Roman Empire.

The NHS [National Health Service] has neglected for too long the need to invest in the skills and potential of staff that do not have a professional qualification.
Jan Goldsmith
Goldsmith J. Developing strategies to support educational and career pathways for NHS support workers. *Work Based Learn Prim Care.* 2007; 5(1): 12–23(12).

Professional identity is important because it informs practice and influences our behaviour, operating as the intersection where the outside world meets the individual.
Ann Griffin
Griffin A. 'Designer doctors': professional identity and a portfolio career as a general practice educator. *Educ Prim Care.* 2008; 19: 355–9.

If there be one species of cant more detestable than another, it is that which eulogises what is called the practical man as contradistinguished from the scientific.
William Robert Grove
Grove WR. An address on the importance of the study of physical science in medical education. *BMJ.* 1869; 1(439): 485–7.

The old exhortation at medical school to keep the professional self widely separated from the personal self can only be a recipe for missed opportunities galore.
David Haslam
Haslam D. Haslam on education. *Ed Gen Pract.* 2001; 12: 233–4.

He who desires to practice surgery must go to war.
Hippocrates
Corpus Hippocraticum.

The physician is the servant of the art.
Hippocrates
Epidemics. I.

It is so hard to get anything out of the dead hand of medical tradition!

Oliver Wendell Holmes

Currents and counter-currents in medical science, from *Medical Essays.*

A bold quack soon commands a large practice in all their great towns, and such persons frequently reap golden harvests, while the better educated, but more modest medical man, just makes a living.

Edward Humpage

Humpage E. Notes on America: its medical schools and establishments. *Prov Med Surg J.* 1849; s1–13(19): 525–7.

If professionalism is the expression of a contract between society and medicine, who can say if and when the content of this contract should change?

Samia Hurst

Hurst SA. Teaching medical professionalism. *JAMA.* 2009; 302(12): 1344–5.

The medical establishment has become a major threat to health.

Ivan Illich

Illich I. *Medical Nemesis: the expropriation of health.* London: Calder & Boyars; 1974.

Professional independence is a privilege, not a right.

Donald Irvine

Irvine D. The performance of doctors: I. Professionalism and self regulation in a changing world. *BMJ.* 1997; 314(7093): 1540–2.

Although fitness for practice remains of paramount importance for all medical and non-medical healthcare professionals working in primary care, there is now an increasing emphasis on fitness for purpose.

Neil Jackson

Jackson N. Report of the Asia Pacific Regional Conference 2005, held in Kyoto, Japan: 27–31 May 2005. *Work Based Learn Prim Care.* 2006; 4(1): 92–6(5).

A natural, healthy and transparent relationship between the medical community and pharmaceutical and other medicinal industry has long been needed and requested by all involved: professionals, producers, health officials, the press, and society.

Geir Jacobsen

Jacobsen G. Prevention – early detection – treatment? All of the above, please! *Med Teach.* 2004; 26(7): 591–3.

Although professional knowledge and expertise, which can be tested, is an important component of a doctor's work, I believe the highest quality required from a doctor is honesty and integrity.

Michael Jarmulowicz

Jarmulowicz M. Cheating at medical school. *BMJ.* 2000 August 15. Available at: www.bmj.com/content/321/7258/398/reply#bmj_el_9244?sid=7f1b5b2e-7b0c-43f6-8a46-f45951808b4f (accessed 11 June 2011).

Thus men of more enlighten'd genius and more intrepid spirit must compose themselves to the risque of public censure, and the contempt of their jealous contemporaries, in order to lead ignorant and prejudic'd minds into more happy and successful methods.

John Jones

Introductory lecture to his course on surgery.

The difference between school-life and that of a medical school is so great that, on this ground alone, it would, I think, always be well to have an intermediate stage of pupilage, wherein the student could gather some general ideas of life and professional work, become acquainted with medical and scientific terms, study pharmacy, osteology, and perhaps chemistry.

Walter Lattey

Lattey W. Defects in medical education. *BMJ.* 1882; 2(1127): 238.

Early professional learning sticks very tenaciously, and it is hard to unlearn.

John Launer

Launer J. Reflective practice. *Work Based Learn Prim Care.* 2003; 1(1): 56–8(3).

In a professional culture that is dominated by the notion of outcome as opposed to meaning, professionals in primary care who hold on to an allegiance to the pursuit of meaning may feel that they are becoming an eccentric, even subversive minority.

John Launer

Launer J. Reflective practice and clinical supervision: finding meaning in medicine. *Work Based Learn Prim Care.* 2004; 2(1): 72–4(3).

There are many professionals who believe that one-to-one conversations matter enormously in sustaining reflective practice, and in promoting personal growth and professional endurance.

John Launer

Launer J. Reflective practice and clinical supervision: making sense of supervision, mentoring and coaching. *Work Based Learn Prim Care.* 2006; 4(3): 268–70(3).

Medicine is not a lucrative profession. It is a divine one.

John Coakley Lettsom

Letter to a friend, 6 September 1791.

First, then, the public have a right to demand, that those to whom their health and lives may be entrusted should be fully instructed in the science of medicine and surgery, and that they should be protected from the ignorance and imposition of disqualified and unprincipled persons.

James Macartney

Macartney J. On medical reform and the remodelling the profession. *Prov Med Surg J.* 1841; s1-1(17): 282–5.

'I haven't got time to be sick!' he said. 'People need me.' For he was a country doctor, and he did not know what it was to spare himself.

Don Marquis

Country Doctor.

There is a tolerably general agreement about what a university is not. It is not a place of professional education.

John Stuart Mill

Inaugural address as Rector of St. Andrews, 1867.

You will by this time infer that my ideal surgeon is a man who, with all the general and special professional knowledge and skill of the day, illustrates, perhaps even more than the physician, that state of mind which results from contact with at least a little of every important department of culture; and who is possessed of that rarest and most valuable of all human gifts – the power to put one's self in another's place.

Wesley Mills

Mills W. Some considerations bearing on the surgeon, the patient, the student, and the nurse, based largely on the personal experiences of the writer. *BMJ.* 1910; 1(2568): 682–6.

Medical education is as much a process of enculturation as the sum of knowledge and competencies gained.

Alan Neville

Neville AJ. In the age of professionalism, student harassment is alive and well. *Med Educ.* 2008; 42(5): 447–8.

The well-conducted medical society should represent a clearing house, in which every physician of the district would receive his intellectual rating, and in which he could find out his professional assets and liabilities.

William Osler

Osler W. On the educational value of the medical society. In: Osler W. *Aequanimitas, With Other Addresses to Medical students, Nurses and Practitioners of Medicine.* London; 1904.

To save a huge loss of litigation against NHS we must invest in developing appropriate communication skills in health professionals at all levels.

Arun Patel

Patel AN. Increasing litigations in NHS. *BMJ.* 2002 August 9. Available at: www.bmj.com/content/325/7359/297.2/reply#bmj_el_24708?sid=d5e693ea-0765-423d-ac1d-1c98624d8fdf (accessed 11 June 2011).

The best of healers is good cheer.

Pindar

Nemean Ode. VI.

By professional patriotism amongst medical men I mean that sort of regard for the honour of the profession and that sense of responsibility for its efficiency which will enable a member of that profession to rise above the consideration of personal or professional gain.

Henry Pritchett

Introduction to Abraham Flexner's *Medical Education in the United States and Canada.*

Old habits, it seems, die as hard in the medical profession as they do in any other.

William Russell

Russell W. Medical education, manpower, and unemployment. *BMJ (Clin Res Ed).* 1981; 282(6263): 580.

Reflective practice has the potential to be transformative, with the result that there is change in professional practice and society.

John Sandars

Sandars J. Transformative learning: the challenge for reflective practice. *Work Based Learn Prim Care.* 2006; 4(1): 6–10(5).

Empirics and charlatans are the excrescences of the medical profession.

Frederick Saunders

The Mysteries of Medicine, from *Salad for the Social.*

There is no harder worker in all Scotland, and none more poorly requited, than the village doctor, unless perhaps it be his horse.
Walter Scott
The Surgeon's Daughter. ch. 1.

The fault dear Brutus is not in our stars but in ourselves that we are underlings.
William Shakespeare
Julius Caesar. I, ii.

All professions are a conspiracy against the laity.
George Bernard Shaw
Smith R. Profile of the GMC: the day of judgment comes closer. *BMJ.* 1989; 298(6682): 1241–4.

Education cannot transform practice. Practice is the sum of custom, tradition, professional knowledge and professional aspirations.
George Silver
Silver GA. Personal view: the myth of educational dominance. *Med Teach.* 1980; 2(4): 191–6.

Growth as a clinician requires acknowledging your weaknesses, as well as your strengths.
Jack Springer
Personal correspondence, 21 June 2011.

By raising and improving the standard of general and professional education, I doubt not that a more healthy tone and a greater vigour will be infused into the body medical, and morbid growths will become more rare.
Joseph Stephens
Stephens J. Medical education and medical parasites. *BMJ.* 1864; 1(178): 596–7.

There are worse occupations in the world than feeling a woman's pulse.
Laurence Sterne
A Sentimental Journey.

Engaged, as many of us are, in promoting the best and highest objects of medical practice and teaching, we are too apt to allow our ideas to be magnified of what has been accomplished in both of these directions; and to shut our eyes to some of the shortcomings of our professional system – more especially, it may be, in our own case, to those which arise, not so much from any want of exertion or attention on the part of the members of the profession itself, as from the circumstances which are inseparable from the over-rapid changes occurring in a community and district like ours, where the population has of late years increased with transatlantic rapidity.
Allen Thomson
Thomson A. An address on the history, constitution, and objects of the British Medical Association: and on medical organisation in Glasgow. *BMJ.* 1876; 2(811): 69–72.

It is in the nature of every profession to set itself an ideal character and attempt to impose it as best it can on new entrants. It is also in the nature of humanity to fail that ideal most of the time.
Polly Toynbee
Toynbee P. Between aspiration and reality. *BMJ.* 2002; 325(7366): 718.

Few things are harder to put up with than the annoyance of a good example.
Mark Twain
Pudd'nhead Wilson. 1894.

It is my opinion that it is not desirable to emphasize in a student's course the more purely professional part of his life's work.
Swale Vincent
Vincent S. Medical research and education. *BMJ*. 1920; 2(3119): 562–5.

It was his part to learn the powers of medicine and the practice of healing, and careless of fame, to exercise the quiet art.
Virgil
Aeneid.

It is therefore reasonable to think that anyone who has spent a long professional life in medicine must have something to hand on – however small or modest.
Francis Martin Rouse Walshe
Walshe FMR. The changing and the unchanging face of medicine. *Can Med Assoc J*. 1952; 67(5): 395–7.

Now, as a liberal and classical education was in its place a good thing in professional men, so an elevated scientific training is even a better thing.
John Wood
Wood J. Observations on medical education. *BMJ*. 1879; 2(970): 162–6.

20. ETHICS

> Intellectual honesty is hard to teach, and personal integrity can be shown only by example.
> **John Ellis**

With the increasing pressures on doctors following the various recent scandals, in all of which dishonesty plays a part, perhaps personal ethics needs to take a high priority in medical education.
Michael Addison
Addison M. Dishonest student: honest doctor. *BMJ*. 2001 February 2. Available at: www.bmj.com/content/322/7281/0.1/reply#bmj_el_12390?sid=bfae656f-d7d3-4ae5-abb6-1b0e432b89b5 (accessed 11 June 2011).

It is time the medical profession took full responsibility for educating prescribers about prescription drugs, instead of abdicating it to drug companies.
Marcia Angell
Angell M. Relationships with the drug industry: keep at arm's length. *BMJ*. 2009; 338: b222.

The time has come to stop mixing politics with education: let us get on with the task in hand.
Jamie Bahrami
Bahrami J. Summative assessment for general practitioner registrars. *BMJ*. 1995; 311(7019): 1573.

American medical education has become sternly introspective and, for all I know, none too soon.

William Bean

Bean WB. Money and medical schools. *Arch Intern Med.* 1963; 111(6): 841–2.

Of all the lessons which a young man entering upon the profession of medicine needs to learn, this is perhaps the first – that he should resist the fascination of doctrines and hypotheses till he has won the privilege of such studies by honest labour and faithful pursuit of real and useful knowledge.

William Beaumont

Notebooks.

In the spirit of things, the title "student doctor" is both ethically and legally permissible because it does clearly imply that the bearer of the title is not qualified.

Simon Benson

Benson SD. An ethical issue out of nothing. *BMJ.* 2005 September 13. Available at: www.bmj.com/content/331/7515/523.1/reply#bmj_el_116399?sid=cb764c2a-ad1a-4f84-a8c4-88b3568c267c (accessed 11 June 2011).

Good communication can either prevent moral dilemmas from arising or make them easier to resolve, while an ability to analyse ethical issues clearly (and to assess other people's arguments fairly) can greatly assist good communication.

Kenneth Boyd

Boyd KM. Helping future doctors learn how to break bad news. *Med Teach.* 1994; 16(4): 297–301.

Ethics and Science need to shake hands.

Richard Clarke Cabot

Introduction to *The Meaning of Right and Wrong.*

If we are to eliminate the pharmaceutical industry as a payer for medical education, we need to be very sure there are others able and willing to pick up the responsibility.

Rebecca Drayer

Drayer RA. Putting our money where our mouths are. *BMJ.* 2008 April 4. Available at: www.bmj.com/content/336/7647/742.3/reply#bmj_el_193074?sid=cc42d2f3-132f-4665-a8cf-736696b01452 (accessed 11 June 2011).

Intellectual honesty is hard to teach, and personal integrity can be shown only by example.

John Ellis

Ellis J. Nature and purpose of medical education. *BMJ.* 1958; 2(5096): 598.

Medical ethics teaching offers considerable potential for the integration of the biomedical and psychosocial aspects of medicine in a relevant context.

Christine Ewan

Ewan C. Teaching ethics in medical school. *Med Teach.* 1986; 8(2): 103–10.

If we cannot be clever, we can always be kind.

Alfred Fripp

Emergencies in Medical Practice.

Most physicians are like athletes who aspire to victory in the Olympic Games without doing anything to deserve it; for they praise Hippocrates as first in the art of healing but make no attempt to resemble him.

Galen

Medicus Philosophus.

There have been physicians, the disgrace of their profession, who seem to have considered themselves, in studying Medicine, as studying not a liberal science, but a mere art for the acquisition of money and have thence been solicitous to acquire an insight rather into the humours than into the diseases of mankind.

Thomas Gisborne

The Duties of Physicians.

It's time for the profession to take a lead. This means saying no to gifts and hospitality, ensuring that research and clinical collaborations are transparent and unbiased in their design and reporting, refusing to be a guest or ghost author, declining the role of paid opinion leader, paying our way for information and education, and refusing industry support unless it is entirely transparent and in patients' or the public's best interests.

Fiona Godlee

Godlee F. Doctors, patients, and the drug industry. *BMJ*. 2009; 338: b463.

The profession of medicine, Gentlemen, is not only one of the most important, one of the most honorable, and one of the most responsible, but the most difficult which offers itself to your choice.

William Guy

Guy WA. Introductory lecture: delivered at King's College, October 1, 1842. *Prov Med J Retrsp Med Sci*. 1842; s1–5(106): 23–32.

The present system of medical education has many virtues, and many of its evils are inherent in the variable natures of individual students and professors.

Jerome Head

Head JR. John Brown on medical education. *Arch Surg*. 1929; 18(4): 1562–9.

To consider dear to me, as my parents, him who taught me this art; to live in common with him and, if necessary, to share my goods with him; To look upon his children as my own brothers, to teach them this art.

Hippocrates

The Hippocratic Oath.

Communication and social interaction skills as well as bioethical dilemmas urgently need to be emphasized and explicitly worked on and taught in medical schools if quality of care is honestly sought.

Claudia Infante

Infante C. Communication and bioethical dilemmas have to be explicitly taught. *BMJ*. 2003 March 20. Available at: www.bmj.com/content/326/7389/569.2/reply#bmj_el_30593?sid=7f27ee1c-bc1e-486c-bc82-03a5164885cc (accessed 11 June 2011).

I doubt that any one paid by a company will talk against the drug of that particular company or say anything positive about the competitor even if the competitor drug is better.

Abid Jameel

Jameel A. Key opinion leaders or drug pushers? *BMJ.* 2008 September 3. Available at: www.bmj.com/content/336/7658/1405/reply#bmj_el_201434?sid=cc42d2f3-132f-4665-a8cf-736696b01452 (accessed 11 June 2011).

Whenever a man has cast a longing eye on offices, a rottenness begins in his conduct.

Thomas Jefferson

Letter to Coxe, 1799.

Whoever wills the end, wills also (so far as reason decides his conduct) the means in his power which are indispensably necessary thereto.

Immanuel Kant

Fundamental Principles of the Metaphysics of Ethics. 1785.

How many doctors can honestly hold their hand up and say they never cheated, in any form, at medical school?

Joanna Knight

Knight J. Cheating at medical school. *BMJ.* 2000 August 15. Available at: www.bmj.com/content/321/7258/398/reply#bmj_el_9244?sid=7f1b5b2e-7b0c-43f6-8a46-f45951808b4f (accessed 11 June 2011).

Legal reasoning is largely based on statutes and case laws, whilst ethical reasoning is based on philosophical and theological principles. It is essential that students have a basic understanding of both approaches.

Wai-Ching Leung

Leung WC. Ethics is given excess emphasis over law in the proposed curriculum. *BMJ.* 1998 June 1. Available at: www.bmj.com/content/316/7145/1623/reply#bmj_el_210?sid=6a4ef178-62d7-4865-ac37-192d0fd43924 (accessed 11 June 2011).

Most sensible individuals agree that the process of obtaining informed consent or authorization for the use of human tissues for education or research needs to be improved, clarified and properly implemented.

David Levison

Levison DA. Autopsy teaching: a dying art? *Med Teach.* 2004; 26(4): 293–4.

No man can succeed in our profession unless he has acquired an honest self-reliance based on an exact knowledge and a true estimate of his own powers and capabilities, as well as on a consciousness that he is in the path of duty.

Alexander Macalister

Macalister A. An address on fifty years of medical education: delivered at the opening of the winter session at King's College, London. *BMJ.* 1908; 2(2492): 957–60.

Oral examinations also give birth to the system of what is called grinding, which is equally dishonest in all the parties concerned.

James Macartney

Macartney J. On medical reform and the remodelling the profession. *Prov Med Surg J.* 1841; s1–1(17): 282–5.

Medical reform groups and student associations are calling for disentanglement from pharmaceutical companies and independent education and sources of information.

Ray Moynihan

Moynihan R. Who pays for the pizza? Redefining the relationships between doctors and drug companies: 2. Disentanglement. *BMJ*. 2003; 326(7400): 1193–6.

I am not suggesting that cheating should be considered anything but wrong – but perhaps the systems which brought the candidate to do it is what is wrong.

Gary Nicholls

Nicholls GJ. Dismayed by 'research': teach and they may learn something. *BMJ*. 2005 May 19. Available at: www. bmj.com/content/330/7499/1064/reply#bmj_el_107288?sid=1e069fc1-8837-4789-925c-3c1714669644 (accessed 11 June 2011).

At the outset appreciate clearly the aims and objects each one of you should have in view – a knowledge of disease and its cure, and a knowledge of yourselves. The one, a special education, will make you a practitioner of medicine; the other, an inner education, may make you a truly good man, four square and without a flaw.

William Osler

Osler W. An address on the master-word in medicine: delivered to medical students on the occasion of the opening of the new laboratories of the Medical Faculty of the University of Toronto, October 1st, 1903. *BMJ*. 1903; 2(2236): 1196–200.

Clinical practice of medicine involves a complex commodity: humans. The entanglement of the emotion and ethics (characteristics of our humanity) with scientific knowledge makes an incongruous partnership.

Rani Pal

Pal R. Humanity and health for humans. *BMJ*. 2000 June 21. Available at: www.bmj.com/content/320/7247/1483.1/reply#bmj_el_8569?sid=7f1b5b2e-7b0c-43f6-8a46-f45951808b4f (accessed 11 June 2011).

Medicine rests upon four pillars – philosophy, astronomy, alchemy, and ethics. The first pillar is the philosophical knowledge of earth and water; the second, astronomy, supplies its full understanding of that which is of fiery and airy nature; the third is an adequate explanation of the properties of all the four elements – that is to say, of the whole cosmos – and an introduction into the art of their transformations; and finally, the fourth shows the physician those virtues which must stay with him up until his death, and it should support and complete the three other pillars.

Paracelsus

Das Buch Paragranum. 1529–30.

Causing distress in learners is unethical and never permissible.

Zoë-Jane Playdon

Playdon Z. Thinking about teaching? *BMJ*. 1999; 318(7196): S2.

The responsibility for medical education should be entirely in the hands of the medical profession and funding should not compromise, or even call into question, the integrity and independence of what is taught or of the physicians who teach.

Arnold Relman

Relman AS. Industry support of medical education. *JAMA*. 2008; 300(9): 1071–3.

Let us show the world that a difference of opinion upon medical subjects is not incompatible with medical friendships; and in so doing, let us throw the whole odium of the hostility of physicians to each other upon their competition for business and money.

Benjamin Rush

Letter to David Hosack, 15 August 1810.

To be learned effectively, bioethics, decision analysis, demographics, medical sociology, and many other important topics must be attached to a patient-centered problem; separate lectures and seminars are insufficient.

Irwin Schatz

Schatz IJ. Changes in undergraduate medical education: reply. *Arch Intern Med.* 1994; 154(1): 109.

The issue of intimate examinations is the tip of a much larger iceberg related to ethical challenges in medical education.

Peter Singer

Singer PA. Intimate examinations and other ethical challenges in medical education: medical schools should develop effective guidelines and implement them. *BMJ.* 2003; 326(7380): 62–3.

To most doctors the GMC [General Medical Council] is a remote body that spells trouble: it is best ignored.

Richard Smith

Smith R. Profile of the GMC: the day of judgment comes closer. *BMJ.* 1989; 298(6682): 1241–4.

One of the problems of the General Medical Council (GMC) is its size. Another problem is the perception that it has insufficient lay representation and hence is not sufficiently accountable to the public.

Richard Smith

Smith R. The GMC: size and public accountability. *BMJ.* 1993; 306(6889): 1356–7.

Passing a student who is found cheating and failing to offer an adequate explanation for the action damages the culture of medicine.

Richard Smith

Smith R. Cheating at medical school: justice must be done and seen to be done. *BMJ.* 2000; 321(7258): 398.

Physicians do not become morally better persons simply by pursuing a course of study, but the nature of the work requires that they be held to a higher degree of moral accountability.

Daniel Sulmasy

Sulmasy DP. Medical education, virtue, and patient trust. *BMJ.* 2000 August 13. Available at: www.bmj.com/content/321/7258/398/reply#bmj_el_9244?sid=7f1b5b2e-7b0c-43f6-8a46-f45951808b4f (accessed 11 June 2011).

There is no situation, no profession, intrinsically dignified; dignity depends solely upon the individual's own character and conduct.

Thomas Turner

Turner T. Mr. Turner's introductory lecture: to the students at the Royal School of Medicine and Surgery, Pine-Street, Manchester, for the winter session of 1840–41. *Prov Med Surg J.* 1840; 1(3): 33–8.

We must never forget, in connexion with education, the importance of early habits, early impressions, and early associations; for we shall find that the false colourings with which the notions of men are tinged in after life, are in the majority of instances dependent upon early impressions on the mind, and we find generally, that if the mind be directed into right channels of observation in youth, it will pass on to virtue and maturity of judgment in riper years.

Thomas Turner

Turner T. Mr. Turner's introductory lecture: to the students at the Royal School of Medicine and Surgery, Pine-Street, Manchester, for the winter session of 1840–41. *Prov Med Surg J.* 1840; 1(3): 33–8.

Reprimand a resident who errs – fire the one who lies.

Unknown

Funding of medical education programs, sophisticated marketing techniques, and direct-to-consumer advertising are just a few, but important, modalities through which drug companies exert significant influence and pressure on physicians' prescribing habits.

Bernd Wollschlaeger

Wollschlaeger B. Hooked: ethics, the medical profession, and the pharmaceutical industry. *JAMA.* 2008; 300(22): 2675–6.

In short, 'success' (i.e. high grades) in clinical attachments is often best attained by students who apply ethics selectively: pay lip service to the theory of ethics but if put in an ethically dubious position by an arrogant teacher, do not question, do not rock the boat, and 'do as they say to secure that grade-A'.

Alan Woodall

Woodall A. Applications of these principles are difficult in practice. *BMJ.* 2001 March 23. Available at: www.bmj.com/content/322/7288/685/reply#bmj_el_13965?sid=bfae656f-d7d3-4ae5-abb6-1b0e432b89b5 (accessed 11 June 2011).

21. KNOWLEDGE AND WISDOM

> The objection I have to much of my medical education is not that I memorised things, but that I memorised the wrong things.
>
> **David Smyth**

Miss not the discourse of the elders.
Eccles. 8.9.

And further, my son, be admonished: of making many books there is no end; and much study is a weariness of flesh.
Eccles. 12.12.

Days should speak, and multitude of years should teach wisdom.
Job 32.7.

Receive my instruction, and not silver, and knowledge rather than choice gold.
Prov. 8.10.

In the multitude of counsellors there is safety.
Prov. 11.14, 24.6.

There is no short cut, nor 'royal road' to the attainment of medical knowledge.
John Abernethy
Hunterian oration, 1819.

It appears, then, that the function of university education is not instruction in the special lines of a profession or trade, however these ends may incidentally be promoted, but in expanding and enlarging the mind and making it a more and more perfect instrument of knowledge and progress, whatsoever its destination.
Thomas Clifford Allbutt
Allbutt TC. An address on medical education in London: delivered at King's College Hospital on October 3rd, 1905, at the opening of the medical session. *BMJ.* 1905; 2(2337): 913–18.

To me the ideal doctor would be a man endowed with profound knowledge of life and of the soul, intuitively divining any suffering or disorder of whatever kind, and restoring peace by his mere presence.
Henri Amiel
Journal Intime. 1873 August 22.

Medical education has metamorphosed into a superior form of technical training which demands compliant apprenticeship, not intellectual development.
HJN Andreyev
Andreyev HJN. Personal view. *BMJ (Clin Res Ed).* 1988; 296(6632): 1326.

All men by nature desire to know.
Aristotle
Metaphysics.

The roots of education are bitter, but the fruit is sweet.
Aristotle
Laertius D. *Lives of Philosophers.*

The kings of modern thought are dumb.
Matthew Arnold
Stanzas from the Grande Chartreuse.

To speak as the common people do, to think as wise men do.
Roger Ascham
Dedication to all the gentlemen and yeomen of England. *Toxophilus.* 1545.

The errors which arise from the absence of facts are far more numerous and more durable than those which result from unsound reasoning respecting true data.
Charles Babbage
On the Economy of Machinery and Manufactures. 1832.

Man, as the servant and interpreter of nature, does and understands as much as his observations on the order of nature, either with regard to things or the mind, permit him, and neither knows or is capable of more.
Francis Bacon
Organum Novum. bk I.

If a man will begin with certainties, he shall end in doubts; but if he will be content to begin with doubts; he shall end in certainties.

Francis Bacon

The Advancement of Learning. 1605.

Medicine is a science which hath been (as we have said) more professed than labored, and yet more labored than advanced: the labour having been, in my judgement, rather in circle than in progression. For I find much iteration, but small addition.

Francis Bacon

The Advancement of Learning. 1605.

As the general public becomes every day better informed upon scientific questions bearing on medicine, it is of paramount importance that medical men should be at least equally well informed, or, without doubt, we shall not retain the respect of the public.

Lionel Beale

Beale LS. Dr. Beale on medical education. *BMJ*. 1864; 1(174): 484–5.

In science one must search for ideas. If there are no ideas, there is no science. A knowledge of facts is only valuable in so far as facts conceal ideas: facts without ideas are just the sweepings of the brain and the memory.

Vissarion Grigorievich Belinskii

Collected Works. 1948.

The experimenter who does not know what he is looking for will never understand what he finds.

Claude Bernard

Attributed.

True science teaches us to doubt and, in ignorance, to refrain.

Claude Bernard

Introduction to the Study of Experimental Medicine. 1865. pt I, ch. I.

From the time of Hunter to the present day, English surgery has about it something noble. Surgery owes its great revolution in the nineteenth century to its attempt to unite all medical knowledge in itself; the surgeon who succeeds in this . . . may feel that he has attained the highest ideal in medicine.

Theodor Billroth

Billroth T. *General Surgical Pathology and Therapeutics*. Hackley CE, trans. 4th ed. London: H K Lewis; 1871.

It does seem strange, that in the improving condition of society, in the advancement of intellectual knowledge, and in the increasing respect paid to real acquirements in science and art, our profession should be repeatedly subjected to disesteem and depreciation.

James Black

Black J. Dr. Black on medical reform. *Prov Med Surg J*. 1840; s1–1(9): 147–9.

Nobody leaves medical school with sufficient knowledge to be "safe"; the unsafe ones are paradoxically those who believe they have "learnt" the most.

Scott Blackwell

Blackwell S. There is no need for a literary component to medical education. *BMJ.* 2005 December 23. Available at: www.bmj.com/content/331/7530/1482/reply#bmj_el_124558?sid=cb764c2a-ad1a-4f84-a8c4-88b3568c267c (accessed 11 June 2011).

Responsibility is, indeed, a master in the art of teaching, no master so thorough as he; books and theory sink into insignificance beside him; ten years under such a master, and the knowledge of men and manners, of what is called life, with the general reading which every thoughtful man would undertake during that period is, to my mind, an education and cultivation not equal with, but far, very far, superior, to that of the University graduate, who is deficient in such training, but who, perhaps, had even distinguished himself in the acquisition of theoretical knowledge.

Robert Bowles

Bowles RL. The general practitioner of medicine: his position and education. *BMJ.* 1879; 2(970): 166–8.

Progress in science depends on new techniques, new discoveries and new ideas, probably in that order.

Sydney Brenner

Attributed.

When I think of the responsibilities attending the practice of medicine or surgery, and think again of the amount and variety of knowledge required to enable a man to solve the complicated problems presented by disease; when I reflect that after more than thirty years of more or less continuous work I find that I have still much to learn, I am tempted to exclaim "Who is sufficient for these things?"

William Broadbent

Broadbent WH. On the clinical side of medical education. *BMJ.* 1890; 2(1553): 777–81.

Learning will be cast into the mire, and trodden down under the hoofs of a swinish multitude.

Edmund Burke

Reflections on the Revolution in France. 1790. p117.

Knowledge is not happiness, and science
But an exchange of ignorance for that
Which is another kind of ignorance.

Byron

Manfred.

The tree of knowledge is not that of life.

Byron

Manfred.

Any man may make a mistake; none but a fool will stick to it. Second thoughts are best as the proverb says.

Cicero

Philippicæ. XII. 2.

Not only is there an art in knowing a thing, but also a certain art in teaching it.
Cicero
De Legibus. II. 19.

The portfolio helps us to focus – and is consequently a bridge between informal learning derived from practice and the enhancement of practice itself.
Mark Cole
Cole M. The practice of developing practice: facilitating the capture and use of informal learning in the workplace. *Work Based Learn Prim Care.* 2004; 2(1): 1–5(5).

I want to suggest that the tacit act of moving from being informed – able to marshal packets of information – to one of being knowledgeable – possessed of the ability to make sense of how the information links together and might be deployed in practice – gives some insight into the act of learning, particularly when we speak of learning being informal.
Mark Cole
Cole M. The exam first, the lesson afterwards: an exploration and celebration of the nature of informal learning. *Work Based Learn Prim Care.* 2005; 3(4): 325–38(14).

It is almost as difficult to make a man unlearn his errors, as his knowledge. Malinformation is more hopeless than non-information: for error is always more busy than Ignorance. Ignorance is a blank sheet on which we may write; but error is a scribbled one on which we first erase. Ignorance is contented to stand still with her back to the truth; but error is more presumptuous, and proceeds, in the same direction. Ignorance has no light, but error follows a false one. The consequence is, that error, when she retraces her footsteps, has farther to go, before we can arrive at the truth, than ignorance.
Charles Caleb Colton
Lacon. 1820.

To understand a science it is necessary to know its history.
Auguste Comte
Positive Philosophy. 1832–42.

Learning without thinking is useless,
Thinking without learning is dangerous.
Confucius
Analects. bk II, ch. XV.

Learning without thought is labor lost; thought without learning is perilous.
Confucius
Analects. bk II, ch. XV. 15.

There is the love of knowing without the love of learning; the beclouding here leads to dissipation of mind.
Confucius
Analects.

When you know a thing, to hold that you know it; and when you do not know a thing, to allow that you do not know it; this is knowledge.
Confucius
Analects. bk II.

I hear and I forget. I see and I remember. I do and I understand.
Confucius
Richards P. Choosing a medical school. *BMJ (Clin Res Ed).* 1983; 287(6389): 409–11.

Seek to delight, that they may mend mankind,
And, while they captivate, inform the mind.
William Cowper
Hope.

The sounding jargon of the schools.
William Cowper
Truth.

To overload the memory with a mass of facts which never become fairly organised into its structure, and which, never being revived, fade gradually but surely into oblivion is a wasteful and exhausting process.
James Cuming
Cuming J. Address in medicine. *BMJ.* 1892; 2(1648): 230–6.

Three fifths of the practice of medicine depends on common sense, a knowledge of people and of human reactions.
Harvey Cushing
Medicine at the crossroads, from *The Medical Career and Other Papers.*

I would like to see the day when somebody would be appointed surgeon somewhere who had no hands, for the operative part is the least part of the work.
Harvey Cushing
Letter to Dr Henry Christian, 20 November 1911.

Practice should always be based upon a sound knowledge of theory.
Leonardo da Vinci
Dell' Anatomia. vol. II, ch. 29.

It must never be forgotten that we exist not only to pursue knowledge, but to show the application of that knowledge in the world of action.
Bertrand Dawson
Dawson B. An address on the future of the medical profession: being the concluding part of the Cavendish Lecture, delivered before the West London Medico-Chirurgical Society on July 11th. *BMJ.* 1918; 2(3003): 56–60.

It is good to rub and polish our brain against that of others.
Michel de Montaigne
Essays.

Now, what I want is, Facts. Teach these boys and girls nothing but Facts. Facts alone are wanted in life. Plant nothing else. And root out everything else. You can only form the minds of reasoning animals upon Facts: nothing else will ever be of any service to them. This is the principle on which I bring up my own children, and this is the principle on which I bring up these children. Stick to Facts, sir!
Charles Dickens
Hard Times.

To be conscious that you are ignorant is a great step to knowledge.
Benjamin Disraeli
Sybil. bk I, ch. V.

While an unreliable test can never be valid, a reliable one may also be invalid if it fails to measure the intended skills and knowledge.
Hilton Dixon
Dixon H. The multiple-choice paper of the MRCGP examination: a study of candidates' views of its content and effect on learning. *Educ Prim Care*. 2005; 16: 655–62.

When a doctor does go wrong he is the first of criminals. He has nerve and he has knowledge.
Arthur Conan Doyle
The Adventure of the Speckled Band.

A man should keep his little brain attic stocked with all the furniture that he is likely to use, and the rest he can put away in the lumber room of his library, where he can get it if he wants it.
Arthur Conan Doyle
The Adventures of Sherlock Holmes. 1892.

The stress is greatest for the general internist trying to keep up with the enormous expansion of medical knowledge.
George Dunea
Dunea G. Continuing education. *BMJ*. 1978; 2(6138): 679–81.

[M]edical education cannot escape the responsibility of inculcating many facts; students cannot think about nothing in a factless vacuum.
Derrick Dunlop
Dunlop D. Internal medicine. *BMJ*. 1968; 1(5589): 433.

Where is the wisdom we have lost in knowledge?
Where is the knowledge we have lost in information?
TS Eliot
The Rock. 1934.

I hate quotations. Tell me what you know.
Ralph Waldo Emerson
Diary, May 1849.

It is the worst of madness to learn what has to be unlearnt.
Desiderius Gerhard Erasmus
De Ratione Studii.

If youth knew; if age could.
Henri Estienne
Les Premices. 1594.

I think the advantages of a good classical education early, to a man entering our profession, cannot be over-rated.

George Cooper Franklin

Franklin GC. President's address: delivered at the Seventy-Third Annual Meeting of the British Medical Association. *BMJ.* 1905; 2(2326): 221–6.

Action is the proper fruit of knowledge.

Thomas Fuller

Gnomologia. 1732.

The fact is that those who are enslaved to their sects are not merely devoid of all sound knowledge, but they will not even stop to learn!

Galen

On the Natural Faculties. bk 1, sect. 13; cited from Arthur John Brock (trans.). *On the Natural Faculties.* London: Heinemann, 1963.

Another point is to be borne in mind – namely, that the teaching should aim at producing a good type of general practitioner; competent to deal with the ordinary ailments, and possessing in respect of certain special diseases that modicum of knowledge necessary for their diagnosis and required for a first treatment before passing the case on to a specialist.

Piero Giacosa

Giacosa P. The international problem of medical education. *BMJ.* 1920; 2(3126): 824–6.

I feel as stupid, from all you've said
As if a mill-wheel whirled in my head.

Goethe

Faust. I. Schulerszene.

I've studied now Philosophy
And Jurisprudence, Medicine
And even, alas, Theology
From end to end with labor keen;
And here, poor fool; with all my lore
I stand no wiser than before.

Goethe

Faust. I. Night.

And still they gazed, and still the wonder grew,
That one small head could carry all it knew.

Oliver Goldsmith

The Deserted Village.

The relatively short half-life of medical knowledge has led to recognition of the importance of instilling the value and the skills of life-long learning as a core piece of medical education.

Robert Golub

Golub RM. Medical education theme issue 2008: call for papers. *JAMA.* 2007; 298(22): 2677.

Self-reflection is the school of wisdom.
Baltasar Gracian
The Art of Worldly Wisdom.

I wish, also, that it were possible for the universities and schools to make more complete and satisfactory arrangements for post-graduate instruction, so that old students might return to the alma mater, and pick up in the course of a few weeks instruction as to new methods and new facts whereby they might keep themselves more abreast of modern progress.
Thomas Grainger Stewart
Grainger Stewart T. President's address: delivered at the Sixty-Sixth Annual Meeting of the British Medical Association. *BMJ.* 1898; 2(1961): 281–6.

The newly qualified man will have received much too little of that technical training essential to the doctor licensed to practise; all doctors entering upon practice will still have to teach themselves, after qualifying, many if not most of the methods used in the detection of disease and in its cure; the doctors will, as of old, continue to compete with one another for honorary posts in order that they may obtain opportunities for the acquisition of knowledge and skill and for the advantage the appropriate and accompanying advertisement gives; and the public will gain no adequate or efficient medical service.
Joseph Griffiths
Griffiths J. A solution of the hospital problem. *BMJ.* 1920; 2(3123): 720–1.

Unfortunately certifying exams, in the quasi totality of cases, verify mainly the power to memorise factual knowledge.
Jean-Jacques Guilbert
Guilbert JJ. The medical teacher's job: "Working together to zero in on patient safety, and zero out preventable errors" (Clinton 1999). *Med Teach.* 2004; 26(4): 299–300.

It would appear to be one of the faults of the medical education of to-day, which this movement may in some degree correct, to lay undue weight upon ultimate facts, whilst we neglect those which are near; to indoctrinate the student with the belief, for instance, that if he can run off upon his fingers the supposed ultimate constitution of the gastric juice (about which we are still very ignorant), that he has learned something respecting the digestive process; or that, by reciting the atomic composition of an organic substance, as muscle, he has learned, something about it, though, in fact, nothing but what appertains equally to mere dead substance.
William Gull
Gull WW. An address on the collective investigation of disease. *BMJ.* 1883; 1(1152): 141–4.

It is my earnest wish that the knowledge you acquire should not merely be book-work, but that, in every respect, the instruction you receive should be made as practical as possible.
David Hamilton
Hamilton DJ. An address on the study of pathology. *BMJ.* 1882; 2(1142): 977–80.

One of the chief faults with our present medical education is that teaching is far too much concentrated on the human being as a biological organism.
Ole Harlem
Harlem OK. Personal view. *BMJ.* 1968; 1(5589): 441.

I think there can be no doubt that every student, before he enter at a medical school, should have some knowledge of chemistry, physics, botany, and zoology; but, at the present time, few of the examining bodies care what his knowledge is at the commencement of his career, so long as he comes up to their standard when presenting himself before them for examination; this strongly tends to produce, if it does not necessitate, a system of cramming.
William Haslam
Haslam WF. The conjoint scheme. *BMJ.* 1885; 2(1297): 895.

Every student who enters upon a scientific pursuit, especially if at a somewhat advanced period of life, will find not only that he has much to learn, but much also to unlearn.
John Frederick William Herschel
Outlines of Astronomy. 1871.

A great part, I believe, of the Art is to be able to observe.
Hippocrates
Corpus Hippocraticum.

A physician who is a lover of wisdom is the equal to a god.
Hippocrates
Decorum. V.

Science is the father of knowledge, but opinion breeds ignorance.
Hippocrates
The Canon Law. VI.

It is the province of knowledge to speak and it is the privilege of wisdom to listen.
Oliver Wendell Holmes
The Poet at the Breakfast-Table. 1872.

I prefer to be called a fool for asking the question, rather than to remain in ignorance.
John Homans
Boston Med Surg J. 1872; 87: 1.

Dare to be wise.
Horace
Epistles. I. 2. 40.

In labouring to be concise, I become obscure.
Horace
Ars Poetica.

One cannot know everything.
Horace
Carmina. IV. 4. 22.

The challenge for medical education is how to capture and deliver the knowledge needed to do the job, rather than just to regurgitate textbooks.
Tom Hughes
Hughes T. Big surprise? *BMJ.* 2003 May 9. Available at: www.bmj.com/content/326/7397/1011/reply#bmj_el_32264?sid=7f27ee1c-bc1e-486c-bc82-03a5164885cc (accessed 11 June 2011).

An invasion of armies can be resisted; an invasion of ideas cannot be resisted.
Victor Hugo
Histoire d'un Crime.

But to produce its best results, knowledge should minister, and be subordinated, to thought.
George Murray Humphry
Humphry G. An address delivered at the opening of the section of physiology. *BMJ.* 1873; 2(658): 160–3.

Too much attention cannot be paid to facts; yet too many facts crowd the mind without advantage, any further than they lead us to establish principles.
John Hunter
Humphry GM. The Hunterian oration. *BMJ.* 1879; 1(947): 259–64.

To acquire knowledge and to communicate it to others has been the pleasure, the business and the ambition of my life.
William Hunter
Sampson Handley W. Makers of John Hunter. *BMJ.* 1939; 1(4076): 313–17.

Those of us who have the duty of training the rising generation of doctors . . . must not inseminate the virgin minds of the young with the tares of our own fads. It is for this reason that it is easily possible for teaching to be too "up to date". It is always well, before handing the cup of knowledge to the young, to wait until the froth has settled.
Robert Hutchison
Hutchison R. An address on fashions and fads in medicine. *BMJ.* 1925; 1(3361): 995–8.

If a little knowledge is dangerous, where is the man who has so much as to be out of danger?
Thomas Huxley
Huxley TH. *On Elementary Instruction in Physiology.*

The great end of life is not knowledge but action.
Thomas Huxley
Technical Education. 1877.

The aim of education is the knowledge not of facts but of values.
William Ralph Inge
Inge WR. The training of the reason. In: Benson AC, editor. *Cambridge Essays on Education.* 1917.

In the case of nutrition and health, just as in the case of education, the gentleman in Whitehall really does know better what is good for people than the people know themselves.
Douglas Jay
The Socialist Case. 1939.

The only sure foundations of medicine are, an intimate knowledge of the human body, and observation on the effects of medicinal subjects on that.
Thomas Jefferson
Letter to Dr Caspar Wistar, 21 June 1807.

It is clinical teaching that brings most closely home to a physician the importance of every advance in our practical knowledge.
William Jenner
Jenner W. Address in medicine. *BMJ.* 1869; 2(448): 114–19.

Who but is conscious of the feeling that, once within these portals, one must acknowledge that the entire universe has contracted itself to the area within these walls, and that one is expected to make the mental surrender to this cosmos before partaking of such gifts as this foundation may confer?
Donald Mcl. Johnson
Johnson DM. A G.P. on his clinical training. *BMJ.* 1950; 2(4677): 493–6.

It is wonderful, when a calculation is made, how little the mind is actually employed in the discharge of any profession.
Samuel Johnson
Boswell J. *Life of Samuel Johnson.* 1791.

All wish to be learned, but no one is willing to pay the price.
Juvenal
Satires. VII. 157.

As a fact both the liberal and utilitarian school aims at the same ideal – practical efficiency – but, whilst the results of the former are more permanent and remote, the outcrop of character, the latter are more immediate, and appeal to the philistine mind.
Arthur King
King A. Universities and medical education. *BMJ.* 1912; 2(2702): 998.

It is not enough to discover and prove a useful truth previously unknown, but that it is necessary also to be able to propagate it and get it recognized.
Jean Baptiste Pierre Antoine de Monet Lamarck
Philosophie Zoologique. 1809.

The Profession of Medicine, in itself and in the things pertaining to it, is running over with knowledge.
Peter Mere Latham
Latham PM. A word or two on medical education: and a hint or two for those who think it needs reforming. *BMJ.* 1864; 1(162): 141–3.

One can seek and gain new knowledge from other people in the space of a few seconds that are snatched between, or even during, consultations.
John Launer
Launer J. Reflective practice. *Work Based Learn Prim Care.* 2003; 1(1): 56–8(3).

The tradition of university lecturing was established at a time when books were scarce and expensive. They are now cheap and numerous; and they contain all the facts that are needed.
Joseph Lauwerys
Lauwerys JA. Methods of education. *BMJ.* 1950; 2(4677): 471–4.

In cases of fracture or dislocation, can the life of a man be safely entrusted to one who has not a knowledge of our exquisite framework?

James Thomas Law

Law JT. Address, delivered at the opening of the present session of Queen's College, Birmingham. *Prov Med Surg J.* 1846; s1–10(41): 485–8.

It is one of the principles of university training that the practical use of what is being learnt is of very secondary importance, and that the chief object in view is to train the mind, leaving the practical knowledge to be obtained elsewhere than at the university.

Robert Lee

Lee R. Medical education. *BMJ.* 1902; 2(2168): 223.

Necropsies have long been recognized as indispensable to medical education and the progress of medical science, yet owing to old prejudices this most reliable source of knowledge has so far been very inadequately tapped.

FE Loewy

Loewy FE. Post-mortem examination. *BMJ.* 1935; 1(3871): 563–4.

What they don't teach you in medical school is at least twice as important for you to learn as all the important things you learn while studying medicine.

Darrell Looney

Personal correspondence, 21 June 2011.

The average lifespan of a physiological truth is three or four years.

Hermann Rudolph Lotze

Attributed.

Diffused knowledge immortalizes itself.

James Mackintosh

Vindiciæ Gallicæ.

The works of Celsus appeared before those of Hippocrates and Galen, and they gave a great impulse to medical education.

George Macleod

Macleod GHB. The four apostles of surgery: an historical sketch. *BMJ.* 1877; 2(873): 403–5.

We live and we learn, but sadly at different rates.

Alan Magid

Personal correspondence, 1 September 2011.

Surgical knowledge depends on long practice, not from speculations.

Marcello Malpighi

Letter to Borghese, 1689.

There is not one of us that does not mourn over innumerable lost opportunities of adding to the common stock of knowledge; opportunities lost, not even recognised, because of the inadequacy and unsuitableness of our initial medical education.

Patrick Manson

Manson P. An address delivered at the opening of the section of tropical diseases: at the Annual Meeting of the British Medical Association at Edinburgh, July, 1898. *BMJ.* 1898; 2(1962): 352–3.

Do we really want future generations of doctors to be mere automatons trained to memorise selected facts just long enough to allow their regurgitation for examination purposes; or should we be nurturing receptive and intelligent individuals who know when and where to look things up?

Andrew Mason

Mason A. Get off your high horse. *BMJ.* 2000 August 19. Available at: www.bmj.com/content/321/7258/398/reply#bmj_el_9244?sid=7f1b5b2e-7b0c-43f6-8a46-f45951808b4f (accessed 11 June 2011).

Once you start studying medicine you never get through with it.

Charles Mayo

Buzzi A. *Dictionary of Medical Quotations with Biographies of Authors.* Duncoe: Sapiens Publishing; 2007. p62.

They should have contented themselves with the perpetual discrepancies in the opinions of the principal master and ancient authors of this science which are known only to those who are well read without showing the common people as well the controversies and inconsistent judgements.

Molière

L'Amour Medicin.

What pleases me most, and in this he is following my example, is that he holds blindly to the ancients, and has never wished to understand or listen to the so-called discoveries of the century on the circulation of the blood and other questions of the same kind.

Molière

Le Malade Imaginaire.

A knowledgeable fool is a greater fool than an ignorant fool.

Molière

Les Femmes savants. 1672.

Grant me an opportunity to improve and extend my training, since there is no limit to knowledge.

Moses ben Maimon (Maimonides)

Mishneh Torah IV.19.

Help me to correct and supplement my educational defects as the scope of science and its horizon widen day by day.

Moses ben Maimon (Maimonides)

Mishneh Torah IV.19.

If we contrast the present state of medicine as a science, with its practical results – the knowledge and acquirements of practitioners – the safety and curative advantages on the score of health, relieved suffering and prolongation of life, now enjoyed by the public, with the general state of the profession previously; the beneficial changes and improvement which have ensued, must be manifest to all, who are old enough to remember the former state of the profession, and capable of appreciating the change.

Albert Napper

Napper A. Sir James Graham's medical bill. *Prov Med Surg J.* 1844; s1–8(23): 355–7.

Knowledge is capable of being its own end.
John Henry Newman
Newman JH. *The Idea of a University*. Ward W, editor. London: Dent; 1915.

The cognitive perspective of learning proposes that learning amounts to interpreting new knowledge in light of what we already know.
Geoff Norman
Norman G. Teaching basic science to optimize transfer. *Med Teach*. 2009; 31(9): 807–11.

It is much simpler to buy books than to read them, and easier to read them than to absorb their contents.
William Osler
Osler W. Remarks on the medical library in post-graduate work. *BMJ*. 1909; 2(2544): 925–8.

A very wise old man said that, it would be well if the youngest amongst us would remember that he is not infallible.
James Paget
Paget J. An address on the collective investigation of disease. *BMJ*. 1883; 1(1152): 144–5.

These great institutions tend to place the disease in far greater prominence than the man who suffers from it; and the error of our times in medical education seems to me to have been just this: cramming the student with abstract knowledge, and leaving him to pick up practical information as he best can.
Joshua Parsons
Parsons J. Medical education. *BMJ*. 1864; 1(168): 326–7.

I still think that the only time one really learns about the science of subjects like physiology and biochemistry is at conventional medical school, and those who argue that a doctor is not primarily a scientist forget how much his practice, especially in these days of specialization, depends on a detailed knowledge of, for example, genetics, biochemistry, and physics.
Alex Paton
Paton A. The physiology of disease. *BMJ*. 1975; 3(5986): 773.

School yourself to demureness and patience. Learn to innure yourself to drudgery in science. Learn, compare, collect the facts.
Ivan Pavlov
Bequest to the academic youth of Soviet Russia, 27 February 1926.

The English approach to ideas is not to kill them, but to let them die of neglect.
Jeremy Paxman
The English: a portrait of a people. 1998.

We must teach the student how to collect the facts, to verify them, to assign a value to them, and how to draw conclusions from them and test those conclusions; in short, how to form a judgment.
George Pickering
Pickering G. Medicine's challenge to the educator. *BMJ*. 1958; 2(5105): 1117–21.

The cure of many diseases is unknown to the physicians of Hellas, because they are ignorant of the whole, which ought to be studied also; for the part can never be well unless the whole is well.

Plato

Charmides.

A little learning is a dangerous thing;
Drink deep, or taste not the Pierian spring;
Their shallow draughts intoxicate the brain,
And drinking largely sobers us again.

Alexander Pope

Essays on Criticism. I. 215.

The proper study of Mankind is Man.

Alexander Pope

An Essay on Man: Epistle II.

'Tis education forms the common mind,
Just as the twig is bent, the tree's inclined.

Alexander Pope

Moral Essays. I, pt II.

Nothing in this world could possibly make sense except in light of one's prior knowledge.

Elapulli Sankaranarayanan Prakash

Personal correspondence, 1 September 2011.

Knowledge without conscience is but the ruine of the soul.

François Rabelais

Gargantua and Pantagruel.

What harm in learning and getting knowledge even from a sot, a pot, a fool, a mitten, or a slipper.

François Rabelais

Gargantua and Pantagruel. III. 16.

Is the purpose of medical training to help doctors acquire as much factual knowledge in a short space of time. Or is an apprenticeship, with students experiencing medical methodology? If the former is the case then surely students would be keen to take short cuts, i.e. cheat.

Asrar Rashid

Rashid A. Medical education-should knowledge be instinctive? *BMJ.* 2000 August 28. Available at: www.bmj.com/content/321/7258/398/reply#bmj_el_9244?sid=7f1b5b2e-7b0c-43f6-8a46-f45951808b4f (accessed 11 June 2011).

Academic departments exist not only to plan and coordinate teaching but also to question and to innovate, to disturb, and to extend knowledge and practice.

Peter Richards

Richards P. University cuts, medicine, and the public interest. *BMJ (Clin Res Ed).* 1984; 288(6416): 507–9.

A scholar knows no ennui.

Jean Paul Richter

Hesperus.

One tries not have one's pockets picked by whoever claims the privilege of specialist knowledge.

Anthony Roberts

Roberts AP. Conjuring tricks. *BMJ*. 2006 December 9. Available at: www.bmj.com/content/333/7580/1226/reply#bmj_el_151876?sid=20523c27-2e0d-443d-a7db-86e43c2767d3 (accessed 15 August 2011).

Science is for those who learn; poetry, for those who know.

Joseph Roux

Meditations of a Parish Priest. 1886.

It is not enough that the student of medicine should be crammed with so many facts about the bodily machinery – it is of infinitely greater importance that he should be really educated in a knowledge thereof.

William Rutherford

Rutherford W. Address in physiology. *BMJ*. 1875; 2(763): 198–200.

All natural science springs from the observation of Nature.

William Rutherford

Rutherford W. An address on the value of practical studies. *BMJ*. 1888; 1(1428): 1002–4.

Communities of practice are recognised as highly valuable resources for creating and sharing tacit knowledge but they require appropriate organisational conditions to enable them to flourish.

John Sandars

Sandars J. Knowledge management: sharing knowledge. *Work Based Learn Prim Care*. 2004; 2(2): 111–17(7).

Social networks offer a useful perspective for understanding and developing work based learning in primary care. They are an integral part of knowledge creation and sharing, a fundamental process for all learning.

John Sandars

Sandars J. Work based learning: a social network perspective. *Work Based Learn Prim Care*. 2005; 3(1): 4–12(9).

The professor must not only teach but must be capable of inspiring a love of learning, to do which he must be himself a student, working at the head of his class, leading the way to new ideas, fresh facts, and broader inductions.

Robert Saundby

Saundby R. An address on modern universities: delivered at the opening of the medical school of University College, Cardiff. *BMJ*. 1898; 2(1971): 1034–8.

Few men make themselves Masters of the things they write or speak.

John Selden

Learning, from *Table Talk*.

Wisdom does not show itself so much in precept as in life – in a firmness of mind and mastery of appetite. It teaches us to do, as well as to talk; and to make our actions and words all of a colour.
Seneca
Epistles. XX.

Learning is but an adjunct to ourself
And where we are our learning likewise is.
William Shakespeare
Love's Labour's Lost. IV. iii.

O this learning, what a thing it is!
William Shakespeare
The Taming of the Shrew. I. ii.

The devil can cite Scripture for his purpose.
William Shakespeare
The Merchant of Venice. I. iii.

Medicine is fast becoming a social science, where scientific knowledge is being trumped by the ability to hug trees and talk to tables.
Niroshan Sivathasan
Sivathasan N. Not joined-up thinking. *BMJ.* 2010 August 28. Available at: www.bmj.com/content/337/bmj.a1279/reply#bmj_el_201654?sid=cc42d2f3-132f-4665-a8cf-736696b01452 (accessed 15 August 2011).

Education is what survives when what has been learned has been forgotten.
Burrhus Frederic Skinner
New Scientist. 1964 May 21.

Oh, don't tell me of facts, I never believe facts; you know, Canning said nothing was so fallacious as facts, except figures.
Sydney Smith
Lady Rolland. *A Memoir of The Reverend Sydney Smith.* 1854.

Facts are stubborn things.
Tobias Smollett
Gil. Glas. x.i.

The objection I have to much of my medical education is not that I memorised things, but that I memorised the wrong things.
David Smyth
Smyth DH. Personal view. *BMJ.* 1978; 2(6144): 1082.

I know nothing except the fact of my ignorance.
Socrates
Laertius D. *Lives of the Philosophers.*

A short saying oft contains much wisdom.
Sophocles
Aletes.

When medical education was less general, the weight of a great name might have influenced the estimation of any new doctrine by the profession, but the mind of every practitioner is now so well stored with information, that the opinions of no man, however distinguished, are likely to be received with any favour, unless founded on a proper investigation of the facts which the subject embraces.

George Southam

Southam G. Ovariotomy: removal of an encysted tumour of the left uterine appendages. *Prov Med Surg J.* 1845; s1–9(37): 561–5.

Science is organized knowledge.

Herbert Spencer

Education: intellectual, moral and physical. 1861.

The doorstep to the temple of wisdom is a knowledge of our own ignorance.

Charles Spurgeon

Gleanings among the Sheaves.

The chapter of knowledge is very short, but the chapter of accidents a very long one.

Philip Dormer Stanhope

Letter to Solomon Dayrolles, February 1753.

Medical education may, after all, be designed to produce physicians who not only have the technical knowledge and skills of their craft, who not only see health and disease as a by-product of personal and social life, but who are at once humane and imaginative educators as well.

Guy Steuart

Steuart GW. The physician and health education. *BMJ.* 1958; 2(5096): 590–2.

Read Don Quixote; it is a very good book; I still read it frequently.

Thomas Sydenham

Blackmore RA. *A Treatise on Syphilis.* 1723. pxi.

Learn to live, and live to learn,
Ignorance like a fire doth burn,
Little tasks make large return.

Bayard Taylor

To My Daughter.

Knowledge comes, but wisdom lingers.

Alfred Tennyson

Locksley Hall.

Wearing all that weight
Of learning lightly like a flower.

Alfred Tennyson

In Memoriam A.H.H.

Discussions on grave human problems cannot be effective on the basis of armchair philosophy. Only the actual situation, in all its complexity, can serve as a basis for action.
Bernard Towers
Towers B. Personal view. *BMJ.* 1972; 4(5840): 606.

It is no matter of wonder that in the past the physician has made good by fiction what he lacked in fact.
Frederick Treves
Treves F. Address in surgery. *BMJ.* 1900; 2(2066): 284–9.

A knowledge of the specific element in disease is the key of medicine.
Armand Trousseau
Introduction to *Clinical Medicine.* vol. 1.

Take care not to fancy that you are physicians as soon as you have mastered scientific facts; they only afford to your understandings an opportunity of bringing forth fruit, and of elevating you to the highest position of a man of art.
Armand Trousseau
Introduction to *Clinical Medicine.* vol. 1.

A physicist learns more and more about less and less, until he knows everything about nothing; whereas a philosopher learns less and less about more and more, until he knows nothing about everything.
Unknown

After this, therefore because of this.
Unknown

Every great scientific truth goes through three states: first, people say it conflicts with the Bible; next, they say it has been discovered before; lastly, they say they always believed it.
Unknown

Experiment adds to knowledge,
Credulity leads to error.
Unknown

Fiction tends to become 'fact' simply by serial passage via the printed page.
Unknown

For most diagnoses all that is needed is an ounce of knowledge, an ounce of intelligence, and a pound of thoroughness.
Unknown

Garbage in, garbage out.
Unknown

Here are the opinions on which my facts are based.
Unknown

It is a mathematical fact that fifty percent of all doctors graduate in the bottom half of their class.
Unknown

Man occasionally stumbles on the truth, but then just picks himself up and hurries on regardless.
Unknown

The ABC's of any morbidity and mortality conference are: Accuse, Blame, Criticize, Defend (yourself), Evade (truth).
Unknown

From one learn all.
Virgil
Aeneid.

Learn, O youth, virtue from me and true labor; fortune from others.
Virgil
Aeneid.

Nature has always had more power than education.
Voltaire
Vie de Molière.

Education is an admirable thing, but it is well to remember from time to time that nothing that is worth knowing can be taught.
Oscar Wilde
Intentions. 1891.

22. COMPETENCE

Competence is a habit.
David Leach

Many of us "soloed" in medicine on Tiger Moths yet find ourselves struggling with the therapeutic equivalent of the Boeing 707, with the prospect of a clinical Concorde to come. Don't we owe it to our passengers to institute periodic examinations of competence?
AL Bussey
Bussey AL. Personal view. *BMJ*. 1968; 4(5625): 250.

Communication skills are a basic part of medicine. As a profession we need to ensure that all doctors are competent at communication.
Peter Davies
Davies P. Ignorance is indefensible. *BMJ*. 2000 November 27. Available at: www.bmj.com/content/321/7270/1233.1/reply#bmj_el_10808?sid=7f1b5b2e-7b0c-43f6-8a46-f45951808b4f (accessed 15 August 2011).

We tend to forget that establishing and maintaining a high quality of relationship between doctor and patient is part of the clinical competence of the doctor and can play an important role in the outcome of treatment.

Charles de Monchy

de Monchy C. More attention should be paid to the formation of attitudes in doctors. *Med Teach.* 1990; 12(3–4): 339–44.

Because high-quality health care depends on both effective clinical decision making and reliable implementation of clinical decisions, efforts to train and ensure the competence of the physician workforce must ensure adequate mastery of both domains of knowledge.

Marvin Dewar

Dewar MA. Assessing competencies of knowledge and process improvement. *JAMA.* 2008; 299(19): 2276.

There is a fine line between the competency framework that emancipates learners and that which prevents their 'expansive learning'.

Tim Dornan

Dornan T. On complexity and craftsmanship. *Med Educ.* 2010; 44(1): 2–3.

The belief that clinical competence in medicine is a rational competence that focuses mainly on the acquisition of medical discipline-based knowledge and technical skills, and the application of evidence-based medicine has turned out to be too narrow minded.

Rijk Gans

Gans ROB. Mentoring with a formative portfolio: a case for reflection as a separate competency role. *Med Teach.* 2009; 31(10): 883–4.

There is widespread agreement that medical graduates need to have intercultural competence (IC); that is, the ability to operate effectively in diverse (and sometimes unfamiliar) cultural contexts, interacting appropriately, comfortably, and in ways compatible with others' expectations, values and communication styles.

John Hamilton

Hamilton J. Intercultural competence in medical education: essential to acquire, difficult to assess. *Med Teach.* 2009; 31(9): 862–5.

An overemphasis on competence-as-knowledge may lead to 'hidden incompetence' such as poor integration of knowledge with performance, a lack of appropriate interpersonal behaviours and poor technical abilities.

Brian Hodges

Hodges B. Medical education and the maintenance of incompetence. *Med Teach.* 2006; 28(8): 690–6.

Common sense is in medicine the master workman.

Peter Mere Latham

General Remarks on the Practice of Medicine. ch. 5.

Competence is a habit.

David Leach

Leach D. Competence is a habit. *JAMA.* 2002; 287(2): 243–4.

Physicians need to have the integrity, motivation, and capacity to discern good learning and good health care but should be restless until they get it right.

David Leach

Leach DC. Competence is a habit. *JAMA*. 2002; 287(2): 243–4.

Over the years society has seen the advantage of maintaining the independence of the medical profession, while at the same time developing a structure by which it could be assured of a standard of competence.

Walpole Lewin

Lewin W. Medicine in society. *BMJ*. 1975; 3(5982): 523–6.

Protocol-driven practitioners may be competent at their craft, but their work is formulaic, predictable and unoriginal.

Stephen Lurie

Lurie S. Towards greater clarity in the role of ambiguity in clinical reasoning. *Med Educ*. 45(4): 326–8.

The practitioners of medicine and surgery, when competently educated, will have a right to exact all the respect and consideration which are due to the most enlightened and humane of the professions.

James Macartney

Macartney J. On medical reform and the remodelling the profession. *Prov Med Surg J*. 1841; s1–1(17): 282–5.

It is almost impossible to trust any professional whose competence is in question.

David Pendleton

Tate P. What are we training for? *Educ Prim Care*. 2002; 13: 416–18.

If one is judging competence it is important that the examination should test that and not something else.

George Pickering

Pickering G. Against multiple choice questions. *Med Teach*. 1979; 1(2): 84–6.

There is alas no law against incompetency; no striking example is made.

Pliny the Elder

Greek physicians, from *Historia Naturalis*.

Training should not be time limited but competency based.

Umesh Prabhu

Prabhu U. Modernisation must be for better! *BMJ*. 2004 May 15. Available at: www.bmj.com/content/328/7449/1158.7/reply#bmj_el_59513?sid=3f545f3a-8b62-4679-979a-2c0b244a4cd7 (accessed 12 July 2011).

Competence in medicine is recognisable and incompetence even more so.

Philip Rhodes

Rhodes P. Incompetence in medical practice. *BMJ (Clin Res Ed)*. 1986; 292(6531): 1293–4.

The public must be protected, which is a duty of the profession, but doctors also have the duty of caring for their colleagues when they need help, as they most certainly do if they are demonstrably incompetent in practice.

Philip Rhodes

Rhodes P. Incompetence in medical practice. *BMJ (Clin Res Ed)*. 1986; 292(6531): 1293–4.

Medicine is both science and art; small wonder, then, that clinical competence – a blend of knowledge, intellect, attitudes, wisdom, and practical skills – is not precisely measurable.

Peter Richards

Richards P. Clinical competence and curiosity. *BMJ (Clin Res Ed)*. 1986; 292(6534): 1481–2.

At present, the notion of competencies is highly popular; many curricula have redefined their outcomes in the form of competencies.

Lambert Schuwirth

Schuwirth L. The need for national licensing examinations. *Med Educ*. 2007; 41(11): 1022–3.

Definitions of specific medical competencies to be acquired by medical students in the course of their studies may be derived from the juxtaposition of a list of generic competencies with a list of appropriate subject areas.

David Stone

Stone DH. A method of deriving definitions of specific medical competencies: a framework for curriculum planning and evaluation. *Med Teach*. 1987; 9(2): 155–9.

Competency-based medical education (CBME) is a general approach to fostering the professional development of physicians at every stage of learning, from the undergraduate years through practice.

Susan Swing

Swing SR. Perspectives on competency-based medical education from the learning sciences. *Med Teach*. 2010; 32(8): 663–8.

Why is kindness a taboo subject in medical education and regulation, even though we all want kindness in our own doctors as well as competence? Are we embarrassed by it, perhaps because we are unsure how well we would score as individuals if it could be measured?

John Temple

Temple J. Medicine's lost word? *BMJ*. 2008 October 17. Available at: www.bmj.com/content/337/bmj.a1993/reply#bmj_el_203277?sid=392b60de-c94a-4a2b-a544-84cd8481e0fd (accessed 19 July 2011).

Medical training could change from fixed-length variable-outcome programmes to fixed-outcome variable-length programmes.

Olle ten Cate

ten Cate O. Entrustability of professional activities and competency-based training. *Med Educ*. 2005; 39(12): 1176–7.

Adequate performance includes the ability and inclination to apply competence in a way that optimises the outcome of professional activities.

Olle ten Cate

ten Cate O. Medical education: trust, competence, and the supervisor's role in postgraduate training. *BMJ*. 2006; 333(7571): 748–51.

Cultural competence is not about generalising on the contraceptive needs of Roman Catholics, or about learning what Somali refugees eat for breakfast on Thursdays. Becoming culturally competent firstly requires learning a great deal about oneself.

Elspeth Webb

Webb E. Pigeon-holing, victim blaming, and stereotyping. *BMJ*. 2000 February 1. Available at: www.bmj.com/content/320/7230/323.1/reply#bmj_el_6505?sid=7f1b5b2e-7b0c-43f6-8a46-f45951808b4f (accessed 19 August 2011).

It is easy to understand why the public criticises doctors for their lack of understanding and compassion since the long and arduous training process engenders technical and theoretical competence but ignores the basics of human nature.

Gavin Yamey

Yamey G. Sexual health: medical training must acknowledge sexuality. *BMJ*. 1993; 307(6902): 500.

23. BEHAVIOUR

> A young man, in whose air and countenance appeared all the uncouth gravity and supercilious self-conceit of a physician piping hot from his studies.
>
> **Tobias Smollett**

Of course, Behaviourism 'works'. So does torture. Give me a no-nonsense, down-to-earth behaviourist, a few drugs, and simple electrical appliances, and in six months I will have him reciting the Athanasian Creed in public.

WH Auden

A Certain World. 1970.

I was not unpopular [at school] . . . It is Oxford that has made me insufferable.

Max Beerbohm

More: Going back to school. 1899.

It has been suggested to me in the past that a proportion of would-be doctors would not enter any training program which does not guarantee them a place in medical school. Candidates with such an attitude are arguably not those to whom places should be offered.

Kenneth Campbell

Campbell K. Common introductory course for medical and related professions. *BMJ*. 2002 August 30. Available at: www.bmj.com/content/324/7347/1170/reply (accessed 29 July 2011).

Of course, the impulse towards jargon is very much a matter of character; and it is likely that you can no more cure a naturally pompous person than you can reflower a virgin.

Alistair Cooke

Cooke A. The doctor in society. *BMJ*. 1981; 283(6307): 1652–5.

The conditions necessary for the surgeon are four; first, he should be learned: second, he should be expert: third, he must be ingenious, and fourth, he should be able to adapt himself.

Guy de Chauliac

Ars Chururgica.

Oh, well, I don't know much about his ability; but he's got a very good bedside manner!

George du Maurier

Punch. 1884 March 15.

The recent debacles within the medical profession can be traced to the widening gap between attitudes that are acceptable to the profession and those that are acceptable to the public. We were all members of the public once, if only we could remember what it was like!

Michel Erlewyn-Lajeunesse

Erlewyn-Lajeunesse M. Teaching correct attitudes. *BMJ.* 2000 July 6. Available at: www.bmj.com/content/321/7252/59.2/reply#bmj_el_8633?sid=7f1b5b2e-7b0c-43f6-8a46-f45951808b4f (accessed 2 September 2011).

My grouse about the teaching is the paperwork it generates. After an hour long tutorial with a group of 8 new students, I am expected to fill in a detailed questionnaire about the performance of each participant.

Charles Fox

Fox C. Observations from a DGH. *BMJ.* 2004 July 13. Available at: www.bmj.com/content/329/7457/92/reply#bmj_el_66954?sid=3f545f3a-8b62-4679-979a-2c0b244a4cd7 (accessed 9 July 2011).

That physician will hardly be thought very careful of the health of others who neglects his own.

Galen

Of Protecting the Health. bk 5.

A physician ought to be extremely watchful against covetousness, for it is a vice imputed, justly or unjustly, to his Profession.

Thomas Gisbourne

The Duties of Physicians.

A good performance at a seminar or conference may do more for a young man's career than any number of well handled clinical problems on the shop floor when no one is watching.

JC Griffiths

Griffiths JC. Personal view. *BMJ (Clin Res Ed).* 1983; 286(6383): 2058.

A man's character is his fate.

Heraclitus

On the Universe.

As to diseases, make a habit of two things – to help, or at least to do no harm.

Hippocrates

Epidemics.

For where there is love of man, there is also love of the art.

Hippocrates

Precepts. sect. VI.

A man of very moderate ability may be a good physician, if he devotes himself faithfully to the work.

Oliver Wendell Holmes

Scholastic and bedside teaching, from *Medical Essays*.

Every man should measure himself by his own standard.

Horace

Epistles.

The pretension is nothing: the performance is everything.

Leigh Hunt

The Story of Rimini. 1832.

Medicine is a "way of life" and combines that rather nebulous feeling of wanting to help and care with the more exact principles of science and logical thought.

Parveen Kumar

Kumar P. The joy of discovery. *BMJ*. 2006; 333(7582): 1321–2.

Men are vain only about themselves; but about their clan, their calling, their profession, they are more – they are vainglorious.

Peter Mere Latham

Latham PM. General remarks on the practice of medicine. *BMJ*. 1861; 2(41): 377–80.

Physicians are prime candidates for burnout. We tend to be hard working and to have high standards, and we are frequently perfectionistic.

Mark Linzer

Linzer M. Preventing burnout in academic medicine. *Arch Intern Med*. 2009; 169(10): 927–8.

Never be dogmatic about anything in medicine. What we hold as best thing since sliced bread today, we'll be laughing at in 5 years and what we are shunning as folly now, we'll be singing its praise in 5 years.

Joe Nemeth

Personal correspondence, 21 June 2011.

The most dangerous physicians are those who can act in perfect mimicry of the born physician.

Friedrich Nietzsche

Human, All Too Human. pt II.

In remembering those with whom I was year after year associated, and whom it was my duty to study, nothing appears more certain than that the personal character, the very nature, the will of each student had far greater force in determining his career than any helps or hindrances whatever.

James Paget

Cullingworth CJ. An address on the importance of personal character in the profession of medicine: delivered at the opening of Yorkshire College, Leeds. *BMJ*. 1898; 2(1971): 1038–40.

Students will only begin to report unacceptable behaviour by senior doctors if they are taught themselves that it is unacceptable – otherwise it will continue to be seen as an inevitable part of training to be a doctor.

Philip Peacock

Peacock P. Culture change is needed. *BMJ.* 2004 October 10. Available at: www.bmj.com/content/329/7469/770/reply#bmj_el_77707?sid=3f545f3a-8b62-4679-979a-2c0b244a4cd7 (accessed 6 June 2011).

Cured yesterday of my disease,
I died last night of my physician.

Matthew Prior

The Remedy is Worse than the Disease.

The best thing to learn early in your careers is humility. If you do not learn it the easy way, you will surely be taught it the hard way.

Rick Redalen

Personal correspondence, 28 June 2011.

Society in general demands the best of its doctors in knowledge, skills, and attitudes, which together make up education.

Philip Rhodes

Rhodes P. Educating the doctor: postgraduate, vocational, and continuing education. *BMJ.* 1985; 290(6484): 1808–10.

Social networks comprise interactions between groups of individuals. The importance of social networks has been recognised in student support and performance, organisational learning and online networks.

John Sandars

Sandars J. Work based learning: a social network perspective. *Work Based Learn Prim Care.* 2005; 3(1): 4–12(9).

Doctors need to know what they are trying to do and how well they are doing it to maintain their enthusiasm; otherwise they develop rituals and their performance declines.

TPC Schofield

Schofield TP. Continued medical education must not be an optional extra. *BMJ.* 1987; 294(6571): 526–7.

The case for the definition and use of behavioural objectives has been fervently made by their advocates, with more than a whiff of ideological extremism, especially amongst those who do not get involved in writing and using objectives regularly.

Michael Simpson

Simpson MA. Controversy: objections to objectives. *Med Teach.* 1980; 2(5): 229–31.

The difficulty and expense of getting poor performers back on track may mean that cash strapped health authorities will be unwilling to foot the bill.

Richard Smith

Smith R. The GMC on performance. *BMJ.* 1992; 304(6837): 1257–8.

A young man, in whose air and countenance appeared all the uncouth gravity and supercilious self-conceit of a physician piping hot from his studies.

Tobias Smollett

The Adventures of Peregrine Pickle. ch. 42.

A "problem" junior may be a learner who does not meet expectations because of problems in one of three areas: knowledge, attitudes, or skills.

Yvonne Steinert

Steinert Y. Teaching rounds: the "problem" junior; whose problem is it? *BMJ.* 2008; 336: 150–3.

The need to strengthen the behavioural aspects of medical education and practice has been widely recognised in recent years, but it has proved very difficult to translate good intentions into practical effect.

Ian Tait

Tait I. Behavioural medicine. *BMJ.* 1975; 4(5987): 41.

The road to success in the practice of our art lies not only in knowing how to deal with disease, but how to deal with men and women while they suffer from it.

Lawson Tait

Tait L. Address in surgery. *BMJ.* 1890; 2(1544): 267–73.

Get the attitude right by thinking, then let instinct, experience and evolution take over and the results are almost magical. John Lennon was wrong, all you need is attitude, but it has to be the right one, and there is the rub.

Peter Tate

Tate P. Tate on training. *Educ Prim Care.* 2001; 12: 461–3.

It is in the earliest days of medical school and residency that physicians' values and attitudes toward their profession are most influenced.

James Todd

Todd JS. Health care reform and the medical education imperative. *JAMA.* 1992; 268(9): 1133–4.

Put simply "good enough" is not good enough. Rather, in the interests of the health and wealth of the nation, we should aspire to excellence.

John Tooke

Tooke J. *Aspiring to Excellence: findings and recommendations of the independent inquiry into Modernising Medical Careers.* London: MMC Inquiry; 2007.

To cure sometimes, to relieve often, to care, always.

Unknown

I learn to relieve the suffering.

Virgil

Aeneid. I.

The best thing for being sad . . . is to learn something.

Terence Hanbury White

The Sword in the Stone. 1938.

Teaching

24. TEACHERS AND TEACHING

> Whoever it was who claimed to have been educated mainly during the holidays must have been an Old Boy of my medical school.
>
> **Michael Simpson**

Give instruction to a wise man, and he will be yet wiser: teach a just man, and he will increase in learning.
Prov. 9.9.

A teacher affects eternity; he can never tell where his influence stops.
Henry Brooks Adams
The Education of Henry Adams. 1907.

It is always in season for old men to learn.
Aeschylus
Agamemnon.

Until recently, practitioners were considered to be the experts who imposed their expertise and frames of understanding upon patients and the role of patients in medical education was passive, with them acting as interesting teaching 'material' – often no more than a medium through which or about which teachers taught.
Alka Ahuja
Ahuja AS. Patient and carer involvement in medical education. *BMJ*. 2006 September 8. Available at: www.bmj.com/content/333/7567/544/reply#bmj_el_142089?sid=20523c27-2e0d-443d-a7db-86e43c2767d3 (accessed 1 November 2011).

The concept of expertise is widely embraced but poorly defined in surgery.
David Alderson
Alderson D. Developing expertise in surgery. *Med Teach*. 2010; 32(10): 830–6.

Education, as contrasted with instruction, is a drawing forth of faculties, a quickening, enlarging, and refining of them when brought out, and an establishment of them in habits, so that virtue and reason become easy and pleasant to us.
Thomas Clifford Allbutt
Allbutt TC. An address on medical education in London: delivered at King's College Hospital on October 3rd, 1905, at the opening of the medical session. *BMJ*. 1905; 2(2337): 913–18.

One wouldn't expect a junior doctor to carry out a procedure without training, and I believe the same argument could and should be said of teaching.

Asif Bachlani

Bachlani AM. Being an effective clinical teacher. *BMJ*. 2009 November 15. Available at: www.bmj.com/content/339/bmj.b4554/reply#bmj_el_225824?sid=c01598e6-7fa7-4552-bbff-d3bc10847fd9 (accessed 9 July 2011).

Consultants and senior registrars are not rewarded for teaching and seldom have been trained in educational methods.

Maureen Baker

Baker M. Enhancing the educational content of SHO posts. *BMJ*. 1993; 306(6881): 808–9.

Why in the face of so much evidence to the contrary should it be thought that doctors are effective educators?

SL Barley

Barley SL. Medical education. *BMJ (Clin Res Ed)*. 1984; 288(6431): 1690.

Teaching resuscitation presents a unique problem in medical education because those who need to be taught are not a nicely circumscribed bunch with a basically similar educational background.

Peter Baskett

Baskett PJF. The way we teach . . .: resuscitation. *Med Teach*. 1981; 3(1): 14–19.

The quality of teaching is not likely to become optimal until the instructors themselves are schooled in the science of imparting knowledge.

Malcolm Bateson

Bateson MC. Teaching the teachers. *BMJ*. 1968; 4(5622): 59.

Teachers change, while examiners remain; and, indeed, it must be confessed that among the latter, at least in the case of the most popular board, are to be found but a small minority who have, for many years, contributed to the advancement of science and to the development of those continually advancing subjects without which there can be no real progress in medicine.

Lionel Beale

Beale LS. Lecture on medical progress: in memoriam R. B. Todd. *BMJ*. 1870; 1(489): 485–8.

Reports of teaching institutes, the kind of thing that the linguistically destitute cheerfully call workshops, often are about as inspiring as a workshop.

William Bean

Bean WB. Report of the First Institute on Clinical Teaching: report of the 6th AAMC Teaching Institute. *Arch Intern Med*. 1961; 107(3): 465.

Spastic introspection characterizes our time. Ours is the age of steel-trap narcissism and medical teachers are strongly affected. Taking into account the compulsive self-catechizing of teachers in the higher realm, it is not surprising that many institutes, "workshops," symposia, colloquia, and other exercises so often mark and sometimes mar the contemporary scene.

William Bean

Bean WB. Report of the Second Institute on Clinical Teaching. *Arch Intern Med*. 1963; 112(2): 286–8.

There is no objective measure of teaching performance; all sources of evidence are fallible.

Ronald Berk

Berk RA. Using the 360° multisource feedback model to evaluate teaching and professionalism. *Med Teach.* 2009; 31(12): 1073–80.

If we want to attract more national or academic authorities to the process of reorienting medical education, and involve them in strengthening and improving it, our work in changing medical education may need to be more systematic, and more objective methods may need to be applied.

Charles Boelen

Boelen C. A call for systematic action for changing medical education: reaction of working partners. *Med Teach.* 1990; 12(2): 131–41.

That which is repeated too often becomes insipid and tedious.

Boileau

L'Art Poétique.

Given that one of the main goals of medical education is to develop clinical diagnostic thinking, how does your teaching contribute to this goal?

George Brown

Brown G. Studies of student learning: implications for medical teaching. *Med Teach.* 1983; 5(2): 52–6.

Although the clinical value of these skills has been known for many years, it has traditionally been difficult for many doctors to accept the idea that something as supposedly intuitive as communication could or should be influenced by teaching or training.

Robert Buckman

Buckman R. Communications and emotions: skills and effort are key. *BMJ.* 2002; 325(7366): 672.

The success of a workshop depends on the participants being comfortable and working not only in a group but as a group.

David Bullimore

Bullimore D. Running a workshop on clinical bedside teaching: a practical guide. *Med Teach.* 1993; 15(1): 49–55.

For clinical expertise to be developed, particular skills are needed, which can only be provided if part of the learning is through case-based teaching.

Jonathan Burton

Burton J. Expertise and case-based teaching in primary care. *Work Based Learn Prim Care.* 2006; 4(2): 130–40(11).

To be trained is to have arrived; to be educated is to continue to travel.

Kenneth Calman

Calman K. The profession of medicine. *BMJ.* 1994; 309(6962): 1140–3.

The assumption underlying faculty development is that prevention is preferable to remediation.

Robert Carroll

Carroll RG. Implications of adult education theories for medical school faculty development programmes. *Med Teach.* 1993; 15(2–3): 163–70.

The very intellectual strength of Hippocrates as a physician was a source of weakness in the promulgation of his teaching after he had passed away.

Alfred Carter

Carter AH. Presidential addresses delivered at the Annual Meetings of the Branches of the British Medical Association: rationalism in the study and practice of physic: delivered at the Annual Meeting of the Birmingham and Midland Counties Branch on June 13th, 1895. *BMJ*. 1895; 2(1804): 186–9.

A good teacher delivers education at a level, in a style and at a time, at which the learner is ready and will gain most benefit.

Ruth Chambers

Chambers R. Teaching and education should be relevant to the needs of the learner, patients and the NHS as a whole. In: Chambers R, Wall D, editors. *Teaching Made Easy: a manual for health professionals*. Oxford: Radcliffe Medical Press; 2000. pp1–27.

It makes sense for all teachers and learners to maintain a portfolio that describes the evidence of the learning that has taken place, starting from a plan arising from learning objectives, the process of gaining the knowledge or skills and demonstration of competence.

Ruth Chambers

Chambers R. Teaching and education should be relevant to the needs of the learner, patients and the NHS as a whole. In: Chambers R, Wall D, editors. *Teaching Made Easy: a manual for health professionals*. Oxford: Radcliffe Medical Press; 2000. pp1–27.

It sanctions imperfect and even vicious methods of teaching. The student is told, not taught.

Andrew Clark

Clark A. The address delivered in the section of medicine. *BMJ*. 1879; 2(971): 222–5.

Many things will be required from the teacher which it will be hard for him in his circumstances to give; things which, indeed, it would be impossible for him to give in any worthful measure without a loving interest in the work and in the workers.

Andrew Clark

Clark A. An address on medical education and the duty of the community with regard to it. *BMJ*. 1888; 2(1449): 747–50.

Although some clinicians are born teachers and some, however eminent in their profession, are abject failures as teachers, most clinicians who possess certain natural attributes can be trained in the art and methods of teaching.

Henry Cohen

Cohen H. Methods and men in the teaching of clinical medicine. *BMJ*. 1950; 2(4677): 478–81.

The good teacher must be able to sense the response of his class so that he knows when to repeat, to emphasize, or to remodel his explanations.

Henry Cohen

Cohen H. Methods and men in the teaching of clinical medicine. *BMJ*. 1950; 2(4677): 478–81.

We have failed to secure coherence, continuity, and interdependence in our teaching.

Henry Cohen

Cohen H. Medicine, science, and humanism. *BMJ*. 1950; 2(4672): 179–84.

Universities must start putting the 'school' back into medical school and reward teachers – avoid the research vs teaching dilemma which has driven many good academics out of the profession.

Kate Collins

Collins K. Personal interest. *BMJ*. 2004 July 27. Available at: www.bmj.com/content/329/7457/92/reply#bmj_el_68712?sid=3f545f3a-8b62-4679-979a-2c0b244a4cd7 (accessed 19 June 2011).

Clinical teaching now needs a new orientation which will involve the abandonment of the infallibility myth and some loss of independence for the teacher.

Beryl Corner

Corner BD. Clinical teaching. *BMJ*. 1955; 2(4942): 789.

As part of your electronic presentation you should incorporate blank slides as required. This will clear the screen allowing the audience to concentrate solely on the speaker.

Joy Crosby

Crosby J. Twelve tips for effective electronic presentation. *Med Teach*. 1994; 16(1): 3–8.

I think our perceptions of relevance and irrelevance alter significantly throughout our careers. It follows that to expect students to immediately appreciate the relevance of all that they are taught is somewhat optimistic.

Peter Davies

Davies PG. Si jeunesse savait, si villesse pouvait. *BMJ*. 2006 October 17. Available at: www.bmj.com/content/333/7572/813.1/reply#bmj_el_144957?sid=20523c27-2e0d-443d-a7db-86e43c2767d3 (accessed 19 June 2011).

But it has always appeared to me that there is one, and that perhaps the main, branch of education which is in danger of being sacrificed in this attempt to instruct, and that is, teaching a student the uses and powers of his own mind.

Campbell de Morgan

de Morgan C. An address on the improvement of medical education. *BMJ*. 1871; 1(526): 84–5.

The student should be given the opportunity of becoming acquainted with and developing the rational attitude of mind. He should be encouraged in the attitude of intelligent scepticism as distinct from that of constant acquiescence in dogmatic teaching.

Frederick Dillon

Dillon F. Methodology in the curriculum. *BMJ*. 1945; 2(4418): 334.

Practical teaching is usually better given by juniors than by consultants, unless the consultant has a special delight in teaching or acting a part.

George Discombe

Discombe G. Medical education. *BMJ*. 1988; 297(6640): 68.

Students and teachers alike have an aversion to massive portfolios whether on paper or on screen.

Erik Driessen

Driessen E. Portfolio critics: do they have a point? *Med Teach*. 2009; 31(4): 279–81.

I am Jesuitical enough to think that if we have done our work adequately in the Junior Course, then what happens subsequently is of less concern.

HAE Dudley

Dudley HAE. The way we teach: how I did and how I should teach surgery. *Med Teach.* 1979; 1(3): 121–5.

Everything should be made as simple as possible, but not simpler.

Albert Einstein

Attributed.

There is no teaching until the pupil is brought into the same state or principle in which you are; a transfusion takes place; he is you, and you are he; there is a teaching; and by no unfriendly chance or bad company can he ever quite lose the benefit.

Ralph Waldo Emerson

Essays and Lectures.

The secret of education lies in respecting the pupil. It is not for you to choose what he shall know, what he shall do. It is chosen and foreordained and he only holds the key to his own secret.

Ralph Waldo Emerson

Emerson RW. Education. In: Emerson RW, editor. *The Complete Works of Ralph Waldo Emerson. Lectures and Biographical Sketches.* Boston: Houghton Mifflin; 1883. pp125–59.

Educators can take on the task of helping trainees become more mindful by explicitly modelling their means for cultivating awareness.

Ronald Epstein

Epstein RM. Mindful practice. *JAMA.* 1999; 282(9): 833–9.

The good practitioner is, and should be, the busy practitioner; the teacher, however, needs leisure – more leisure than the practitioner – to read, study and investigate.

Abraham Flexner

Flexner A. Medical education, 1909–1924. *JAMA.* 1924; 82(11): 833–8.

How far it is consistent with the public interest or with the dignity of the medical profession that branches of medicine should be practised without being taught, your readers can judge.

R Fortescue Fox

Fortescue Fox R. Post-graduate teaching and the university of London. *BMJ.* 1918; 2(3024): 669.

It seems to me that the importance of the education of the medical man or woman of to-day is greater than ever it was, and the responsibilities of those who are engaged in teaching are also greater than ever.

George Cooper Franklin

Franklin GC. President's address: delivered at the Seventy-Third Annual Meeting of the British Medical Association. *BMJ.* 1905; 2(2326): 221–6.

That leaves education and research to consider, and most of us know of colleagues who scamp teaching and concentrate on research; on the other hand, there are not a few whose main value to their respective departments lies in their teaching power.

Kenneth Franklin

Franklin KJ. Adult education: for the preclinical scientist. *BMJ.* 1955; 2(4938): 507–9.

Instruction does not prevent waste of time or mistakes; and mistakes themselves are often the best teachers of all.

James Anthony Froude

Education, from *Short Studies on Great Subjects.*

A teacher is paid to teach, not to sacrifice rats and hamsters.

Edward Gall

Gall GA. The three faces of medicine. *J Med Educ.* 1961; 36: 275–81.

It is the system, then, that I consider responsible for the present unsatisfactory state of things, and not the students, the teachers, or the examiners as such, but only so far as they may be councillors of the several colleges and still permit such a reprehensible system to continue.

George Gascoyen

Gascoyen GG. The coming race. *BMJ.* 1871; 2(573): 743.

Doctors have this time-honoured requisite to teach their followers, but not all want to.

David Gibson

Gibson DR. Learning to teach. *BMJ.* 2009 November 24. Available at: www.bmj.com/content/339/bmj.b4554/reply#bmj_el_225824?sid=c01598e6-7fa7-4552-bbff-d3bc10847fd9 (accessed 19 June 2011).

Grand Medical Rounds has an imperialistic ring reminiscent of Victorian Britain.

JAL Gilbert

Gilbert JAL. Against the grand medical round. *Med Teach.* 1979; 1(6): 314–15.

Evidence-based medicine (EBM) is like safe sex: talked about a lot, preached (taught) a little and practiced infrequently.

Paul Glasziou

Glasziou P. What is EBM and how should we teach it? *Med Teach.* 2006; 28(4): 303–4.

In medicine we still assume that if someone is an expert in his subject he is automatically qualified to teach it. This is of course a fallacy: teaching is a separate skill that one acquires by personal inclination or application, and is different from the skills inherent in removing a gall bladder or cultivating a bedside manner.

Stephen Golding

Golding S. Fellowship in medical communication? *BMJ.* 1978; 1(6119): 1056.

There is no need for me to speak to this audience of what medical education has now become, but I wish that all teachers could manage to make their instruction a training of the powers and mastering of the methods, rather than a loading of the memory with unnecessary facts and transient theories.

Thomas Grainger Stewart

Grainger Stewart T. President's address: delivered at the Sixty-Sixth Annual Meeting of the British Medical Association. *BMJ.* 1898; 2(1961): 281–6.

I believe that a specific barrier to reform of medical education is the inertia of the medical teachers themselves.

James Grant

News. *BMJ.* 1993; 307: 463.

Teaching and medicine are natural partners and their rewards often similar, including keeping up to date, humanism, reflection, and enjoyment from helping others learn.

Ann Griffin

Griffin A. 'Designer doctors': professional identity and a portfolio career as a general practice educator. *Educ Prim Care.* 2008; 19: 355–9.

Example is contagious, and descends from teacher to pupil.

William Gull

Gull WW. Introductory address on the study of medicine. *BMJ.* 1874; 2(718): 425–9.

The first suggestion as to how we can improve PowerPoint presentations therefore, is to forget about PowerPoint in the initial planning for the presentation.

Ronald Harden

Harden RM. Death by PowerPoint: the need for a 'fidget index'. *Med Teach.* 2008; 30(9–10): 833–5.

Questioning is one of the most powerful teaching tools and is accessible by all clinical teachers.

Richard Hays

Hays R. Clinical teaching skills. In: Hays R. *Teaching and Learning in Clinical Settings.* Oxford: Radcliffe Publishing; 2006. pp31–56.

While clinical teachers are employed to help students learn clinical knowledge and skills, it is no longer sufficient to just have technical expertise in individual patient care.

Richard Hays

Hays R. Developing as a learner and a teacher. In: Hays R. *Teaching and Learning in Clinical Settings.* Oxford: Radcliffe Publishing; 2006. p5.

Good doctoring, just like good teaching, is built on the relationship between two particular people. Its effectiveness depends on the identity and integrity of the doctor: on it being a form of happiness.

Iona Heath

Heath I. From my diary. *Educ Prim Care.* 2007; 18: 544–5.

While teachers themselves may be born with a natural inclination to educate others, those who also administer graduate medical education (GME) must be amenable to a gruelling learning process that no amount of talent can circumvent.

Hannah Hedrick

Hedrick HL. Guide to graduate medical education. *JAMA.* 1995; 274(9): 773–4.

The powerful driving effect of psychometrically reliable, summative examinations means the role of teachers often falls in line with examination preparation.

Brian Hodges

Hodges B. Medical education and the maintenance of incompetence. *Med Teach.* 2006; 28(8): 690–6.

A good clinical teacher is himself a Medical School.

Oliver Wendell Holmes

Scholastic and bedside teaching, from *Medical Essays.*

The bedside is always the true center of medical teaching.

Oliver Wendell Holmes

Scholastic and bedside teaching, from *Medical Essays.*

Instruction enlarges the natural powers of the mind.
Horace
Carmina. IV. 4. 33.

There are already many students who will 'never forget a good teacher': many of their memories are of patients, and most of the rest are of their primary care tutors.
Amanda Howe
Howe A. Has a decade made a difference? The contribution of UK primary care to basic medical training in 2004. *Educ Prim Care.* 2005; 16: 10–19.

Were teachers satisfied that their students would only be asked straightforward, practical questions, I feel sure they would willingly endeavour to prepare their pupils not merely in view of examinations, but for the practice of their profession.
Alfred Hughes
Hughes AW. The address in surgery. *BMJ.* 1890; 2(1546): 422.

Learning depends on several factors, but a crucial step is the engagement of the learner.
Linda Hutchinson
Hutchinson L. ABC of learning and teaching: educational environment. *BMJ.* 2003; 326(7393): 810–12.

At all times, however, it should be held in mind, that in the comprehensive subjects they had to teach, the best and most accomplished teachers are still students – still, like themselves, learners, the only difference being, that the former were no longer beginners, but had made some progress in their course, so that imperfections and deficiencies were to a certain extent unavoidable.
J Ingham Ikin
Ingham Ikin J. Introductory lecture on the opening of the medical session. *Prov Med Surg J.* 1844; s1–8(30): 455–60.

To encourage group interaction consider breaking a larger group into smaller groups of five or six students; organise membership on a heterogeneous or random basis to prevent cliques forming.
David Jaques
Jaques D. ABC of learning and teaching in medicine: teaching small groups. *BMJ.* 2003; 326(7387): 492–4.

Students are influenced not so much by what they have been taught about how to be clinicians, but rather by the teachers' styles as teachers: the way they teach results in many of their students becoming clinicians who bring those same characteristics to their style of health care.
Hilliard Jason
Jason H. Teaching is messy. *Med Teach.* 1979; 1(20): 61–3.

Self directed learning can be viewed as a method of organising teaching and learning in which the learning tasks are largely within the learners' control.
David Kaufman
Kaufman DM. ABC of learning and teaching in medicine: applying educational theory in practice. *BMJ.* 2003; 326(7382): 213–16.

A difficulty for the current generation of communication skills teachers is that many of us have not had the experience of being formally taught communication skills ourselves.

Maureen Kelly

Kelly M. A practical guide for teachers of communication skills: a summary of current approaches to teaching and assessing communication skills. *Educ Prim Care.* 2007; 18: 1–10.

Communication skills can be taught.

Maureen Kelly

Kelly M. A practical guide for teachers of communication skills: a summary of current approaches to teaching and assessing communication skills. *Educ Prim Care.* 2007; 18: 1–10.

Communications skills teaching is most effective when it is consistent and complementary with clinical teaching.

Maureen Kelly

Kelly M. A practical guide for teachers of communication skills: a summary of current approaches to teaching and assessing communication skills. *Educ Prim Care.* 2007; 18: 1–10.

Organizing and running rotational training schemes have caused most of my grey hairs. They are activities I recommend only to those with square jaws and very thick skins.

David Kerr

Kerr DNS. How to . . . organize rotational training schemes in medicine. *Med Teach.* 1984; 6(3): 86–91.

Ask any Medical Illustration Department what they consider to be the greatest problem in slide preparation and you will hear these words 'too much information to fit on a slide'.

Jennifer Laidlaw

Laidlaw JM. Twelve tips on preparing 35 mm slides. *Med Teach.* 1987; 9(4): 389–93.

Leave the exhibition area as you found it otherwise you might jeopardise your chances of being invited back!

Jennifer Laidlaw

Laidlaw JM. Exhibitions: twelve tips for exhibitors. *Med Teach.* 1988; 10(2): 133–7.

It is healthy to observe each other's teaching: we can learn many tricks of the trade and if we are frank we can advise each other how to improve.

John Last

Last JM. Personal view. *BMJ (Clin Res Ed).* 1985; 290(6485): 1900.

So, if you would teach a man medicine and its practice, you must not begin with half a dozen philosophies, or with any philosophy at all, but you must put, as it were, his alphabet into his hand at once, and bid him learn its simple characters one by one, and then help him to join them together and make the best sense of them he can.

Peter Mere Latham

Latham PM. A word or two on medical education: and a hint or two for those who think it needs reforming. *BMJ.* 1864; 1(162): 141–3.

Reformers have urged that the success of a teacher anywhere is to be measured, not by the number of words or verbal formulations which his pupils learn, but by the degree of purposive mental activity which he arouses in them.

Joseph Lauwerys

Lauwerys JA. Methods of education. *BMJ.* 1950; 2(4677): 471–4.

I consider that clinical medicine is, for many reasons, the most difficult of subjects to teach, and that some training in it is of paramount importance.
Robin Lawrence

Lawrence RD. The training of clinical teachers. *BMJ.* 1950; 2(4677): 481–4.

The teacher is becoming an advisor, a guide.
Emilio Ledezma

Ledezma EP. The palm top medical education: the becoming of a new era. *BMJ.* 2003 March 11. Available at: www.bmj.com/content/326/7388/543/reply#bmj_el_30315?sid=7f27ee1c-bc1e-486c-bc82-03a5164885cc (accessed 19 June 2011).

Teaching is a fundamental part of being a doctor, but, as with the other skills that are needed, it must be learnt.
Sam Leinster

Leinster S. Reviving academic medicine in Britain. *BMJ.* 2000; 321(7259): 511.

It appears to me that the great object of reform in medical education should be to simplify the teaching without curtailing the material of the science itself.
Percy Leslie

Leslie P. Medical education. *BMJ.* 1864; 1(168): 327.

The result was that there was a tendency to distract the attention of the students from work under their teachers to making special preparations for the examinations.
Joseph Lister

Barnes R. The relations of the graduates and convocation of the University of London to the proposed reform of the university. *BMJ.* 1890; 1(1518): 267–8.

No proper review of an education system should ignore the role of the teachers. But in medical education the teachers are not easy to define.
Stella Lowry

Lowry S. Medical education: teaching the teachers. *BMJ.* 1993; 306(6870): 127–30.

Teaching excellence should be rewarded, and there should be real penalties for individuals or units if they fail to fulfil their teaching obligations.
Stella Lowry

Lowry S. Medical education: teaching the teachers. *BMJ.* 1993; 306(6870): 127–30.

Teachers should be selected on account of their knowledge of the subject, and their materials for communicating that knowledge to their pupils.
James Macartney

Macartney J. On medical reform and the remodelling the profession. *Prov Med Surg J.* 1841; s1–1(17): 282–5.

I am well aware that in these days, when a student must be converted into a physiologist, a physicist, a chemist, a biologist, a pharmacologist, and an electrician, there is no time to make a physician of him.
Andrew MacPhail

MacPhail A. An address on the source of modern medicine. *BMJ.* 1933; 1(3767): 443–7.

It seems to him that his teachers are like the giants of old, and, in their attempts to scale the heavens, are heaping Ossa on Pelion, and inadvertently crushing his prostrate form beneath the superincumbent weight.

Howard Marsh

Marsh H. An address on the education of the student of medicine: delivered at the opening of the winter session (1910–1911), in the Medical Department of the University of Leeds. *BMJ*. 1910; 2(2598): 1105–8.

Education should be a two way process since this will help promote mutual understanding of different roles and functions within the medical profession.

Martin Marshall

Marshall MN. Qualitative study of educational interaction between general practitioners and specialists. *BMJ*. 1998; 316(7129): 442–5.

To generate educational insight at a medical school is a long-term undertaking.

Dick Martenson

Martenson D. Educational development in an established medical school: facilitating and impeding factors in change at the Karolinska Institute. *Med Teach*. 1989; 11(1): 17–25.

I hope you enjoy the absence of pupils . . . the total oblivion of them for definite intervals is a necessary condition for doing them justice at the proper time.

James Clerk Maxwell

Letter to Lewis Campbell, 1862.

Begin with an arresting sentence; close with a strong summary; in between speak simply, clearly, always to the point; and, above all, be brief.

William Mayo

Cope Z. William and Charles Mayo. *BMJ*. 1955; 1(4929): 1516.

Medicine, once the most respected of all the professions, is coming under increasing attack as it is currently practiced and taught.

Ernest Mazzaferri

Mazzaferri EL. Bedside teaching in the preparation of physicians for the 21st century. *Arch Intern Med*. 1986; 146(10): 1912.

Effective all-round flexible teachers demonstrate creative, innovative and novel solutions to the practical problems of teaching in clinical settings, which are based on critique of the literature as well as original thought.

Kay Mohanna

Mohanna K. The all-round flexible and adaptable teacher. In: Mohanna K, Chambers R, Wall D. *Your Teaching Style: a practical guide to understanding, developing and improving*. Oxford: Radcliffe Publishing; 2008. pp23–9.

Good teachers recognise that learners differ.

Kay Mohanna

Mohanna K. The all-round flexible and adaptable teacher. In: Mohanna K, Chambers R, Wall D. *Your Teaching Style: a practical guide to understanding, developing and improving*. Oxford: Radcliffe Publishing; 2008. pp23–9.

Teachers vary in their preference for one or another style of teaching, just as learners demonstrate differences in learning styles.

Kay Mohanna

Mohanna K. The importance of variation in teaching styles. In: Mohanna K, Chambers R, Wall D. *Your Teaching Style: a practical guide to understanding, developing and improving*. Oxford: Radcliffe Publishing; 2008. pp1–12.

It is necessary that a plan be marked out for directing students, and that they should be taught a regular course of every distinct branch of medicine; the infant state, and the want of professed teachers, have hitherto clogged medical pursuits in America with innumerable obstacles.

John Morgan

Morgan J. *A Discourse upon the Institution of Medical Schools in America.* Philadelphia; 1765. p19.

The major advantage of a profiling system is that it enables teachers to generate a framework within which observations of learners' progress and achievements can be made.

Helen Mulholland

Mulholland H. What is . . . a profile? *Med Teach.* 1988; 10(3–4): 277–82.

Discussion in class, which means letting twenty young blockheads and two cocky neurotics discuss something that neither their teacher nor they know.

Vladimir Nabokov

Pnin. 1957.

The Socratic method is a game at which only one (the professor) can play.

Ralph Nader

The High Citadel. 1978.

If there is a deep desire to learn, a student can learn on his own even without the help of a teacher. Such a student will be a life long learner.

Satheesha Nayak

Nayak S. What is the reason for yawning in the class? *BMJ.* 2005 July 10. Available at: www.bmj.com/content/331/7508/105.2/reply#bmj_el_111907?sid=cb764c2a-ad1a-4f84-a8c4-88b3568c267c (accessed 19 June 2011).

Students now worship teachers who make them laugh in the class, the teacher who leaves them early and asks easy questions in the exams.

Satheesha Nayak

Nayak S. "Student and education" today. *BMJ.* 2005 July 18. Available at: www.bmj.com/content/331/7509/151/reply#bmj_el_112486?sid=cb764c2a-ad1a-4f84-a8c4-88b3568c267c (accessed 19 June 2011).

It has become almost a truism to draw parallels between the interpersonal dynamics of the doctor-patient relationship and those operating in the educational domain between teacher and learner.

Roger Neighbour

Neighbour R. Reflections on the ethics of assessment. *Educ Prim Care.* 2003; 14: 406–10.

To discover and to teach are distinct functions; they are also distinct gifts, and are not commonly found united in the same person.

John Henry Newman

Discourses on the Scope and Nature of University Education: addressed to the Catholics of Dublin. 1852.

For, remember, and it is a fact which can never be too prominently brought before the minds of students, that be the talents of the teachers ever so great, or the means and appliances of the place of education unsurpassed, the permanent reputation of the school, college, or university, can only be maintained by the character and acquirements of those whose education has been received, and whose characters have been formed, within its precincts.

Thomas Nunneley

Nunneley T. Introductory lecture: delivered at the Leeds School of Medicine, October 4th, 1852. *Prov Med Surg J.* 1852; s1–16(21): 525–9.

Teacher training requirements in Britain mean that university graduates who wish to teach their subject undergo a year of teacher training.

Graham O'Byrne

O'Byrne G. Are doctors born teachers? *BMJ.* 1988; 296(6625): 838–9.

A blank board can be simultaneously a daunting and a creative venue for artistic teaching.

Jay Orlander

Orlander JD. Twelve tips for use of a white board in clinical teaching: reviving the chalk talk. *Med Teach.* 2007; 29(2–3): 89–92.

Once a week, over a little "beer and bacey," I meet my clinical clerks in an informal conference upon the events of the week. For half an hour I give a short talk on one of the "Masters of Medicine," in which, as far as possible, the original editions of the works are shown.

William Osler

Osler W. A note on the teaching of the history of medicine. *BMJ.* 1902; 2(2167): 93.

Nothing drives adult learning like a practical demonstration of the 'need to know' in a real-life setting.

Elisabeth Paice

Paice E. Foreword. In: Hays R. *Teaching and Learning in Clinical Settings.* Oxford: Radcliffe Publishing; 2006. pv.

Good teaching cannot be reduced to technique; good teaching comes from the identity and integrity of the teacher.

Parker Palmer

Palmer P. *The Courage to Teach: exploring the inner landscape of a teacher's life.* San Francisco: Jossey-Bass; 1998. p10.

We could do with more good teachers; we could certainly do with fewer bad ones – boring, self satisfied, bullying, sarcastic, insensitive, lazy, or otherwise lacking in the capacity to inspire and support.

James Parkhouse

Parkhouse J. Book review: medicine and books. *BMJ.* 1985; 290: 230.

The true aim of the teacher should be to impart an appreciation of method rather than a knowledge of facts.

Karl Pearson

Pickering G. Medicine's challenge to the educator. *BMJ.* 1958; 2(5105): 1117–21.

People tend to learn best from those who love their subject, and although this love is nothing without the ability to understand it, there is a balance to be struck.

Michael Peckitt

Peckitt MG. Three B's: balance to be struck. *BMJ*. 2006 August 28. Available at: www.bmj.com/content/333/7565/453.2/reply#bmj_el_140577?sid=20523c27-2e0d-443d-a7db-86e43c2767d3 (accessed 19 June 2011).

A true educator must have certain innate characters. He must be intelligent and thoughtful; he must be interested in the material he is using for teaching, and in the minds of those taught.

George Pickering

Pickering G. Medicine's challenge to the educator. *BMJ*. 1958; 2(5105): 1117–21.

Teaching requires a different methodology from training: teacher education is different from training the trainers.

Zoë-Jane Playdon

Playdon Z. Thinking about teaching? *BMJ*. 1999; 318(7196): S2.

Until the status of teaching improves in the medical profession it seems unlikely that doctors in training will choose to make the efforts necessary to acquire teaching skills.

Bill Plummer

Plummer B. Medical education. *BMJ*. 1993; 306(6875): 456.

Men must be taught as if you taught them not,
And things unknown propos'd as things forgot.

Alexander Pope

Essay on Criticism.

The formal ward round is perceived unfavourably because the juggling act of assessing, teaching and comforting at the same time is beyond the capacity of most physicians.

Solomon Posen

Posen S. *The Doctor in Literature: satisfaction or resentment.* Oxford: Radcliffe Publishing; 2005. pp210–11.

As long as teaching is perceived as an activity which is relatively unimportant in comparison to clinical work and research, those who teach will be at a disadvantage because they will have less time to devote to activities with more tangible rewards.

Anisur Rahman

Rahman A. Teaching medical students: whose job is it anyway; author's response. *BMJ*. 2005 February 1. Available at: www.bmj.com/content/330/7483/153.1/reply#bmj_el_95074?sid=1e069fc1-8837-4789-925c-3c1714669644 (accessed 19 June 2011).

Physical examination (PEx) skills are declining among medical trainees, yet many institutions are not teaching these systematically and effectively.

Subha Ramani

Ramani S. Twelve tips for excellent physical examination teaching. *Med Teach*. 2008; 30(9–10): 851–6.

In hospitals every doctor seems to think that he is ordained to teach, though sometimes he has little idea of what this requires. Only rarely do any of them formally learn something of the techniques of teaching.

Philip Rhodes

Rhodes P. Postgraduate education in general practice. *BMJ (Clin Res Ed)*. 1983; 286(6379): 1725–7.

Teaching, of course, is not to be equated with learning. The teacher's message may be accepted and modified (which is learning, and perhaps education), or it may be rejected or ignored.

Philip Rhodes

Rhodes P. Teaching. *BMJ (Clin Res Ed)*. 1983; 286(6375): 1426–7.

Students who are trained primarily as diagnosticians can potentially find the reality of medicine a huge culture chock. Valiant efforts are being made to address these problems centrally, but clinical students often face teachers who still expect and teach older philosophies.

Jason Roach

Roach JO. Seeds of unhappiness are sown in medical school. *BMJ*. 2002 April 27. Available at: www.bmj.com/content/324/7341/835/reply#bmj_el_21047?sid=d5e693ea-0765-423d-ac1d-1c98624d8fdf (accessed 19 June 2011).

There are so many crises at the moment that the word has lost some of its emphasis, but globally there do seem to be significant difficulties in recruiting medical practitioners into academic careers.

Trudie Roberts

Roberts TE. Catch them early. *Med Teach*. 2010; 32(3): 193–4.

While there is extensive literature on the qualities that are perceived by trainees to make a good clinical teacher, there is also evidence of the presence of poor role models among clinical teaching faculty.

Sue Roff

Roff S. New resources for measuring educational environment. *Med Teach*. 2005; 27(4): 291–3.

Students are seeking a model for a good doctor and they look for one in their teachers.

Mikko Roine

Roine MA. Doctor as a member of a team. *Med Teach*. 1986; 8(4): 377–81.

The basis of a good medical school is good teaching by those who are interested in their subject and alive to the needs and problems of the students.

Edward Rossiter

Rossiter EJR. The student and the clinical curriculum. *BMJ*. 1958; 2(5096): 608, 609–10.

There is only one person really capable of assessing teachers, and that is the student, who is on the receiving end.

Edward Rossiter

Rossiter EJR. The student and the clinical curriculum. *BMJ*. 1958; 2(5096): 608, 609–10.

He cannot be educated unless you assume that he has a right to question your statements, and to demand from you a demonstration of the truth of what you say.

William Rutherford

Rutherford W. Address in physiology. *BMJ*. 1875; 2(763): 198–200.

Although the preclinical teachers are primarily concerned with education, the clinical teachers, whose vision is, or should be, constantly broadened by practice, are hampered in their duty to the student by many other public and private claims upon their energy, and sometimes by a very real mental weariness.

John Ryle

Ryle JA. "The student in irons". *BMJ.* 1932; 1(3716): 587.

The general physician has practically disappeared from the clinical teaching staff.

Richard Scott

Scott R. Undergraduate education and the general practitioner. *BMJ.* 1958; 2(5096): 577–80.

Even while they teach, men learn.

Seneca

Epistulae Morales.

There is growing support for academics to transform their approaches to learning and teaching to one where the emphasis is on supporting students to become independent learners.

Madeleine Shanahan

Shanahan M. Learning centred approach for developing the electronic information search processes of students. *Med Teach.* 2009; 31(11): 994–1000.

I'll teach you differences.

William Shakespeare

King Lear. I. iv.

Those that do teach young babes, Do it with gentle means and easy tasks.

William Shakespeare

Othello. II. ii.

When I am forgotten, as I shall be,
And sleep in dull cold marble,
Say, I taught thee.

William Shakespeare

Henry VIII. III. ii.

I am not a teacher: only a fellow-traveller of whom you asked the way. I pointed ahead – ahead of myself as well as of you.

George Bernard Shaw

Getting Married.

Teach him to think for himself: Oh, my God, teach him rather to think like other people!

Mary Wollstonecraft Shelley

On her son's education. In: Arnold M. *Essays in Criticism.* 1888.

We had many fine teachers at Guy's, and most of them spent much of the day in bed – the patients taught me a great deal (as they still do).

Michael Simpson

Simpson MA. A study in irrelevancy. *Med Teach.* 1979; 1(2): 94–6.

Whoever it was who claimed to have been educated mainly during the holidays must have been an Old Boy of my medical school.

Michael Simpson

Simpson MA. A study in irrelevancy. *Med Teach.* 1979; 1(2): 94–6.

Be prepared to be opportunistic in clinical teaching, since cases never occur in a logical order.

Avtar Singh

Singh A. Practical teaching tips. *BMJ.* 2009 November 23. Available at: www.bmj.com/content/339/bmj.b4554/reply#bmj_el_225824?sid=c01598e6-7fa7-4552-bbff-d3bc10847fd9 (accessed 19 June 2011).

Dissatisfaction with medical education runs deep among teachers and students, and it is unusual to meet young doctors who talk glowingly of their education.

Richard Smith

Smith R. Profile of the GMC: the day of judgment comes closer. *BMJ.* 1989; 298(6682): 1241–4.

I have often thought it would be important to instruct physicians how to behave in cases of incurable disease; not so much to tell them what to do, but rather what not to do.

Johann Stieglitz

Letter to Dr Karl FH Marx, 15 December 1826.

Looking back, clinical education, largely centralized in the hospital ward since the 1900s, has focused on the diagnosis and treatment of acute disease.

John Stoeckle

Stoeckle JD. The market pushes education from ward to office, from acute to chronic illness and prevention: will case method teaching-learning change? *Arch Intern Med.* 2000; 160: 273–80.

The shortcomings of hospital teaching are easily seen but readily tolerated.

Octavius Sturges

Sturges O. Dissolution of the Medical Teachers' Association. *BMJ.* 1876; 2(834): 840.

Residents play an important part in the education of students and other residents, and they need to be supported in this activity.

James Tacci

Tacci JA. The resident as teacher: a neglected role. *JAMA.* 1998; 280(10): 934.

Unfortunately, residents often assume teaching responsibilities with little formal preparation, and few programs set aside time and other resources to develop residents' teaching skills.

James Tacci

Tacci JA. The resident as teacher: a neglected role. *JAMA.* 1998; 280(10): 934.

Experiential learning seeks active participation by the student and changes the role of faculty to emphasize facilitating student learning rather than teaching with a unidirectional flow of information to the students.

Roger Thomas

Thomas RE. Methods of teaching medicine using cases. *Med Teach.* 1993; 15(1): 27–34.

At the conclusion of an apprenticeship, an examination ought to prove the acquirements of the student, and, at the same time guarantee the title of his master to be a teacher of the elements at least of his profession.

Spencer Thomson

Thomson S. Medical education and apprenticeship. *BMJ.* 1885; 2(1283): 228.

It is commonly said that one of the chief objects of medical education should be to make the student think scientifically. The saying is perhaps as good an example as could be found of the need in which medicine stands for the exercise of the critical mind.

Wilfred Trotter

Trotter W. General ideas in medicine. *BMJ.* 1935; 2(3900): 609–14.

See one do one teach one.

Unknown

There's nothing so unequal as the equal treatment of unequals.

Unknown

Those who can do. Those who can't teach. Those who can't teach become educationalists. Those who can't become educationalists become medical educationalists.

Unknown

In education we are overly inclined to rely on our own tradition and intuition and to over-state the uniqueness of our particular circumstances (think of the thousands of teachers with their own stock of test questions in their drawer).

Cees van der Vleuten

van der Vleuten C. Improving medical education. *BMJ.* 1993; 306(6873): 284–5.

It is, I suppose, impossible to instruct a person without in some degree educating him, or to educate without in some degree instructing him.

Willoughby Francis Wade

Wade WF. President's address, delivered at the Fifty-Eighth Annual Meeting of the British Medical Association. *BMJ.* 1890; 2(1544): 259–62.

One reason, perhaps, why instruction and education are so often used as if they were synonymous terms is that no hard and fast line can be drawn between them.

Willoughby Francis Wade

Wade WF. President's address, delivered at the Fifty-Eighth Annual Meeting of the British Medical Association. *BMJ.* 1890; 2(1544): 259–62.

The teacher, the organisations in which we work, society and others are key stakeholders in the business of teaching and learning.

David Wall

Wall D. Determining your teaching style. In: Mohanna K, Chambers R, Wall D. *Your Teaching Style: a practical guide to understanding, developing and improving.* Oxford: Radcliffe Publishing; 2008. pp13.

Concept maps are a useful way for the teacher to elicit and externalize their teaching and learning strategies.

Gordon Watson

Watson GR. What is . . . concept mapping? *Med Teach.* 1989; 11(3–4): 265–9.

Come forth into the light of things,
Let Nature be your Teacher.
William Wordsworth
The Tables Turned. 1798.

I have read many persuasive reports about medical education, but they generally overlook
the essential point, that if you have first-class students and first-class teachers the rest
matters very little.
Samson Wright
Wright S. Remuneration of teachers. *BMJ.* 1948; 2(4565): 47–8.

25. LECTURES

> John Hunter never had more than 20 students at his lectures, and at the beginning, when a
> solitary student presented himself, he had to ask the attendant to bring in the skeleton, so that
> he might address them as "Gentlemen".
>
> **William Macewen**

My speech shall distil as the dew, as the small rains upon the tender herb, and as the
showers upon the grass.
Deut. 32.2.

Surely medical education has failed to achieve its aims when at a revision lecture on
valvular heart disease two weeks before finals 95% of the year's students wrote down the
lecturer's opening words: "The murmur of aortic stenosis is heard in systole."
HJN Andreyev
Andreyev HJN. Personal view. *BMJ (Clin Res Ed).* 1988; 296(6632): 1326.

Again in the habits and regulations of schools, universities and the like assemblies,
destined for the abode of learned men and the improvement of learning, everything is
opposed to the progress of the sciences; for the lectures and exercises are so ordered, that
anything out of the common track can scarcely enter the thoughts and contemplations
of the mind.
Francis Bacon
Organum Novum. bk I, para 90.

He that desires to learn truth should teach himself by facts and experiments; by which
means he will learn more in a year than by abstract reasoning in an age.
Hermann Boerhaave
Academical Lectures on the Theory of Physic. vol. I. 1751.

Video excerpts can be used as an illustrative medium in lectures, seminars or laboratory
classes and thereby enrich the teaching and expose the students to experiences which are
not readily available.
George Brown
Brown GA. How to make and use video in teaching. *Med Teach.* 1985; 7(2): 139–49.

A lecture format allows one expert to share his or her expertise with a great many learners in a short time; it is relatively cheap in terms of resources – one room and one expert serve many learners.

Ruth Chambers

Chambers R. The one-off teacher. In: Mohanna K, Chambers R, Wall D. *Your Teaching Style: a practical guide to understanding, developing and improving.* Oxford: Radcliffe Publishing; 2008. pp69–75.

No observant lecturer can fail to notice that, so long as he is dealing with abstract principles, general statements, bare descriptions, and dry facts slightly associated, it is difficult to secure the attention of his students.

Robert Christison

Christison R. President's address, delivered at the Forty-Third Annual Meeting of the British Medical Association. *BMJ.* 1875; 2(762): 155–63.

The reading of a lecture is usually uninspiring, and the student may pointedly ask, If the lecturer has not learnt the subject, why should I?

Henry Cohen

Cohen H. Methods and men in the teaching of clinical medicine. *BMJ.* 1950; 2(4677): 478–81.

A sophistical rhetorician, inebriated with the exuberance of his own verbosity.

Benjamin Disraeli

Speech at the Riding School, 1878.

If we insist on a rigid, Victorian classroom-style approach to higher education – we will by definition, encourage well-mannered but 'infantile' practitioners.

Harry El-Sayeh

El-Sayeh HG. A problem with problem-based learning. *BMJ.* 2004 July 30. Available at: www.bmj.com/content/329/7457/92/reply#bmj_el_69225?sid=3ccbd2b2-6802-483a-8a14-9c933f373379 (accessed 19 June 2011).

The most prominent requisite to a lecturer, though perhaps not really the most important, is a good delivery; for though to all true philosophers science and nature will have charms innumerable in every dress, yet I am sorry to say that the generality of mankind cannot accompany us one short hour unless the path is strewn with flowers.

Michael Faraday

Advice to a Lecturer.

As an anesthesiologist, I am always trying to ensure that my subjects are asleep during surgery, while hoping that my residents are awake during my lectures.

Thomas Fuhrman

Fuhrman T. The study of NOELs. *CMAJ.* 2005; 172(12): 1540.

You do not come here as passive receptacles to be filled through books and lectures with a complement of so-called knowledge which shall fit you to answer questions.

William Gull

Gull WW. Introductory address on the study of medicine. *BMJ.* 1874; 2(718): 425–9.

During a great part of the time that he is engaged in attending lectures, and in acquiring a practical knowledge of the subjects which I have mentioned, the student must be in attendance, during some hours of every day, in the wards of the hospital, where he is to acquire such a knowledge of disease as shall enable him to enter upon the practice of his profession with honor to himself, and with safety to the public.

William Guy

Guy WA. Introductory lecture: delivered at King's College, October 1, 1842. *Prov Med J Retrosp Med Sci.* 1842; s1–5(106): 23–32.

Let the pupil, then, aim at the formation of habits of steady application, attending his lectures with scrupulous punctuality, adopting a strict method in his private studies, giving to all laispractical pursuits a zealous and sustained attention and setting his face steadily against all temptations, whether from within or from without, which would allure him from the straight path into which his duty, no less than his interest, have led him.

William Guy

Guy WA. Introductory lecture: delivered at King's College, October 1, 1842. *Prov Med J Retrosp Med Sci.* 1842; s1–5(106): 23–32.

They can scarcely pass a day in the wards of the hospital without perceiving the vast difference which exists between the best descriptions of disease which they have read in books, or heard in the lecture-room, and disease itself.

William Guy

Guy WA. Introductory lecture: delivered at King's College, October 1, 1842. *Prov Med J Retrosp Med Sci.* 1842; s1–5(106): 23–32.

The lecture, as an example of pedagogy, has been a much derided (and much employed) educational tool for the attempted transfer of knowledge from, usually, one individual to many others assumed to be at a lower educational level.

Peter Herbert

Herbert P. The educator is expert; the learner is expert. *Work Based Learn Prim Care.* 2004; 2(3): 280–4(5).

The most essential part of a student's instruction is obtained . . . not in the lecture-room, but at the bedside.

Oliver Wendell Holmes

Scholastic and bedside teaching, from *Medical Essays.*

It has been said that lectures occasion loss of time to the student, and that better information is to be obtained by private reading and reflection.

John Hughes Bennett

Hughes Bennett J. Professor Bennett on medical education. *BMJ.* 1864; 1(180): 649.

It is scarcely necessary to remark upon what is known to all, that the museums of our forefathers were very heterogeneous, and that they oftened catered as much for the love of what is curious as for the love of knowledge.

Jonathan Hutchinson

Hutchinson J. The Bradshaw lecture on museums in their relation to medical education and the progress of knowledge. *BMJ.* 1888; 2(1458): 1257–65.

The process of lecturing is often caricatured as the transferring of the lecturer's notes to the students' notepads without any intervening thinking.
Geoff Isaacs
Isaacs G. Lecture note-taking, learning and recall. *Med Teach.* 1989; 11(3–4): 295–302.

I suspect that the students end up knowing just about the same whether or not they have formal lectures, notes handed out, slide shows, tapes, films, and so forth.
WPU Jackson
Jackson WPU. Personal view. *BMJ.* 1970; 3(5717): 281.

I Think That I Shall Never See, A Lecture Room That's Made for Me.
Charles Johnson
Johnson CF. I think that I shall never see, a lecture room that's made for me: the lecture arena. *Med Teach.* 1986; 8(3): 217–23.

The human classroom of the hospital is obsolete; the lecture format lacks efficiency and may be outmoded.
Jerome Kassirer
Voelker R. AMA, AAMC say reform needed across continuum of US medical education. *JAMA.* 2005; 294(4): 416–17.

Few of us have escaped the dreary experience of dry, disconnected facts being poured out monotonously as flat as dish-water and served up tepid as a lecture.
Arthur King
King A. Universities and medical education. *BMJ.* 1912; 2(2702): 998.

Through handouts, lectures can become portable and enduring.
Kurt Kroenke
Kroenke K. Handouts: making the lecture portable. *Med Teach.* 1991; 13(3): 199–203.

The start of a lecture is most important so do not waste your first sentence by apologising for your presentation or content.
Jennifer Laidlaw
Laidlaw JM. Twelve tips for lecturers. *Med Teach.* 1988; 10(1): 13–17.

Most people tire of a lecture in ten minutes; clever people can do it in five. Sensible people never go to lectures at all.
Stephen Leacock
My Discovery of England. 1922.

Traditional didactic lecture-based teaching is increasingly replaced by problem- or scenario-based learning.
Paul Lee
Lee P. Directile dysfunction. *Med Teach.* 2010; 32(5): 422–4.

John Hunter never had more than 20 students at his lectures, and at the beginning, when a solitary student presented himself, he had to ask the attendant to bring in the skeleton, so that he might address them as "Gentlemen".
William Macewen
Address to the British Medical Association, 1923.

Use handouts as advance organizers which help the students orientate themselves to the purpose of the next lecture and suggest how they can prepare themselves for it.

Ilse Maclean

Maclean I. Twelve tips on providing handouts. *Med Teach.* 1991; 13(1): 7–12.

Hermann Boerhaave lectured five hours a day; his hospital contained only twelve beds, but by Sydenham's method he made of it the medical centre of Europe.

Andrew MacPhail

MacPhail A. An address on the source of modern medicine. *BMJ.* 1933; 1(3767): 443–7.

You can wander about, you can indulge in irritating mannerisms, you can hum and haw, you can remain glued to a desk, you can twiddle your fingers, you can commit all the crimes on the statute book (the latter would make entertaining reading if someone would write it: "The Deadly Sins of the Lecture Theatre"), and you can get away with all of them if, only you have the one supreme virtue. What is that virtue? The name I would give it is vitality.

G Patrick Meredith

Meredith GP. The art of lecturing. *BMJ.* 1950; 2(4677): 475–7.

It is a tiresome way of speaking, when you should despatch the business, to beat about the bush.

Plautus

Mercator.

For the mind does not require filling like a bottle, but rather, like wood, it only requires kindling to create in it an impulse to think independently and an ardent desire for the truth.

Plutarch

Moralia. sect. 48. On listening to lectures.

If I was aware that a lecture on impotence was being given by a urologist whose department was funded by Rhino Horn International my own interpretation of his recommendations would take that into account.

Pawan Randev

Randev P. Competing interests are relevant to lectures approved for PGEA. *BMJ.* 1999; 319(7213): 855.

At my first lecture at medical school, the first lecturer to say anything to us said, "You're extremely privileged to attend this medical school because 70% of you are going to be hospital consultants," and I think this ethos still exists.

Richard Savage

Carnall D. Training for excellence in the inner city: an interview with Richard Savage and Clare Vaughan. *BMJ.* 1996; 313(7056): 544–6.

What is the short meaning of this long harangue?

Friedrich Schiller

Piccolomini.

I will set down what comes from her, to satisfy my remembrance the more strongly.

William Shakespeare

Macbeth. V. i.

Many of my lecturers were content to do little more than churn out standard textbook material, and their manner of presentation was too often repetitive, inaudible, and somniferous.

Michael Shepherd

Shepherd M. Miscellaneous lectures and lecturers. *BMJ.* 1988; 297(6664): 1682–3.

As I am in the mood to proffer advice – enjoy being students – get a stupid hair cut at least once – perhaps even a eyebrow piercing – you must go out at the very least twice a week – dodge a few lectures – don't bother with distinctions or merits they will seem pointless in twenty years – avoid the seriously dull.

Des Spence

Spence D. Dramatic effect. *BMJ.* 2006 August 28. Available at: www.bmj.com/content/333/7565/453.2/reply#bmj_el_140577?sid=20523c27-2e0d-443d-a7db-86e43c2767d3 (accessed 19 June 2011).

In a word, so soon as the learner recognises the fact that he has always within easy reach and awaiting his leisure, not only concise text-books, but the very highest authorities upon every point that his teacher can bring before him, systematic lectures unaccompanied by demonstration sink inevitably into mere routine.

Octavius Sturges

Sturges O. Dissolution of the Medical Teachers' Association. *BMJ.* 1876; 2(834): 840.

The much lectured pupil petrifies or reads a book; the teacher learns to be blind; the Medical Council is ready with sympathy; nothing is done.

Octavius Sturges

Sturges O. Dissolution of the Medical Teachers' Association. *BMJ.* 1876; 2(834): 840.

The great evil of modern medical education is, that it has become a preparation, not for discharging the duties of a profession, but merely for passing examinations which, for the most part, imply neither an accurate knowledge of facts nor the possession of sound principles, being simply affairs of memory loaded with dry terminology, to be thrown overboard at the earliest opportunity.

James Syme

Syme J. Concluding lecture of a winter course on clinical surgery. *BMJ.* 1868; 1(381): 371.

An expert surgeon: someone more than fifty miles from home with a carousel of slides.

Unknown

The formal lecture without demonstrations is a pitiable anachronism. It is a survival from the days when there were no textbooks.

Swale Vincent

Vincent S. Medical research and education. *BMJ.* 1920; 2(3119): 562–5.

Symposia, like hard liquor, should be taken in reasonable measure, at appropriate intervals.

Francis Martin Rouse Walshe

Walshe FMR. *Perspect Biol Med.* 1959; 2: 197.

My own belief is that taking notes is valuable because a second reading of them, not more than a day or two later, stamps the impress of the lecture on the mind, but an accumulation of notes can become an incubus.

Leslie Witts

Witts LJ. Traditional tutorial wisdom. *BMJ.* 1960; 1(5185): 1550, 1551.

Why lecture? Why be lectured? Why, since printing presses have been invented these many centuries, should he [the lecturer] not have printed his lecture instead of speaking it? ... Why continue an obsolete custom, which not merely wastes time and temper, but incites the most debased of human passions – vanity, ostentation, self-assertion and the desire to convert? Why encourage your elders to turn themselves into prigs and prophets, when they are ordinary men and women? Why not abolish prigs and prophets?

Virginia Woolf

Woolf V. Why? In: Woolf V. *The Death of the Moth.* London: Hogarth Press; 1942.

26. SUPERVISION AND MENTORING

Supervision does not have to be solemn.

John Launer

Mentoring encourages constructive reflection before exploring alternative courses of action.

Robert Alliott

Alliott R. Facilitatory mentoring in general practice. *BMJ.* 1996; 313: S2–7060.

Mentoring in general practice facilitates personal/professional development looking at both educational and pastoral issues as a mentee's agenda dictates.

Robert Alliott

Alliott R. Facilitatory mentoring in general practice. *BMJ.* 1996; 313: S2–7060.

The essential requirements for any improvement in the preregistration period must include at least the following: protected time for teaching by senior staff; the continuous availability of senior staff for supervision and support at all times; a well designed rotational scheme of training during the preregistration period; effective formative assessment; enhancement of the teaching skills of consultants and senior grade staff; and regular appraisal of posts by the postgraduate dean or the dean's representatives, or both, and the doctors in training.

Jamie Bahrami

Bahrami J. Improving preregistration training. *BMJ.* 1992; 304(6840): 981.

While medication errors are a significant and perhaps reducible form of error, a virtually unmentioned and at least as significant source of error, are those committed by poorly supervised, sleep deprived, and chronically fatigued juniors/resident physicians.

Bertrand Bell

Bell BM. Poorly supervised juniors (residents) are a significant cause of error. *BMJ.* 2001 March 3. Available at: www.bmj.com/content/322/7285/0.1/reply#bmj_el_12965?sid=bfae656f-d7d3-4ae5-abb6-1b0e432b89b5 (accessed 22 September 2011).

A significant cause of serious errors, including deaths among hospitalized patients, can be attributed to resident physicians who work in GME [graduate medical education] programs that feature as part of their educational structure sleep deprivation, chronic fatigue, and poor supervision.

Bertrand Bell

Bell BM. Reforming graduate medical education. *JAMA.* 2002; 287(6): 715.

Is it right to be involved both with assessing underperformers and recommending and supervising the educational part of their remediation?

Reed Bowden

Bowden R. The underperforming doctor. *Educ Prim Care.* 2002; 13: 223–7.

Personal learning contracts with mentoring is a promising new technique with the potential for general practitioners to recapture personal control over and responsibility for their continuing education.

Peter Burrows

Burrows P. Continuing medical education does not guarantee standards. *BMJ.* 1995; 311(6997): 129.

There appear to be four aspects to work based learning, which takes place when new professionals come into the healthcare workforce. These four aspects are to do with attitude, expertise, collaborative learning and the giving and receiving of what is called variously supervision and mentorship.

Jonathan Burton

Burton J. Changing roles in health care: implications for learning. *Work Based Learn Prim Care.* 2005; 3(2): 95–8(4).

Your relationship as a mentor with your mentee should be one of mutual trust and respect in a supportive yet challenging relationship.

Ruth Chambers

Chambers R. Providing supervision and support. In: Chambers R, Wall D, editors. *Teaching Made Easy: a manual for health professionals.* Oxford: Radcliffe Medical Press; 2000. pp145–61.

May I make a counter suggestion: that we go back to the kind of education that Jenner received – that is, apprenticeship first and science second, when he had become aware of what he needed to know in order to do his job properly.

John Davis

Davis JA. University cuts. *BMJ.* 1982; 285(6347): 1050.

Not surprisingly, unsupervised service experience seems to be no substitute for supervised training.

Sue Dowling

Dowling S. Junior doctors' confidence in their skill in minor surgery. *BMJ.* 1991; 302(6784): 1083.

There is a conflict between service and training. Senior house officers should be able to have their training supervised by consultants instead of learning by the process of see one, do one, teach one.

Donal Duffin

Dillner L. Senior house officers: the lost tribes. *BMJ.* 1993; 307(6918): 1549–51.

In my view asking questions does not merely generate answers, but stimulates thinking and reflection and can be carried out in a way that provides support and care for the practitioner as an integral aspect of clinical supervision.

Helen Halpern

Halpern H. Experience of clinical supervision workshops for general practitioners. *Educ Prim Care*. 2008; 19(1): 90–3.

Some clinicians seem to find it easy to muster their curiosity in order to generate a wide range of questions to use in supervision, while others struggle to maintain a questioning stance and tend to rush in with advice and problem solving.

Helen Halpern

Halpern H. Supervision and the Johari window: a framework for asking questions. *Educ Prim Care*. 2009; 20: 10–14.

The answer to optimising performance is regular compulsory continuing medical education and continuing professional development supported by audit and mentoring, combined with a fair but robust independent inspectorate that can be alerted by safe whistleblowing.

Stephen Hayes

Hayes SF. Where next with revalidation? Make CME and CPD compulsory with support of audit and mentoring. *BMJ*. 2005; 331(7512): 352–3.

Implementing effective role modeling and mentorship involves a wide array of necessary elements that I will not expand on other than to say that the educational environment requires the philosophical, physical, and monetary support of the leadership. From where does the last of these, money, become available?

William James

James WD. Sponsorship of graduate medical education: one successful model. *Arch Dermatol*. 2007; 143(9): 1211–13.

Many so-called 'postmodern' thinkers argue that discovering reality is not an activity like peeling away the layers of an onion, but more like weaving a conversational tapestry, and that truth is largely a matter of consensus rather than exceptional insight.

John Launer

Launer J. Reflective practice and clinical supervision: to delve or not to delve. *Work Based Learn Prim Care*. 2003; 1(2): 147–9(3).

Approaches such as clinical supervision – based on reflection, self-inquiry and mutuality – do not sit comfortably with notions like performance monitoring, assessment, accreditation or revalidation.

John Launer

Launer J. Redefining supervision. *Work Based Learn Prim Care*. 2004; 2(2): 160–2(3).

Fellow educators all seem to understand that training and supervision must incorporate standards if they are to mean anything at all.

John Launer

Launer J. Reflective practice and clinical supervision: developing supervision skills. *Work Based Learn Prim Care*. 2004; 2(3): 264–6(3).

Supervising others exposes you to different minds, different belief systems, and different ways of working. Supervision is therefore an opportunity to allow oneself to be perturbed as well as to perturb others.

John Launer

Launer J. Training GP educators in clinical supervision. *Work Based Learn Prim Care.* 2004; 2(4): 366–9(4).

Feelings have a place in supervision but not an exclusive one, and certainly not to the detriment of thoughts, impressions, intuitions and information.

John Launer

Launer J. Reflective practice and clinical supervision: emotion and interpretation in supervision. *Work Based Learn Prim Care.* 2006; 4(2): 171–3(3).

Much teaching of supervision, and virtually all the literature on the subject, emphasises the importance of understanding supervision as a process of 'bringing forth' rather than 'holding forth'.

John Launer

Launer J. Reflective practice and clinical supervision: neutrality and honesty. *Work Based Learn Prim Care.* 2006; 4(4): 384–6(3).

Supervision does not have to be solemn.

John Launer

Launer J. Reflective practice and clinical supervision: emotion and interpretation in supervision. *Work Based Learn Prim Care.* 2006; 4(2): 171–3(3).

Supervision is not therapy. Supervisors should not aspire to produce personal transformation in their clients, and should actively resist any implied invitation from clients to attempt this.

John Launer

Launer J. Reflective practice and clinical supervision: emotion and interpretation in supervision. *Work Based Learn Prim Care.* 2006; 4(2): 171–3(3).

Supervisors, just like appraisers, often need to reflect on how to manage dilemmas about their authority and their accountability, and what to do if there are concerns about a supervisee's performance.

John Launer

Launer J. Reflective practice and clinical supervision: teaching supervision skills to GP appraisers. *Work Based Learn Prim Care.* 2007; 5(1): 51–4(4).

If you would learn to do a thing, you go to one who does it well; you watch, you listen, and your own first attempts are made under supervision.

Thomas Lewis

Lewis T. The Huxley lecture on clinical science within the university. *BMJ.* 1935; 1(3873): 631–6.

A mentorship then is a fortuitous relationship that fosters the development of the adult learner.

Mark Longhurst

Longhurst MF. The mentoring experience. *Med Teach.* 1994; 16(1): 53–9.

To participate actively in mentoring students, faculty must value that role, seeing it as both rewarding and rewarded.

Mary Pat Mann

Mann MP. Faculty mentors for medical students: a critical review. *Med Teach.* 1992; 14(4): 311–19.

Supervised clinical practice forms a substantial element in most training schemes for the health care professions, yet no straightforward method exists to allow for the exchange of information necessary to promote best practice for training across disciplines.

Celia McCrea

McCrea C. The quality delivery process: a useful framework for quality improvement initiatives in training? *Med Teach.* 1996; 18(4): 300–3.

The improvement in students is largely due to the increased personal contact of the students with their teachers, and to the greater extent of personal supervision by the teachers of the studies of each student.

Norman Moore

Moore N. Medical education in London. *BMJ.* 1878; 2(928): 581.

For various reasons, some contractual and some personal, consultants find it scarcely possible to do much about the poorly performing trainee doctor except to restrict his areas of work and supervise him closely until he moves on and becomes someone else's problem.

Philip Rhodes

Rhodes P. Incompetence in medical practice. *BMJ.* 1986; 292(6531): 1293–4.

The challenge for each teaching institution that wants to survive is to find the changes in structure, schedules, supervision, and education that will help residents provide quality and efficiency in patient care.

Terrill Rosborough

Rosborough TK. Doctors in training: wasteful and inefficient? Not if the training is properly structured and supervised. *BMJ.* 1998; 316: 1107.

E-mentoring is effective, enhances face-to-face interaction with colleagues and should be driven by learning needs and educational principles.

Markus Schichtel

Schichtel M. A conceptual description of potential scenarios of e-mentoring in GP specialist training. *Educ Prim Care.* 2009; 20(5): 360–4.

Problems arise when the teacher, mentor or tutor is also responsible for assessment, a situation that now exists within the GP registrar-trainer relationship.

Jill Thistlethwaite

Thistlethwaite J. Reflection on 'reflections on the ethics of assessment'. *Educ Prim Care.* 2004; 15: 125.

The appointment of clinical supervisors and the introduction of structured education and training will be effective only if there are profound conceptual changes in the understanding of the purpose of the preregistration year, if there are contractual agreements to enable the educational supervisor to fulfil the role, and if there is financial provision for the training of trainers and regular formative assessment of the trainees.

David Wilson

Wilson DH. Education and training of preregistration house officers: the consultants' viewpoint. *BMJ.* 1993; 306(6871): 194–6.

What does the patient think about a surgical trainee performing his first unsupervised appendectomy or his first unsupervised bowel resection? Yet, conversely does the patient want a fully qualified surgeon who has never operated unsupervised whilst training?

Kenneth Wong

Wong K. The ethics of medical training. *BMJ.* 2003 August 9. Available at: www.bmj.com/content/327/7410/326/reply#bmj_el_35607?sid=7f27ee1c-bc1e-486c-bc82-03a5164885cc (accessed 22 September 2011).

27. LEADERSHIP AND CHANGE

> Somewhere betwixt and between the extremes of the dynamic power seeker who triples his efforts as he loses sight of his goals and the ineffectual one driven about by every casual breeze, we find good deans of good medical schools who produce the inspiration and leadership as well as exert the firm hand of the helmsman in just the right combination.
>
> **William Bean**

Deans of medicine must be born. They are certainly not made.

Donald Acheson

Acheson D. University, medical school, and community. *BMJ.* 1970; 2(5711): 683–7.

Deans need to focus on the broad scope and to translate their dreams into applied institutional operations and functions.

Bharat Bassaw

Bassaw B. Determinants of successful deanship. *Med Teach.* 2010; 32(12): 1002–6.

Deans are harassed by demands for space, money, beds, teaching, research, with a groundswell of complaints from those in practice that doctors are getting "too scientific."

William Bean

Bean WB. Money and medical schools. *Arch Intern Med.* 1963; 111(6): 841–2.

Somewhere betwixt and between the extremes of the dynamic power seeker who triples his efforts as he loses sight of his goals and the ineffectual one driven about by every casual breeze, we find good deans of good medical schools who produce the inspiration and leadership as well as exert the firm hand of the helmsman in just the right combination.

William Bean

Bean WB. Fundamentals of medical education. *Arch Intern Med.* 1965; 115(4): 500–1.

It is high time those who are in charge of medical education took into account the aspirations of those for whom the education is intended.

Donald Bowers

Bowers DM. Career structure and casualty departments. *BMJ.* 1972; 1(5792): 114.

No academic person is ever voted into the chair until he has reached an age at which he has forgotten the meaning of the word 'irrelevant'.

Francis Cornford

Microcosmographia Academica. 1908.

Humility may clothe an English dean.

William Cowper

Truth.

There is so much change for change's sake in education that we should be very careful to do only what is likely to prove good and useful in changing our educational system.

TC Dann

Dann TC. Interviews for prospective students. *BMJ*. 1972; 2(5808): 293.

If we want things to stay as they are, things will have to change.

Giuseppe di Lampedusa

The Leopard. 1957.

In the country of the blind will managers with an understanding of clinical concepts be the one eyed?

Liam Donaldson

Donaldson L. Book review: medicine and books. *BMJ*. 1993; 307: 572.

It is encouraging that medical schools have started to change their curricula to include communication skills training, but many still use inappropriate teaching methods.

Lesley Fallowfield

Fallowfield LJ. Things to consider when teaching doctors how to deliver good, bad and sad news. *Med Teach*. 1996; 18(1): 27–30.

It would not be at all a bad thing if the elite of the medical world would be a little less clever, and would adopt a more primitive method of thinking, and reason more as children do.

Georg Groddeck

Letter XII, from *The Book of the It*.

There must always be an aristocracy in every profession.

Henry Holland

Edin MD. The present influence of Oxford upon medical education. *BMJ*. 1878; 1(893): 214.

And in the case of Mr. Brudenell Carter, who represents the Apothecaries' Society, we have the unedifying spectacle of a seat on the General Medical Council being occupied by a man who is sent there by a handful of City grocers who have not a particle of medical education about them.

Victor Horsley

Horsley V. The Direct Representatives' Meeting at Newcastle. *BMJ*. 1899; 2(2030): 1501–11.

Professors must live: to live they must occupy themselves with practice, and if they occupy themselves with practice, the pursuit of the abstract branches of science must go to the wall.

Thomas Huxley

Huxley TH. *Critiques and Addresses*. London: Macmillan; 1873. p66.

The difficulty is that a large portion of our pedagogues and so-called learned men know nothing else than Greek and Latin, and are anxious to continue earning an easy livelihood by teaching them.

William Ireland

Ireland WW. A universal language for medical men. *BMJ*. 1895; 1(1782): 447–8.

By the time a man has attained some weight in the profession he may (happily it is not always the case) have lost interest in those fundamental studies which form the secure foundation of medical knowledge.

Ray Lankester

Lankester ER. Biology and medical students. *BMJ*. 1885; 2(1279): 42–3.

That state of resentful coma . . . dons dignify by the name of research.

Harold Laski

Letter to Oliver Wendell Holmes.

Hippocrates and Maimonides still abide, but the vast changes in situation and circumstance since they spoke create the need for other canons.

Jennifer Leaning

Leaning J. Human rights and medical education: why every medical student should learn the Universal Declaration of Human Rights. *BMJ*. 1997; 315: 1390–1.

A medical school is a vibrant place. Such a powerhouse of intellect and achievement needs a firm hand inside the supple glove of deanship if ideas are to be converted into opportunities and students are to become the doctors the country needs.

Brian Livesley

Livesley B. Book review: medicine and books. *BMJ*. 1989; 299: 1172.

We frequently hear that the United States has one of the best – if not the best – medical education systems in the world. However, with the same frequency, detractors complain about the system's resistance to improvements and change.

Carlos Martini

Martini CJM. Partnerships in medical education. *JAMA*. 1991; 266(7): 996–1000.

GERONTE: It seems to me you are locating them wrongly: the heart is on the left and the liver is on the right.

SGANARELLE: Yes, in the old days that was so, but we have changed all that, and we now practise medicine by a completely new method.

Molière

La Medecin malgre lui. 1667.

In short the teacher in a university is the pivot of the method. He must be learned in his subject, skilled in craft, competent in administration, experienced in research, and catholic in mind. He should reach his post not by favour, by merit of age or seniority, by social convention, but chiefly because he is a teacher and a leader of men.

George Newman

Newman G. *Some Notes on Medical Education in England: a memorandum presented to the president of the board.* London: HMSO; 1918. p24.

Would you know the signs by which in man or an institution you may recognise old fogeyism? They are three: First, a state of blissful happiness and contentment with things as they are; secondly, a supreme conviction that the condition of other people and other institutions is one of pitiable inferiority; thirdly, a fear of change which not alone perplexes but appals.

William Osler

Osler W. An address on the importance of post-graduate study: delivered at the opening of the museums of the Medical Graduates College and Polyclinic, July 4th, 1900. *BMJ.* 1900; 2(2063): 73–5.

Without effective, dedicated and motivated educational personnel supported by a properly resourced infrastructure, less rather than more educational activity will take place.

John Pitts

Pitts J. Plus ça change . . . course organisers' remuneration today. *Educ Prim Care.* 2002; 13: 18–19.

Immediately I became sub-dean at Barts there was a great stamping of feet into my office, with complaints about everything. I cannot remember half of them, but it was a depressing experience to hear young men and women complaining of all the inadequacies that they perceived in the educational process that they had been through for five years.

Lesley Rees

Lowry S. What's wrong with medical education in Britain? *BMJ.* 1992; 305(6864): 1277–80.

Medical schools face challenges in their missions of education, research, and patient care that call for effective leadership at all levels of the organization.

John Rogers

Rogers J. Aspiring to leadership: identifying teacher-leaders. *Med Teach.* 2005; 27(7): 629–33.

Our profession cannot be and will not be immune from major social change, and history repeatedly shows us that we have a choice: we can either provide leadership that understands society's evolving expectations or have change forced upon us.

Peter Rubin

Rubin P. Christmas 2008: formative years; not what we used to be? *BMJ.* 2008; 337: 2905.

A major question facing the Commons Social Services Committee in its inquiry into medical education is how to change the balance between the number of consultants (currently too few) and the number of junior staff (too many). The committee is all too painfully aware that nobody likes to have his retinue cut and equally that someone who has lived in the expectation of acquiring one in due course does not like being deprived of his hopes.

William Russell

Russell W. Mrs Short tackles the numbers game. *BMJ (Clin Res Ed).* 1981; 282(6267): 916.

Successful change in the behaviour of healthcare workers, to produce more effective and efficient care, requires that these workers have the opportunity to integrate the explicit knowledge with their tacit knowledge.

John Sandars

Sandars J. Knowledge management: we've only just begun! *Work Based Learn Prim Care.* 2004; 2(3): 208–13(6).

Equipping doctors to adapt to change is becoming an increasingly important part of continued education.

Theo Schofield

Schofield TPC. Personal view: the aims of continuing education in general practice. *Med Teach.* 1985; 7(2): 225–30.

There are few activities in which Britain plays a leading world part but academic medicine (along with rock music) is one of them, and destroying that excellence would be very short sighted.

Richard Smith

Smith R. The starving of the medical schools. *BMJ (Clin Res Ed).* 1982; 284(6312): 335–7.

Dispassionate survey of the history of medicine in the nineteenth and early part of the twentieth century leaves no doubt that England compared badly with other countries and Germany assumed the undisputed leadership.

Arthur Thomson

Thomson A. History and development of teaching hospitals in England. *BMJ.* 1960; 2(5201): 749–51.

One change that I would like to propose is that the universities concentrate on running courses in medical science resulting in an honours or pass degree, and leave the teaching of clinical medicine entirely to the National Health Service.

WR Timperley

Timperley WR. Medical education. *BMJ (Clin Res Ed).* 1982; 285(6348): 1121.

From what I have said earlier you will not be surprised to hear that any reform of medical education should, in my view, be aimed at preparing a doctor to live with change – and rapid change at that.

Alexander Todd

Todd A. The doctor in a changing world. *BMJ.* 1968; 4(5625): 207–9.

28. EDUCATIONAL ENVIRONMENT

The connection between teaching and learning is so profound, it is surprising that teaching hospitals are not called learning hospitals.

David Pencheon

The hospital is the only proper College in which to rear a true disciple of Aesculapius.

John Abernethy

Keynes G. The Oslerian tradition. *BMJ.* 1968; 4(5631): 599–604.

Is there not needed in the medical schools not only more training in psychiatry, but an incorporation in the teaching of all branches of medicine of a due appreciation of the emotional background of disease?

Sidney Abrahams

Abrahams S. Just what the doctor ordered. *BMJ.* 1960; 2(5196): 466.

It is unconscionable to continue to insist that junior doctors work 19th century hours in an evolved epoch like today's, where work-home balance and personal health and wellbeing are rightly considered important. "Because we did it" doesn't mean they should.

Margaret Allen

Allen ME. Surgeon training and physician assistants. *BMJ.* 2009 November 10. Available at: www.bmj.com/content/339/bmj.b4488/reply#bmj_el_226755?sid=c01598e6-7fa7-4552-bbff-d3bc10847fd9 (accessed 22 September 2011).

Medical educators have a responsibility to foster a learning environment that equally enables all students to succeed.

Brenda Beagan

Beagan BL. Everyday classism in medical school: experiencing marginality and resistance. *Med Educ.* 2005; 39(8): 777–84.

Anyone who has trained in general and teaching hospitals cannot help but notice the disparity of clinical skills. Without doubt trainees are being trained and taught by those with inadequate skills.

Ian Beales

Beales I. Valuing clinical skills. *BMJ.* 2000 July 11. Available at: www.bmj.com/content/320/7251/1739.1/reply#bmj_el_8533?sid=7f1b5b2e-7b0c-43f6-8a46-f45951808b4f (accessed 22 September 2011).

Medical education should re-examine the emphasis it places on the importance of the integration of mind, body, and spirit and acknowledge the role of social, cultural, and environmental influences and the power of self care and healing.

Brian Berman

Berman BM. Complementary medicine and medical education: teaching complementary medicine offers a way of making teaching more holistic. *BMJ.* 2001; 322(7279): 121–2.

Unless a solution is found, the proposed increase in teaching in the community will probably be on an ad hoc basis, as at present, relying on enthusiasm that may peter out.

DF Bird

Bird DF. Teaching students in the community. *BMJ.* 1994; 309(6963): 1229.

Will students learn paediatrics from one who has never seen the appalling difficulties of the working-class mother trying to rear a baby in one room in a condemned slum?

J Vernon Braithwaite

Braithwaite JV. Damnable heresy? *BMJ.* 1952; 1(4675): 974.

Acute disease must be seen at least once a day by those who wish to learn; in many cases twice a day will not be too often.

Richard Bright

Reports of Medical Cases.

There seems to be a poor person-environment fit in medical education at present.

Chris Bundy

Bundy C. McManus is right but for the wrong reasons. *BMJ.* 2003 January 17. Available at: www.bmj.com/content/325/7368/786/reply#bmj_el_28867?sid=7f27ee1c-bc1e-486c-bc82-03a5164885cc (accessed 22 September 2011).

The true University of these days is a collection of books.

Thomas Carlyle

On Heroes, Hero-Worship, and the Heroic in History. 1841.

Remember that a teacher does not just need sufficient knowledge, skills and resources, but also the right attitudes and understanding of the overall context and cultural environment to be able to make the teaching relevant to the learner's needs.

Ruth Chambers

Chambers R. Teaching and education should be relevant to the needs of the learner, patients and the NHS as a whole. In: Chambers R, Wall D, editors. *Teaching Made Easy: a manual for health professionals.* Oxford: Radcliffe Medical Press; 2000. pp1–27.

It is someone's business in every medical school to teach laboratory methods to the students but it is no one's particular business to teach them how to use medical literature . . . Short talks on the use of the library might well be made an obligatory sectional exercise for students.

Harvey Cushing

Cushing H. Bookshelf browsing: the doctor and his books. *Amer J Surg.* 1928; 4(1): 100–10.

The African continent is short of doctors and the obvious place to train doctors for Africa is in Africa. This requires medical schools. But as soon as these two simple statements are accepted, problems crowd around the scene like bees around a honeypot.

Lindsay Davidson

Davidson L. The setting up of a new medical school. *Postgrad Med J.* 1965; 41: 61–6.

There are more senior house officers than doctors in any other training grade in Britain but nobody knows what they do in hospitals or has a clear idea what skills they should be learning.

Luisa Dillner

Dillner L. Senior house officers: the lost tribes. *BMJ.* 1993; 307(6918): 1549–51.

Medical education is built on the myth of the general physician and surgeon, and students are disproportionately exposed to these subjects.

AB Drake-Lee

Drake-Lee AB. The general surgeon. *BMJ (Clin Res Ed).* 1986; 292(6525): 956.

The domestic relationship between the health care provision system and the content and processes of medical education defies easy classification. It is not even clear that the two are legally married, though there is certainly a common-law union.

H Jack Geiger

Geiger HJ. Educational implications of changing methods of health care provision. *Am J Dis Child.* 1974; 127(4): 554–8.

The world of medical education is far from being a level playing field; it is unfairly angled towards a fortunate few: is the remit of international medical education to level that playing field and correct the infectious and dangerous divide that exists at present?

Trevor Gibbs

Gibbs T. Medical education in Africa: not always a level playing field. *Med Teach.* 2007; 29(9–10): 853–4.

Medical training is "situated learning" – that is, the trainee participates in practice, initially on the periphery and finally as a central and highly skilled practitioner.

Janet Grant

Grant J. The Calman report and specialist training: Calman report builds on the status quo. *BMJ.* 1993; 306(6894): 1756.

Health centres in the teaching of social health correspond to hospitals in the teaching of clinical medicine.

John Grant

Grant JB. Social medicine in the curriculum. *BMJ.* 1948; 1(4546): 333–6.

As a physician who left the profession, I was left with a strong sense that the quality and extent of medical education differs not only between medical schools, but also for individuals within medical schools, dependent on their exposure to the clinical environment in the "firm" system.

Alexander Gray

Gray A. Robust revalidation needs to start with appropriate validation. *BMJ.* 2005 July 5. Available at: www.bmj.com/content/330/7506/1504/reply#bmj_el_111298?sid=cb764c2a-ad1a-4f84-a8c4-88b3568c267c (accessed 22 September 2011).

Reflection on practice, asking why, what and how with a colleague skilled in the coaching function of clinical supervision, in a safe environment is a powerful tool for identifying learning needs and developing practice.

Brenda Greaves

Greaves B. Professional development and nursing: practice nursing. *Work Based Learn Prim Care.* 2004; 2(1): 79–81(3).

Preventive medicine, though of such recent growth, has made such rapid progress and is so powerful for good in the hands of the practitioner, that to send men out of our schools instructed only in the cure of disease, and ignorant of all that is known as to its cause and prevention, seems not only short sighted, but culpable conduct.

John Haddon

Haddon J. The teaching of public medicine. *BMJ.* 1890; 2(1542): 178–9.

Professional expertise relies not only on medical knowledge and skills but also on adequate knowledge of the specificities of the working environment and awareness of teamwork related factors.

Guy Haller

Haller G. Increase in the rate of undesirable events at the beginning of the academic year: a universal problem. *BMJ.* 2009 November 9. Available at: www.bmj.com/content/339/bmj.b3974/reply#bmj_el_225033?sid=c01598e6-7fa7-4552-bbff-d3bc10847fd9 (accessed 22 September 2011).

Medical students can, and almost certainly should, be placed in a diverse range of clinical settings in order to achieve the learning objectives of current medical courses.
Richard Hays

Hays R. Teaching in common clinical settings. In: Hays R. *Teaching and Learning in Clinical Settings.* Oxford: Radcliffe Publishing; 2006. pp57–78.

It seems to me, therefore, that our main object in training is to give our students the intellectual equipment to meet this challenge of our technological society.
Kenneth Hill

Hill KR. Some reflections on medical education and teaching in the developing countries. *BMJ.* 1962; 2(5304): 585–7.

Management training should start with junior doctors so that clinicians are familiar with the organisation developing around them.
Russell Hopkins

Hopkins R. Doctors as general managers: to be or not be. *BMJ (Clin Res Ed).* 1987; 295(6609): 1360–2.

Excessive hours of work hamper rather than help junior doctors in attaining adequate training opportunities, and clearly the opportunity should be taken to ensure optimal training within the context of lower hours of work, emphasising contact with senior staff with formal organised didactic teaching, and with more time available to read and assimilate information.
Stephen Hunter

Hunter S. Commitment vital for new deal. *BMJ.* 1991; 303(6806): 840–1.

In the era of managed health care there never was a clearer need for the medical profession as a whole to have its own strong and coherent sense of direction for medical education.
Donald Irvine

Irvine D. Educating general practitioners. *BMJ.* 1993; 307(6906): 696–7.

Who among those educated at one of the older teaching hospitals can doubt that the monastic tradition has descended in strong measure through the hundreds of years from their early foundation?
Donald Mcl. Johnson

Johnson DM. A G.P. on his clinical training. *BMJ.* 1950; 2(4677): 493–6.

Medical education should not be regarded as a series of separated compartments. Like all other forms of education it is a continuum.
Robert Kilpatrick

Kilpatrick R. Profile of the GMC: portrait or caricature? *BMJ.* 1989; 299(6691): 109–12.

I contend that the proper homes for medical study and medical education are universities.
Ray Lankester

Lankester ER. Introductory address, delivered in the Medical Department of University College, at the opening of the session 1879. *BMJ.* 1878; 2(927): 501–7.

While clinical exposure is necessary for clinical learning, it is not sufficient.
Sam Leinster

Leinster S. Learning in the clinical environment. *Med Teach.* 2009; 31(2): 79–81.

The problem with medical education is that it is delivered by academic subspecialists who generalize their 1–2% referred population experience to our 98–99% general practice experience.

Herschel Lessin

Personal correspondence, 30 June 2011.

The long hours worked by preregistration house officers, the high service commitment, and the low rating given to the educational aspects of the job have led to numerous criticisms of this part of medical education.

Stella Lowry

Lowry S. Medical education: the preregistration year. *BMJ*. 1993; 306(6871): 196–8.

Confessing that no one can learn everything, it becomes a question of selection, and of determining in any given case what is really ad hoc, what is the particular knowledge which the student requires, and how much of this he can be taught in the circumstances in which he is placed.

Howard Marsh

Marsh H. An address on the education of the student of medicine: delivered at the opening of the winter session (1910–1911), in the Medical Department of the University of Leeds. *BMJ*. 1910; 2(2598): 1105–8.

The US graduate medical education system has been strongly criticized by policymakers and by private and public agencies for not being responsive to the population's health needs.

Carlos Martini

Martini CJM. Graduate medical education in the changing environment of medicine. *JAMA*. 1992; 268(9): 1097–105.

Although most patients accept that doctors in training must develop their clinical skills, the presence of a student might add to the arousal that the medical environment already imposes on a patient.

Jan Matthys

Matthys JH. Impact on patients of general practice based, student teaching. *BMJ*. 2005 July 25. Available at: www.bmj.com/content/331/7508/89/reply#bmj_el_112988?sid=cb764c2a-ad1a-4f84-a8c4-88b3568c267c (accessed 22 September 2011).

The education of the preregistration house officer would be greatly improved if he could have seven or eight hours' supervised work each week in the nearest medical school, which would usually be his own.

Harry May

May HB. Day release for house officers. *BMJ*. 1970; 2(5703): 234.

Exposure to primary care allows students to learn the use of clinical skills to make or exclude diagnoses in patients when they first present; demonstrate prevalence of illness in populations and therefore provide more reasonable ideas of probability; and show the natural history of chronic illness and the interactions between disease, person, and environment.

David Metcalfe

Metcalfe D. London after Tomlinson: care in the capital; what needs to be done. *BMJ*. 1992; 305(6862): 1141–4.

The training of the medical school gives a man his direction, points him the way, and furnishes a chart, fairly incomplete, for the voyage but nothing more.
William Osler

Osler W. An address on the importance of post-graduate study: delivered at the opening of the museums of the Medical Graduates College and Polyclinic, July 4th, 1900. *BMJ.* 1900; 2(2063): 73–5.

In no way can a society better help in the education of its members than in maintaining for them a good library.
William Osler

Osler W. On the educational value of the medical society. In: Osler W. *Aequanimitas, With Other Addresses to Medical students, Nurses and Practitioners of Medicine.* London; 1904.

If you want to recruit medical academics you must re-create medical schools and put the scientists out to institutes, or perhaps pasture, the latter being a more useful and cheaper option.
David Paratt

Paratt D. Not just a question of money. *BMJ.* 2000 March 7. Available at: www.bmj.com/content/320/7235/591/reply#bmj_el_6941?sid=7f1b5b2e-7b0c-43f6-8a46-f45951808b4f (accessed 22 September 2011).

It is always difficult to write specifically about medical education while acknowledging its interrelation with service and manpower.
James Parkhouse

Parkhouse J. Stars and stripes: for ever? *BMJ (Clin Res Ed).* 1983; 286(6368): 825–6.

The object of medical education is to make medical practitioners. Now the business of a medical practitioner is, as we full well know, of a highly multifarious kind.
Joshua Parsons

Parsons J. Medical education. *BMJ.* 1864; 1(168): 326–7.

Disconnection between workaday educators in primary care and those responsible for the educational systems and governance is highly detrimental.
Ed Peile

Peile E. Educational management: a neglected area. *Educ Prim Care.* 2009; 20(3): 137–8.

The connection between teaching and learning is so profound, it is surprising that teaching hospitals are not called learning hospitals.
David Pencheon

Pencheon D. Development of generic skills. *BMJ.* 1998; 317(7160): S2.

The present climate in medicine is one in which individualism is to be shunned and replaced by a form of collectivism.
James Penston

Penston J. The intolerant streak in current medical education . . . *BMJ.* 2006 September 13. Available at: www.bmj.com/content/333/7567/518/reply#bmj_el_141733?sid=20523c27-2e0d-443d-a7db-86e43c2767d3 (accessed 22 September 2011).

It is quite rare to find nurses, midwives, radiographers, and physiotherapists, in higher education, who carry a significant clinical workload.
Robert Pittilo

Pittilo RM. Should nurses who teach also practise? *BMJ.* 1998 September 3. Available at: www.bmj.com/content/317/7157/546.1/reply#bmj_el_697?sid=6a4ef178-62d7-4865-ac37-192d0fd43924 (accessed 22 September 2011).

In conclusion, the present system of medical education is one gigantic obstacle race for registration, and it abounds in trickery, triviality, and trash; and the whole organization needs revitalizing ere it can be said to the newly-fledged practitioner, "Thou art a piece of virtue; I doubt not but thy training hath been noble" (Shakespeare).

Dobson Poole

Poole D. Medical education. *BMJ.* 1902; 2(2171): 426.

Although virtue receives some of its excellencies from nature, yet it is perfected by education.

Quintilian

De Institutione Oratoria.

There remains an immature culture within our medical training which is hard to define. GPs might offer "maturity" training.

Peter Reynolds

Reynolds P. GP's might offer "maturity" training. *BMJ.* 2001 March 27. Available at: www.bmj.com/content/322/7288/709/reply#bmj_el_13530?sid=bfae656f-d7d3-4ae5-abb6-1b0e432b89b5 (accessed 22 September 2011).

Are we really prepared to see medical education and science jeopardised by the uncertain outcome of a market environment aimed at solving completely different problems?

Peter Richards

Richards P. University hospitals and the NHS review. *BMJ.* 1990; 300(6718): 138–9.

Well supervised training during limited hours in the front line of service needs to be complemented by withdrawal to an uninterrupted, reflective educational programme.

Peter Richards

Richards P. Improving preregistration training. *BMJ.* 1992; 304(6840): 1510.

The teaching staff of the graduate hospital and school raise some difficult points; its members should be well known for their teaching ability and in the full tide of their energies.

Humphry Rolleston

Rolleston H. The aims and methods of graduate study. *BMJ.* 1920; 1(3081): 77–9.

An interest in disease and all that it means draws men, according to their habit of mind, in one of three directions: (1) to practise medicine, curative and preventive; (2) to investigate the problems of disease; or (3) to teach others.

Humphry Rolleston

Rolleston H. Medicine as a career. *BMJ.* 1930; 2(3642): 699–2.

Here, surely, is a gap in medical education, that we teach so much about man and pay such scant attention to his surroundings.

John Ryle

Ryle JA. To-day and to-morrow. *BMJ.* 1940; 2(4167): 657–9.

Good gracious, you've got to educate him first. You can't expect a boy to be vicious until he's been to a good school.

Saki

Saki: Reginald in Russia. 1910.

The chief, the long-existing and, I grieve to say it, the still prominent evils among us are the neglect of general education, the confounding of instruction with education, and the giving of greater importance to the special training than to the general culture of the student.

William Stokes

O'Brien E. William Stokes 1804–78: the development of a doctor. *BMJ.* 1978; 2(6139): 749–50.

The function of universities, at least those so situated, in relation to medical education especially, should be that of great scientific schools, and not centres for practical clinical study.

William Stokes

Stokes W. The address in surgery. *BMJ.* 1882; 2(1128): 256–61.

In developing a climate of continuous learning and improvement we are in effect building a learning organisation.

Tim Swanwick

Swanwick T. Organisational structure and culture in postgraduate general practice education: implications for the management and leadership of change. *Educ Prim Care.* 2005; 16: 115–28.

I feel that the British method of teaching is the best, and that we should not attempt to copy the foreigner.

John Swift Joly

Swift Joly J. Training of the urologist. *BMJ.* 1930; 1(3603): 171–2.

A human being cannot become intellectual property and her/his freedom of movement cannot be restricted. Thus, both developed and developing countries together have to address the problems that lead to the brain drain.

Guillermo Herrera Taracena

Taracena GAH. Trained to become Westernized. *BMJ.* 2002 March 6. Available at: www.bmj.com/content/324/7336/499/reply#bmj_el_20334?sid=d5e693ea-0765-423d-ac1d-1c98624d8fdf (accessed 22 September 2011).

Shared decision making does need to begin in primary care, but we will need to alter the learning and working environments to ensure a good outcome.

Jill Thistlethwaite

Thistlethwaite JE. Shared decision making: a need for education. *BMJ.* 2004 November 19. Available at: www.bmj.com/content/329/7476/1197/reply#bmj_el_86043?sid=3f545f3a-8b62-4679-979a-2c0b244a4cd7 (accessed 22 September 2011).

Conventional medical training is fine in certain respects but not in the management of uncertainty or setting objectives in functional terms concerning those with chronic illness.

Malcolm Keith Thompson

Thompson MK. Child health surveillance. *BMJ.* 1990; 300(6723): 536.

Climate studies are undertaken in order to determine how students experience the educational environment generated by a curriculum.

Hettie Till

Till H. Identifying the perceived weaknesses of a new curriculum by means of the Dundee Ready Education Environment Measure (DREEM) Inventory. *Med Teach.* 2004; 26(1): 39–45.

As educational climate strongly affects student achievement, satisfaction and success, it is important to get regular feedback from students on how they experience the educational environment.

Hettie Till

Till H. Climate studies: can students' perceptions of the ideal educational environment be of use for institutional planning and resource utilization? *Med Teach.* 2005; 27(4): 332–7.

The dean warned about the dangers of alcohol. And the new students went off to do the "four legged stagger" and vomit themselves witless round Paddington. 0 tempora, 0 Mary's.

Richard Wakeford

Wakeford R. Medicine and the media. *BMJ.* 1986; 293: 127.

A good supportive educational climate is very important in motivating trainees to learn.

David Wall

Wall D. Educational concepts: the theory behind the practical aspects of teaching and learning. In: Chambers R, Wall D, editors. *Teaching Made Easy: a manual for health professionals.* Oxford: Radcliffe Medical Press; 2000. pp29–57.

A hospital is an institution absolutely essential to a medical school, and one which would afford relief and comfort to thousands of the sick and miserable.

John Collins Warren

Fundraising letter, 20 August 1810.

In many universities now students receive little by way of teaching from the faculty, so consumed are the latter with grant writing and pursuing their own, often esoteric, interests. This has led to severe myopia on the part of academia as a whole; it has simply lost sight of the big picture, its members living out a life of unreality in their own respective ivory towers.

Neil Watson

Watson N. New directions for academic medicine. *BMJ.* 2003 November 21. Available at: www.bmj.com/content/327/7422/1001/reply#bmj_el_39485?sid=7f27ee1c-bc1e-486c-bc82-03a5164885cc (accessed 22 September 2011).

The stress placed on American graduate medical education is merely a symptom of a health care system continually being asked to do more with less.

Peter Watson

Watson PY. The working and learning environment for physicians in training in the US. *BMJ.* 2003; 327: 88.

Airline pilots are a modern trade, born into a modern age with sophisticated citizens and a strong legislative framework, even back when airlines first started and more so today. Doctors share this environment now but medicine developed as a profession with unsophisticated citizens, a much weaker framework of government and legislation and much greater emphasis on self-employment.

Peter West

West PA. Pilots, doctors and the history of the job. *BMJ.* 2002 August 9. Available at: www.bmj.com/content/324/7345/1105.1/reply#bmj_el_21991?sid=d5e693ea-0765-423d-ac1d-1c98624d8fdf (accessed 3 August 2011).

It is a defect in our medical education that the student entering medicine, usually with the idea of general practice, is kept for six to nine years in an artificial environment and is not shown the variety of work available.

Leslie Witts

Witts LJ. Happy at work. *BMJ.* 1952; 2(4782): 478.

29. AMBULATORY CARE AND GENERAL PRACTICE

Clinical medicine is best learnt through apprenticeship, and general practice offers an ideal opportunity for this.

Raymond Hoffenberg

The young medical man who intends, from the moment of qualification, or from the day on which he finishes his term of duty on the hospital house staff, to live by general practice knows little or nothing of the prejudices of patients, and not very much of minor maladies or prescribing, unless he be the son of a doctor.

Senex Adolescens

Adolescens S. Curriculum and apprenticeship. *BMJ.* 1888; 2(1454): 1075.

And the family physician needs something more than technical education; he needs a larger and less wasteful life.

Thomas Clifford Allbutt

Allbutt TC. Medical education in England: a note on Sir George Newman's memorandum to the president of the Board of Education. *BMJ.* 1918; 2(3005): 113–15.

Our system of medical education continues to produce physicians for speciality practice rather than for the delivery of primary or continuing comprehensive care.

Joel Alpert

Alpert JJ. Educating the physician toward a solution. *Arch Intern Med.* 1971; 127(1): 85–8.

Regulations for vocational training have served us well in the past, but it is now time to move on by revoking all of these and allowing general practice, like any other medical discipline, to decide for itself, through its college, what system of education it should have.

Jamie Bahrami

Bahrami J. General practice must decide on its own education system. *BMJ.* 1998; 316(7139): 1246.

To be a good general practitioner a young doctor must himself experience the conditions of general practice, guided at first by an older man, but free to improve on his predecessor.

Geoffrey Barber

Barber G. Education in general practice. *BMJ.* 1952; 2(4782): 490–1.

Whilst student preparedness is highly desirable for all clinical learning, it is particularly important that those in ambulatory care settings are sufficiently well-prepared to allow them to make good use of both their time and that of their teachers.

Sharon Buckley

Buckley SG. Teaching in ambulatory care settings: further issues to consider. *BMJ.* 2008 September 30. Available at: www.bmj.com/content/337/bmj.a1156/reply#bmj_el_202624?sid=90b7a8a2-7af4-4018-b137-261049bb6944 (accessed 3 August 2011).

Now, we are all agreed (and we should be allowed to have an opinion) that it is indispensible for the public good, that the general practitioner should be in every respect as thoroughly educated as possible.

James Cole

Cole J. Proposal to incorporate the eighteen thousand licentiates of the hall into a royal college of medicine and midwifery. *Prov Med Surg J.* 1845; s1–9(2): 29–31.

As with most attitudes and prejudices, education and personal experience may change the sometimes judgmental attitudes towards general practice of newly qualified house officers, particularly those intending to enter hospital practice.

David D'Cruz

D'Cruz DP. Preregistration rotation including general practice. *BMJ.* 1985; 291(6490): 280–1.

Those of us who teach in the increasingly important setting of general practice indeed find that a great deal of what we demonstrate is caring for chronic illness.

James Dickinson

Dickinson J. SNAPPS becomes SINAPPS in general practice teaching. *BMJ.* 2003 December 15. Available at: www. bmj.com/content/327/7428/1393/reply#bmj_el_44830?sid=7f27ee1c-bc1e-486c-bc82-03a5164885cc (accessed 3 August 2011).

Learning organisational culture can help to provide the adaptability which allows general practice to respond to continuous change within the NHS [National Health Service].

Craig Dobson

Dobson C. Can the key characteristics of a learning organisation be found in our general practice? *Educ Prim Care.* 2008; 19: 74–9.

It is vital that developments in education, research, and the practical delivery of primary care continue, not in any spirit of competition with other medical disciplines or the allied professions, but with appropriate collaboration and interdependence.

PR Evans

Evans PR. Education and debate medicine in Europe: the changing scene in general practice in Europe. *BMJ.* 1994; 308(6929): 645–8.

One of the primary aims of medical education should be that the newly qualified man is not an agglomeration of embryonic consultants, but is well instructed in the fundamentals of general practice.

Thomas Hammond

Hammond TE. The surgeon and the public. *BMJ.* 1925; 2(3382): 768.

The general practitioner must not entrust his interests to the hands of others; he must not allow any other grade to interfere in his education, or acknowledge any power to control his practice that does not emanate from members of his own rank.

Alfred Hardwicke

Hardwicke A. Statement of the Society of Apothecaries. *Prov Med Surg J.* 1844; s1–8(10): 145.

The most important factor that will preserve the quality of medical student teaching in general practice and allow for expansion is the engagement of enthusiastic GP teachers.

Adrian Hastings

Hastings A. Undergraduate learning: never mind the quality, feel the width! Medical student teaching in general practice. *Educ Prim Care.* 2010; 21: 56–8.

There is good evidence that doctors whom students encounter as role models have a strong influence on their future career choices and that this can change in a positive direction during a general practice placement.

Adrian Hastings

Hastings A. Undergraduate learning: never mind the quality, feel the width! Medical student teaching in general practice. *Educ Prim Care.* 2010; 21: 56–8.

Giving students the opportunity to care for ambulatory patients allows them to learn valuable lessons absent from the inpatient experience.

William Hensel

Hensel WA. Graduate medical education confronted. *JAMA.* 1988; 259(18): 2695.

For general practice it is clearly not sensible to stipulate that the competent practitioner would know all or something about everything, but rather they know about processes, the important patient safety issues, political imperatives, common problems and human illness behaviour.

Arthur Hibble

Hibble A. The GP curriculum: three years, five years, or life? *Educ Prim Care.* 2009; 20: 83–6.

When the content of the job of general practice is potentially 'anything from anyone' in many locations then clearly learning the job is not finished until it is finished.

Arthur Hibble

Hibble A. The GP curriculum: three years, five years, or life? *Educ Prim Care.* 2009; 20: 83–6.

With the current changes to the health service the time has come to take stock and ask whether we are performing as well as we should be or whether vocational training is joining that long list of things that – like tennis and parliamentary democracy – may have been developed here but now seem to be done better elsewhere.

Roger Higgs

Higgs R. Vocational training in general practice. *BMJ.* 1991; 303(6801): 480–1.

Clinical medicine is best learnt through apprenticeship, and general practice offers an ideal opportunity for this.

Raymond Hoffenberg

Hoffenberg R. What price academic general practice? *BMJ (Clin Res Ed).* 1986; 292(6535): 1545–6.

We need to test trainees before they start their vocational training, to measure the needs of entrants so that individual teaching may be offered to every trainee.

Robin Hull

Hull R. Training for general practice. *BMJ.* 1989; 299(6706): 996.

Any process of education is a mixture of theory and practice. I feel sure that it is the function of medical education to present the theory. It is the duty of the student to digest the theory and put it into practice.

Noel Jackson

Jackson NJ. Training for general practice. *BMJ.* 1950; 2(4681): 728.

The "narrow" and uneducated scientist with no view beyond his specialized horizons is a stock figure of educational mythology. In our desire to produce rounded personalities do not let us fall into the heresy of regarding science as in itself narrowing or as anything less than what it is, one of the great channels by which the human spirit may be enriched.

Eric James

James E. General practice and medical education: the education of the scientist. *BMJ.* 1958; 2(5096): 575–6.

The loss of the chance to reflect upon, and therefore learn from, the details of our own professional learning history has the potential to render personal development planning, as currently conceived within GP appraisal and elsewhere, a less satisfying and less valuable experience.

Alex Jamieson

Jamieson A. E-learning: theories of learning and conversations with e-learners. *Work Based Learn Prim Care.* 2004; 2(1): 62–71(10).

Competition in general practice could force education out.

Roger Jones

Jones RH. Competition in general practice could force education out. *BMJ.* 2005 November 30. Available at: www. bmj.com/content/331/7526/1196/reply#bmj_el_122704?sid=cb764c2a-ad1a-4f84-a8c4-88b3568c267c (accessed 3 August 2011).

Not only are educational placements for learners needed in the ambulatory setting, the ambulatory setting itself needs to evolve and become part of the fabric of academic medicine.

Leonard Katz

Katz LA. Where will managed care fit in medical education? *JAMA.* 1997; 277(13): 1038.

Abolish the rank and file mentality. Give everyone the chance for growth.

Marshall Marinker

Handysides S. General practice enriching careers in general practice: building an efficient and healthy practice. *BMJ.* 1994; 308(6922): 179–82.

It has been recognised for some time that, in the general practice setting, improved patient care, better team work and mutual understanding can be met by the introduction of in-house, work based learning programmes.

Richard McDonough

McDonough R. The influence of the new contract on practices as learning organisations. *Work Based Learn Prim Care.* 2004; 2(4): 315–22(8).

The school for the young doctor is a general practice, in which the number and variety of cases will enable him at once to put his methods into daily use.

William Osler

Osler W. An address on the importance of post-graduate study: delivered at the opening of the museums of the Medical Graduates College and Polyclinic, July 4th, 1900. *BMJ.* 1900; 2(2063): 73–5.

Because those who are in power in the health professions are primarily those who represent the hospital services and the biomedical sciences, the likelihood of a major diversion of resources away from these sectors and towards primary care is minimal.

David Pendleton

Pendleton D. Relevant medical education. *Med Teach.* 1983; 5(3): 84–5.

Training general practitioners not only means teaching them the essentials of GP medicine, but also helping them to develop into effective professionals.

Eelco Runja

Runja E. The parallel process in the training of general practitioners. *Med Teach.* 1995; 17(4): 399–408.

Without a proper job description unenthusiastic tutors will not find it difficult to do the bare minimum while conscientious tutors will wear their fingers to the bone and still feel guilty that they have not accomplished all that they might.

MN Ruscoe

Ruscoe MN. Thoughts of a general practice clinical tutor. *BMJ (Clin Res Ed).* 1987; 295(6607): 1175–6.

Apprenticeship is claimed to be a good idea. It is. But if you are going to be a general practitioner, a researcher, or an administrator, what use is being apprenticed (for short spells) to a variety of hospital consultants?

TDS Seddon

Seddon TDS. The preregistration year. *BMJ.* 1994; 308(6933): 921.

The main focus of trainees in their early general practice experience is on coping with clinical practice in a community setting.

Roger Strasser

Strasser RP. Mini research projects for GP trainees. *Med Teach.* 1993; 15(1): 77–81.

It has been argued that a compulsory vocational course will increase the shortage of general practitioners. This may well be but at least the profession will know that once compulsory vocational training is accepted those doctors who then apply to become a partner or principal in general practice will be of the right calibre, and the standard of general practice in this country will inevitably rise.

Bernard Taylor

Taylor B. Vocational training for general practice. *BMJ.* 1968; 2(5598): 174.

All general practitioners must participate in the education process: there should be no practice without education and no education without practice.

MB Taylor

Taylor MB. Unifying academic general practice: approach with caution. *BMJ.* 1993; 307(6913): 1215.

Why do medical students never cease saying 'I suppose I will end up in general practice', while motivated young doctors continue to ask for career advice, pronouncing 'I'd like to be a GP but my consultant says it's a waste; I am too bright'?

Valerie Wass

Wass V. Growing your own. *Educ Prim Care.* 2005; 16: 215–16.

I further remarked, that London would soon cease to be the metropolis of medical education, if students intended for the general practice of their profession had to spend their valuable time and (too commonly) limited means in running from one special hospital to another, to gather piece-meal that competent knowledge which they could acquire under one roof, at either Edinburgh or Dublin.

William Webber

Webber W. Special hospitals. *BMJ.* 1861; 2(36): 267.

Previously left entirely to hospitals, PRHO [preregistration house officer] rotations represent a major new educational challenge for general practice and it can be argued that general practice experience has just as important a part to play in the PRHO year as hospital experience.

Joe Wilton

Wilton J. Identifying appropriate tasks for the preregistration year. *BMJ.* 1999 August 24. Available at: www.bmj. com/content/319/7204/224/reply#bmj_el_4388?sid=3b793041-95a4-4870-a5d9-9fc0c51e668f (accessed 3 August 2011).

So long as we go on expecting to prepare students for general practice in institutions which have a different frame of reference we shall continue to be dissatisfied with the results.

Leslie Witts

Witts LJ. The difficulty in medical education. *BMJ.* 1950; 2(4679): 622.

30. COST AND VALUE IN MEDICAL EDUCATION

> It is arguable whether there are too many doctors being produced in the world. It is certain that they are maldistributed.
>
> **Philip Rhodes**

Medical education is expensive, and, unlike many students in other faculties, medical students do not have lengthy vacations in which to supplement their income.

David Alexander

Alexander DA. Loans for medical students. *BMJ.* 1988; 297(6663): 1561.

But let it be clearly understood that all these betterments of medical education will cost money, and let us not hesitate to say so.

Thomas Clifford Allbutt

Allbutt TC. Medical education in England: a note on Sir George Newman's memorandum to the president of the Board of Education. *BMJ.* 1918; 2(3005): 113–15.

Not for all students then, even students of some promise, may it be worth while to take a university course with its greater cost in time and money; some very valuable members of our profession have a turn for craft rather than for intellectual study.

Thomas Clifford Allbutt

Allbutt TC. The training of the medical student. *BMJ.* 1922; 2(3218): 407–9.

Finance for study leave should be freely available, but the only criterion for granting study leave must be its educational validity.

Andrew Bamji

Bamji A. SHO training: proposals expensive. *BMJ.* 1993; 306(6887): 1274.

The education is so expensive that none enter upon the study except the sons of men of independent fortune.

John Banks

Banks J. Preliminary medical education and the medical curriculum. *BMJ.* 1890; 2(1560) 1213.

Education may not be the sole motive of all consultants taking study leave, but nor is it the entire purpose of the organisations providing it as profit may be vital for them.

John Bennett

Bennett JR. Keeping up to date. *BMJ.* 1993; 306(6893): 1692.

The costs of medical education rise yearly and a large proportion of these costs are met by borrowing. Conventional wisdom suggests that students select higher-paying medical specialties in order to repay the debt.

Daniel Bernstein

Bernstein DS. Medical student indebtedness and choice of specialty. *JAMA.* 1992; 267(14): 1921.

During the past two decades, the traditional approach to undergraduate medical education has come under increased scrutiny by the consumer group (students) and the professionals (medical educators).

Giles Bole

Bole GG. Assessing the effectiveness of residency training programs. *Arch Intern Med.* 1980; 140(11): 1421–2.

A geographic maldistribution of physicians, insufficient funding for education, an imbalance between specialization and general practice, and inadequate mechanisms to evaluate medical competence are serious concerns in many countries today.

Cristyn Carlson

Carlson CA. International medical education: common elements in divergent systems. *JAMA.* 1991; 266(7): 921–3.

An assortment of medical education systems currently operate throughout the world, reflecting variations in populations, histories, societal and cultural traditions, political systems, and stages of economic development.

Cristyn Carlson

Carlson CA. International medical education: common elements in divergent systems. *JAMA.* 1991; 266(7): 921–3.

Medical education is expensive. Medical students expect to be taught by professional teachers, not just professional clinicians.

Yap-Seng Chong

Chong YS. Medical education especially needs help. *BMJ.* 2003 November 2. Available at: www.bmj.com/content/327/7422/1001/reply#bmj_el_39485?sid=7f27ee1c-bc1e-486c-bc82-03a5164885cc (accessed 3 August 2011).

To mount a reliable OSCE [objective structured clinical examination] is an extremely resource-intensive exercise, and to use it to test cognitive skills is wasteful.

Rufus Clarke

Clarke RM. Criterion-referencing: the baby and the bathwater. *BMJ.* 2009 February 24. Available at: www.bmj.com/content/338/bmj.b690/reply#bmj_el_209927?sid=c01598e6-7fa7-4552-bbff-d3bc10847fd9 (accessed 3 August 2011).

Surely it is better for the parents, for the pupil, and for the public that a boy should have some opportunity for seeing what the practice of medicine demands, and for judging whether he is able to make the necessary effort before heavy fees are paid in launching him at a hospital.

Carey Coombs

Coombs C. The five years' curriculum. *BMJ.* 1892; 2(1668): 1363–4.

Owing to the cheapness of medical education, numbers of young men who, in other industrial and less agricultural countries, would turn to business or a handicraft, enter the profession by hundreds, especially in the larger cities.

Gustav Dintenfass

Dintenfass G. The medical profession in Europe and the British colonies: Austria. *BMJ.* 1905; 1(2318): 1204–7.

In the current, cost-constrained environment, those funding the education of our doctors will no longer tolerate an approach of quality at any cost.

Liam Donaldson

Donaldson L. Foreword. In: Walsh K, editor. *Cost Effectiveness in Medical Education.* Oxford: Radcliffe Publishing; 2010. ppvii–viii.

Medical education is increasingly driven by economic models looking to maximise return on investment and other metrics of accountability.

Rachel Ellaway

Ellaway R. eMedical teacher. *Med Teach.* 2008; 30(3): 342–3.

The number of medical students coming from under-privileged communities is decreasing and if the current trend continues, it could shrink to almost zero in three or four years time.

Kate Emmitt

Emmitt K. Broadening access to undergraduate medical education. *BMJ.* 2000 November 29. Available at: www.bmj.com/content/321/7269/1136/reply#bmj_el_11131?sid=7f1b5b2e-7b0c-43f6-8a46-f45951808b4f (accessed 3 August 2011).

Although the cost:benefit ratio is highly dependent on the context in which testing is used, recent literature is burgeoning with suggestions that there may be pedagogical benefits to testing that have been underappreciated and understudied.

Kevin Eva

Eva KW. What the educators are saying: putting the cart before the horse: testing to improve learning. *BMJ.* 2007; 334(7592): 535.

These are public services; and we are sure that all right-minded men will acknowledge that the burden of maintaining high-class medical education which is not self-supporting should be in part borne by the public who profit by it, and not wholly thrown upon a few zealous medical men, who as now give vast time and labour in teaching for most inadequate remuneration.

Alexander Fleming

Fleming A. Observations on the English universities, with reference to affiliation of medical schools. *BMJ.* 1867; 1(322): 217–18.

The business of the medical faculty is to look after patients, students and science. They have no time to hunt money.

Abraham Flexner

Flexner A. Medical education, 1909–1924. *JAMA.* 1924; 82(11): 833–8.

The needs for funding for scholarship in medical education and a better mechanism for promoting clinician-educators are important messages, but they are not new.

Robert Golub

Golub RM. Medical Education 2005: from allegory to bull moose. *JAMA.* 2005; 294(9): 1108–10.

I wonder if the current divide between post graduate and undergraduate medical education has more to do with bureaucracy, finances and power, than the genuine needs of our health system.

Christopher Gunstone

Gunstone CC. Pace of change too slow maybe! *BMJ.* 2004 July 27. Available at: www.bmj.com/content/329/7457/92/reply#bmj_el_68893?sid=3f545f3a-8b62-4679-979a-2c0b244a4cd7 (accessed 3 August 2011).

The cost of medical education has also increased a good deal these last few years, thus affecting those who are putting their sons into the profession.

Arthur Hawkyard

Hawkyard A. Contract practice and the medical profession. *BMJ.* 1910; 2(2597): 1095–6.

Teaching and learning is a mysterious process, much thought and written about, involving a multitude of diverse elements such as the motivation of the learner, the skills of the teacher, adequate protected time and space for the process, the mutual respect or even affection of each for the other, financial incentives, the fear of failure or exposure, peer pressure, and the need for approval and acceptance.

Peter Herbert

Herbert P. The educator is expert; the learner is expert. *Work Based Learn Prim Care.* 2004; 2(3): 280–4(5).

In an era of university budgetary restraint, clinical teaching must become more cost-effective.

David Hill

Hill DA. SCORPIO: a system of medical teaching. *Med Teach.* 1992; 14(1): 37–41.

It is indisputable, that the system of apprenticeship has been much abused, especially in the country, and in towns not possessing recognized medical schools; for a young man not having the opportunity of attending a lecture, or witnessing the practice of a hospital, til a five years' apprenticeship is expired, is a great loss of time, and causes a considerable increase of expenditure.

J Ingham Ikin

Ingham Ikin J. Introductory lecture on the opening of the medical session. *Prov Med Surg J.* 1844; s1–8(30): 455–60.

All physicians leaving a poorer jurisdiction for a richer one should be obligated to pay for the true cost of their education. Or else the receiving county or province or state should pay the state where they had subsidised education and professional training.

Alexander Jablanczy

Jablanczy A. The cost of an MD. *BMJ.* 2001 January 26. Available at: www.bmj.com/content/322/7280/189.2/reply#bmj_el_13184?sid=bfae656f-d7d3-4ae5-abb6-1b0e432b89b5 (accessed 23 May 2011).

Medical education is a form of technical education in the efficiency of which the public, if they only realized it, are interested as much if not more than in many others to which public money is given, inadequately it is true, but without hesitation.

James Kingston Fowler

Kingston Fowler J. Address in medicine: delivered at the Seventy-Sixth Annual Meeting of the British Medical Association. *BMJ.* 1908; 2(2483): 248–54.

If a boy wants to be qualified for practice and in a position to earn his own living as soon as he has finished his medical course, and has obtained his registerable qualification, his education ought from the very first to have been directed to practical purpose.

Robert Lee

Lee R. Medical education. *BMJ.* 1902; 2(2168): 223.

In a country where free market forces operate a product that offers the best value for money will always be purchased by the consumer, whether that product is a meeting or textbook.

Julian Leigh

Leigh JM. Commercialisation of medical education. *BMJ (Clin Res Ed).* 1987; 295(6605): 1064.

Money is the root of all progress.

Iain MacLeod

Nairne P. Green College lectures: the National Health Service; reflections on a changing service. *BMJ.* 1988; 296(6635): 1518–20.

Targetting medical training to local needs might reduce the export value of medical graduates.

Keith Masnick

Masnick K. Migration of health professionals: concerns for developing countries like India. *BMJ.* 2005 February 7. Available at: www.bmj.com/content/330/7485/210/reply#bmj_el_95765?sid=1e069fc1-8837-4789-925c-3c1714669644 (accessed 23 May 2011).

Academic freedom is not a single concept. If it is the freedom to pursue the truth wherever it leads and to express opinions without fear of persecution then the concept is incontestable. But if it is the freedom to use public funds to train professional people who are unable to serve the public need, then the concept cannot be defended.

Ian McWhinney

McWhinney IR. Personal view. *BMJ.* 1972; 2(5806): 162.

Professions exist to serve the public interest and if universities use public funds to train members of professions they must expect to be held accountable.

Ian McWhinney

McWhinney IR. Personal view. *BMJ.* 1972; 2(5806): 162.

The lot of our own medical students is, from a financial standpoint, not a bed of roses, and I have personal recollections of existence for over three years on a diet of cocoa and dry bread, with an occasional kipper for variety, in order to save enough money to pay my hospital fees.

Vincent Norman

Norman V. Assistance to medical students from Austria. *BMJ.* 1938; 1(4042): 1394.

How about the West spending less on armaments and more on medical education so that we can make a large net export of caring professionals rather than on dropping high technology smart bombs.

Jon Orrell

Orrell JM. US lives saved but at what global cost? *BMJ.* 2006 June 11. Available at: www.bmj.com/content/332/7553/1328/reply#bmj_el_135330?sid=20523c27-2e0d-443d-a7db-86e43c2767d3 (accessed 23 May 2011).

Even in comparatively poor countries we find scientific knowledge and trained intellects regarded as sound public investments, and the popular voice applauding a liberal application of public money to secure them.

Isambard Owen

Owen I. One hundred years ago: the future of London medical education. *BMJ*. 2004; 329(7477): 1276.

Medical education is more prolonged and expensive than it has ever hitherto been; the ranks of the profession are overcrowded; the enterprise of chemists is bringing within the command of the public remedies which previously could only be obtained through the prescriptions of qualified medical men; and the blatant and unrestricted pretensions of advertising quacks are appealing more than ever to the credulity of an increasing number of people whose feeble and unstable nerves clamour with unwearying insistence for narcotics, stimulants, sedatives, and, in short, a cheap and quick cure for every imaginable ailment.

Guthrie Rankin

Rankin G. Home hospitals for the middle classes. *BMJ*. 1908; 1(2477): 1474–6.

It is arguable whether there are too many doctors being produced in the world. It is certain that they are maldistributed.

Philip Rhodes

Rhodes P. St George's University School of Medicine, Grenada: benefit or liability? *BMJ (Clin Res Ed)*. 1982; 285(6339): 436–7.

Nearly all the costs of study leave come out of public funds and are an investment in the doctor, who should therefore do his utmost to give a fair return on the investment.

Philip Rhodes

Rhodes P. Arranging for study leave. *BMJ*. 1983; 286(6364): 539–40.

Rather than compensating the more expensive teaching hospitals for (possibly) unnecessary costs we should consider ways of redistributing medical students to the medical schools, teaching hospitals and community teaching settings which have the lowest marginal excess costs.

Trevor Sheldon

Sheldon TA. Don't compensate less efficient teaching hospitals, redistribute clinical medical students. *BMJ*. 1999 October 1. Available at: www.ncbi.nlm.nih.gov/pmc/articles/PMC1117375/ (accessed 1 November 2011).

There is a huge need for more doctors globally. Can we achieve this without burdening the taxpayer? We believe we can and increase the diversity amongst tomorrow's doctors at the same time.

Karol Sikora

Sikora K. University of Buckingham Medical School. *BMJ*. 2005 January 17. Available at: www.bmj.com/content/330/7482/62.1/reply#bmj_el_93013?sid=1e069fc1-8837-4789-925c-3c1714669644 (accessed 23 May 2011).

Education in . . . the liberal professions is . . . tedious and expensive. The pecuniary recompense, therefore [of] physicians ought to be much more liberal; and it is so accordingly.

Adam Smith

The Wealth of Nations. 1776. bk I: X.

The cost of medical education is an important issue and has not been well defined.
Richard Sperry
Sperry RJ. Cost of teaching medical students. *JAMA.* 1995; 273(10): 771.

Let's be a little hopeful and a little unselfish and offer medical education to as many as possible of those who can benefit from it.
David Stevenson
Stevenson D. Too many doctors: or too few? *BMJ.* 1984; 289(6451): 1070.

It is wasteful to train doctors to senior registrar level and not to appoint them to consultant posts.
John Stewart
Stewart JSS. More consultants, fewer juniors. *BMJ (Clin Res Ed).* 1982; 285(6343): 742.

Ready money is ready medicine.
Unknown

Lectures are highly efficient to transmit knowledge with a limited number of teachers but active learning is usually low.
Henk van den Berg
Van den Berg H. Rating of SPICES criteria to evaluate and compare curricula. *Med Teach.* 2004; 26(4): 381–3.

If only the students who are the least well furnished with money were always the least well furnished with brains, well and good. But we all know that it is quite as often the opposite.
Willoughby Francis Wade
Wade WF. President's address, delivered at the Fifty-Eighth Annual Meeting of the British Medical Association. *BMJ.* 1890; 2(1544): 259–62.

Clinical education has always been considered to be more prestigious than its preclinical counterpart, but there seem to be few reasons for its greater cost.
Laurence Wale
Wale LW. University budgets and medical education. *BMJ (Clin Res Ed).* 1981; 282(6282): 2137–8.

So why is clinical education so expensive? The obvious reason is too many staff. Certainly in teaching hospitals this is coupled with too few patients and makes it very difficult to give an all-round education to the undergraduate.
Laurence Wale
Wale LW. University budgets and medical education. *BMJ (Clin Res Ed).* 1981; 282(6282): 2137–8.

I think I may state that without exception it is impossible to carry on satisfactorily any form of scientific instruction, such as is necessary in medicine, on fees which are paid by the student alone.
Holburt Waring
Waring HJ. An address on post-graduate medical education in England: delivered before the Manchester Medical Society. *BMJ.* 1925; 2(3387): 1022–6.

Securing adequate protected time to teach, remuneration and facilities has caused frustrations for a long time.
Val Wass
Wass V. The impact of change in healthcare delivery on medical education. *Educ Prim Care.* 2007; 18: 551–7.

The real issue that needs to be confronted is not the culture shock of evidence-based medical education, but the increasing dissociation between the funds that some hospitals receive for medical education and the ability of clinicians to meet teaching obligations.

Graham Watt

Watt G. Clinical assessment of medical students. *BMJ.* 1998 November 17. Available at: www.bmj.com/content/317/7168/1329.1/reply#bmj_el_1365?sid=35c7ac25-b25d-43e6-9bc0-a5da27e4e533 (accessed 23 May 2011).

There may be plenty of reasons to criticise medical education (and indeed by making students increasingly responsible for meeting the cost of their degree it should be expected that they will become more demanding).

Martin Williams

Williams M. Wide of the mark. *BMJ.* 2004 July 19. Available at: www.bmj.com/content/329/7457/92/reply#bmj_el_67827?sid=3f545f3a-8b62-4679-979a-2c0b244a4cd7 (accessed 23 May 2011).

The expenses of a medical education are already as high as can well be borne by the classes supplying the greatest number of students.

John Wood

Wood J. Observations on medical education. *BMJ.* 1879; 2(970): 162–6.

31. FUTURE

All is now flux in medical education where once all was stasis.

Chris McManus

As regards our own profession, it is in the extension of clinical instruction in hospital wards, and in the extension of practical technical education, such as obtains in physiological laboratories, microscopic rooms, and such like practical work in connection with hospitals, with extension of time for work and study, that future improvements in medical education must lie.

William Aitken

Aitken W. Introductory lecture on the influence of human progress on medical education. *BMJ.* 1872; 1(590): 411–13.

There is no branch of medical education which embraces more points of importance than clinical instruction; certainly no other comprehends so much that is specially valuable and applicable to future practice.

William Basham

Basham WR. A course of lectures on clinical medicine. *Prov Med Surg J.* 1846; s1–10(43): 509–11.

Doctors are increasingly under public scrutiny; maintaining the reputation of the profession in the future is a process that begins in the halls of learning now.

Suneel Bhat

Bhat S. In the hands of students. *BMJ.* 2005 May 19. Available at: www.bmj.com/content/330/7499/1064/reply#bmj_el_107250?sid=1e069fc1-8837-4789-925c-3c1714669644 (accessed 21 September 2011).

When will we as leaders in medical education "get the picture?" When will we comprehend that our programs of graduate medical education have major flaws?

Frederic Burg

Burg FD. Toward a sane and better future in graduate medical education. *Am J Dis Child.* 1987; 141(4): 405–6.

The future of American medical education is, like all other higher developments, simply in the hands of the only aristocracy we strive for – the aristocracy of an enlightened public opinion.

Fielding Garrison

Preface to *Introduction to the History of Medicine.* 2nd ed.

The process of learning, by whatever means, should encourage students to share, discuss and learn, without prejudice; a process that encapsulates their needs for the future, recognising a changing world, its different environments, cultural diversities and varying forms of medicine and healthcare delivery.

Trevor Gibbs

Gibbs T. The place of complementary medicine in modern medical education. *Educ Prim Care.* 2006; 17: 206–12.

We cannot expect every virtue from every doctor, even if that were theoretically desirable, and who can say that what we want from today's doctors will be acceptable in tomorrow's?

Sandra Goldbeck-Wood

Goldbeck-Wood S. Choosing tomorrow's doctors. *BMJ.* 1996; 313(7053): 313.

Declare the past, diagnose the present, foretell the future.

Hippocrates

Epidemics.

The advance of scientific medicine has been so rapid since the war that it tests severely not only the structure of medical practice in this country but also the capacity of the individual to keep pace with it.

Douglas Hubble

Hubble D. Adult education: for the consultant. *BMJ.* 1955; 2(4938): 505–7.

You had better not write down that observation for very likely I will think differently next year.

John Hunter

Paget S. *John Hunter: man of science and surgeon.*

Girls as well as boys often break down quite unnecessarily, not because their health is defective, but because they study in a foolish and headstrong way, ignoring the ordinary laws of hygiene, and destroying their own future by attempting the impossible in the present.

Sophia Jex-Blake

Jex-Blake S. Medical education of women. *BMJ.* 1895; 2(1814): 869.

Provided we are clear on the basic philosophy that guides our great profession we can reach acceptable solutions. But should this philosophy be challenged – if the fire is kindled – we must not fear the flame.

Walpole Lewin

Lewin W. Medicine in society. *BMJ.* 1975; 3(5982): 523–6.

As unpopular as it may be in some quarters, the profession needs to accept that post-training career progression should take the form of a pyramid – rather than the current square, which allows most doctors to progress to the top.

Martin Marshall

Marshall M. The future for trainee doctors. *BMJ.* 2007; 335(7632): 1222–3.

Learning for work is about acquiring the requisite knowledge and skills for the job in hand. Learning from work, also often described as prior experiential learning, should help people to acquire transferable knowledge and skills – in other words to fit them for future tasks and challenges.

Richard McDonough

McDonough R. All fired up about The Apprentice. *Work Based Learn Prim Care.* 2006; 4(3): 209–10(2).

All is now flux in medical education where once all was stasis.

Chris McManus

McManus IC. New pathways to medical education: learning to learn at Harvard Medical School. *BMJ.* 1995; 311(6996): 67.

I understand all too well why the schools would like to sit comfortably outside the NHS [National Health Service] system, but cannot think of anything worse for the education of future NHS doctors.

Elaine Murphy

Murphy E. University hospitals and the NHS review. *BMJ.* 1990; 300(6723): 538.

Essential to any discussion about medical education in the future are the following three topics: the students, the educational process, and its content.

Robert Petersdorf

Petersdorf RG. Medical education. *JAMA.* 1990; 263(19): 2652–4.

My greatest objection to MCQs [multiple-choice questions] is that in my opinion they are a hazard to the future of medical culture.

George Pickering

Pickering G. Against multiple choice questions. *Med Teach.* 1979; 1(2): 84–6.

In an age of precocious specialization we should be ever conscious of the danger that medical education may cease to be informed by its old humanistic tradition.

Harry Platt

Platt H. Medicine in the modern state. *BMJ.* 1950; 1(4652): 503–5.

I believe that competition is the very essence of progress and that the largely increased competition in the matter of medical education is full of good omen for the future of medicine in this country. So long as the competition be really free there is nothing to fear.

George Vivian Poore

Poore GV. Opening of the medical schools: introductory addresses. *BMJ.* 1900; 2(2075): 984–95.

The development of leadership, scholarship and fellowship is needed to sustain general practice in the future.

Tim van Zwanenberg

van Zwanenberg T. GP tomorrow. In: Harrison J, van Zwanenberg T, editors. *GP Tomorrow.* 2nd ed. Oxford: Radcliffe Medical Press; 2002. pp209–23.

Many practitioners, engaged not only in private, but also those in public practice, have even never been within the precincts of any lunatic asylum to study diseases of the mind. In my opinion this feature in modern medical education constitutes a great defect, which ought to be remedied by future legislation at the different licensing colleges in Great Britain.

John Webster

Webster J. The neglected teaching power of our public lunatic asylums. *BMJ*. 1858; 1(65): 251.

Thankfully the world is still populated mostly by altruistic patients who realise that medicine cannot be learned from a book alone, and who know that future doctors need the opportunity to learn practical skills so they maybe can help others in the future. That is all most students ask for.

Alan Woodall

Woodall A. The letter by McCracken defies belief. *BMJ*. 2001 March 26. Available at: www.bmj.com/content/322/ 7288/743.1/reply#bmj_el_13409?sid=bfae656f-d7d3-4ae5-abb6-1b0e432b89b5 (accessed 21 September 2011).